ebsite www.jaypeebrothers.com, for detailed information on nursing books

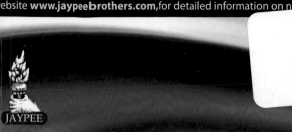

Fundamentals *of*
NURSING
Clinical Procedure Manual

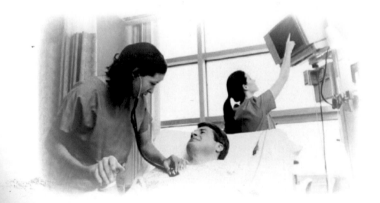

JC Helen Shaji

Foreword
Nalini Jeyavanth Santha

Fundamentals of
NURSING
Clinical Procedure Manual

JC Helen Shaji

MA (Psychology) MSc (Nursing) PhD (Nursing)

Professor
Department of Nursing
College of Applied Medical Sciences, Majmaah University
Kingdom of Saudi Arabia

Ex-Principal and Professor
St. Isabel's College of Nursing
Mylapore, Chennai, Tamil Nadu, India

Foreword
Nalini Jeyavanth Santha

(JAYPEE) *The Health Sciences Publisher*

New Delhi | London | Philadelphia | Panama

Jaypee Brothers Medical Publishers (P) Ltd

Headquarters

Jaypee Brothers Medical Publishers (P) Ltd
4838/24, Ansari Road, Daryaganj
New Delhi 110 002, India
Phone: +91-11-43574357
Fax: +91-11-43574314
Email: jaypee@jaypeebrothers.com

Overseas Offices

J.P. Medical Ltd
83 Victoria Street, London
SW1H 0HW (UK)
Phone: +44 20 3170 8910
Fax: +44 (0)20 3008 6180
Email: info@jpmedpub.com

Jaypee Medical Inc
The Bourse
111 South Independence Mall East
Suite 835, Philadelphia, PA 19106, USA
Phone: +1 267-519-9789
Email: jpmed.us@gmail.com

Jaypee Brothers Medical Publishers (P) Ltd
Bhotahity, Kathmandu, Nepal
Phone +977-9741283608
Email: kathmandu@jaypeebrothers.com

Jaypee-Highlights Medical Publishers Inc
City of Knowledge, Bld. 237, Clayton
Panama City, Panama
Phone: +1 507-301-0496
Fax: +1 507-301-0499
Email: cservice@jphmedical.com

Jaypee Brothers Medical Publishers (P) Ltd
17/1-B Babar Road, Block-B, Shaymali
Mohammadpur, Dhaka-1207
Bangladesh
Mobile: +08801912003485
Email: jaypeedhaka@gmail.com

Website: www.jaypeebrothers.com
Website: www.jaypeedigital.com

© 2015, Jaypee Brothers Medical Publishers

The views and opinions expressed in this book are solely those of the original contributor(s)/author(s) and do not necessarily represent those of editor(s) of the book.

All rights reserved. No part of this publication may be reproduced, stored or transmitted in any form or by any means, electronic, mechanical, photocopying, recording or otherwise, without the prior permission in writing of the publishers.

All brand names and product names used in this book are trade names, service marks, trademarks or registered trademarks of their respective owners. The publisher is not associated with any product or vendor mentioned in this book.

Medical knowledge and practice change constantly. This book is designed to provide accurate, authoritative information about the subject matter in question. However, readers are advised to check the most current information available on procedures included and check information from the manufacturer of each product to be administered, to verify the recommended dose, formula, method and duration of administration, adverse effects and contraindications. It is the responsibility of the practitioner to take all appropriate safety precautions. Neither the publisher nor the author(s)/editor(s) assume any liability for any injury and/or damage to persons or property arising from or related to use of material in this book.

This book is sold on the understanding that the publisher is not engaged in providing professional medical services. If such advice or services are required, the services of a competent medical professional should be sought.

Every effort has been made where necessary to contact holders of copyright to obtain permission to reproduce copyright material. If any have been inadvertently overlooked, the publisher will be pleased to make the necessary arrangements at the first opportunity.

Inquiries for bulk sales may be solicited at: jaypee@jaypeebrothers.com

Fundamentals of Nursing: Clinical Procedure Manual

First Edition: **2015**

ISBN 978-93-5152-637-7

Printed at Repro India Limited

Dedicated to

*The nursing students and registered nurses
who have always been the source of inspiration
and make a difference in patients'
life every day and every moment*

Foreword

It gives me immense pleasure, and it is a great privilege and honor to write the foreword for this book *Fundamentals of Nursing: Clinical Procedure Manual* written by Dr JC Helen Shaji.

The initiative and effort taken toward bringing up this manual is commendable. The contents of the book cover the curriculum prescribed by Indian Nursing Council, which sustains uniform standard of nursing education in the country. The author states that the primary purpose of this work is to provide a textbook for young nursing students who are studying to become qualified professional nurses. This book also serves as a ready reference source for the practicing nurses.

This book has detailed information to understand fundamental and advanced medical and surgical nursing procedures, which would benefit students and graduates to maintain high standard of nursing practice for humanitarian service, and the dignity and status of the profession. In order to enhance the quality of nursing, it is essential to maintain standard of care in nursing education and nursing practice. This manual will help the nursing students to maintain standard and high quality patient care in the healthcare setting. Through this manual, wide knowledge and fine nursing skills can be transferred to the nursing students very effectively.

Nalini Jeyavanth Santha PhD (N)
Principal
Sacred Heart Nursing College, Ultra Trust
Madurai, Tamil Nadu, India

Preface

I am extremely happy to present this book *Fundamentals of Nursing: Clinical Procedure Manual* to the nursing students and registered nurses in India as well as overseas. The primary objective of this book is to prepare competent nurses to meet the challenging situations of nursing, since it is prepared according to the curriculum of Indian Nursing Council as well as the syllabus adopted by various universities overseas. The nursing students will find it as a 'textbook' for learning nursing procedures.

The nurse educators will find it easy to teach their students and prepare them well for the examination. Moreover, the present-day practicing nurses also find this book as a ready reference source for better understanding of basic and advanced medical and surgical nursing procedures. This book will also bring a uniform standard of the nursing education in India.

It will be much appreciated, if readers send their criticism, suggestions and corrections if any for further improvement of this book.

JC Helen Shaji

Acknowledgments

I am highly indebted to Dr Nalini Jeyavanth Santha, for writing the foreword. I am grateful to my husband G David Rajesh, my children Daleesh, Prajol and Sharon, for their invaluable assistance and dedication during the preparation of this book. I am also grateful to some of my colleagues in profession who has encouraged me throughout, for writing this book.

I am thankful to Shri Jitendar P Vij (Group Chairman), Mr Ankit Vij (Group President), Mr Tarun Duneja (Director–Publishing) and all the staff of Bengaluru Branch of M/s Jaypee Brothers Medical Publishers (P) Ltd, New Delhi, India, for bringing out this book in a professional manner.

Contents

Section 2: Advanced and Other Nursing Procedures

Section
1

Basic Nursing Care Procedures

- ❑ Bed Making
- ❑ Checking Vital Signs
- ❑ Performing Hygienic Procedures and Other Basic Procedures
- ❑ Specimen Collection
- ❑ Administration of Medications

Bed Making

MAKING AN UNOCCUPIED BED

Definition

A bed prepared to receive a new patient is an unoccupied bed.

Purposes

1. To provide clean and comfortable bed for the patient.
2. To reduce the risk of infection by maintaining a clean environment.
3. To prevent bed sores by ensuring that there are no wrinkles to cause pressure points.

Equipments Required

- Mattress: 1
- Bed sheets: 2
  - Bottom sheet: 1
  - Top sheet: 1.
- Pillow: 1
- Pillow cover: 1
- Mackintosh: 1
- Draw sheet: 1
- Blanket: 1
- Savlon water or Dettol water in basin
- Sponge cloth: 4
  - To wipe with solution: 1
  - To dry: 1
  - When bed making is done by two nurses, sponge cloth is needed two each.
- Kidney tray or paper bag: 1
- Laundry bag or hamper bag: 1
- Trolley: 1.

Procedure

Bed making procedure is detailed in Table 1.1.

Table 1.1: Bed making procedure

SI No	Care action	Rationale
1.	Explain the purpose and procedure to the client	Providing information fosters cooperation
2.	Perform hand hygiene	To prevent the spread of infection
3.	Prepare all required equipments and bring the articles to the bedside	Organization facilitates accurate skill performance
4.	Move the chair and bedside locker	It makes space for bed making and helps effective action
5.	Clean the bedside locker: • Wipe with wet and dry	To maintain the cleanliness
6.	Clean the mattress: • Stand in right side • Start wet wiping from top to center and from center to bottom in right side of mattress • Gather the dust and debris to the bottom • Collect them into kidney tray • Give dry wiping as same as procedure 2 • Move to left side • Wipe with wet and dry the left side • Move to right side	To prevent the spread of infection

7.	Bottom sheet:
	• Place and slide the bottom sheet upward over the top of the bed leaving the bottom edge of the sheet
	• Open it lengthwise with the center fold along the bed center
	• Fold back the upper layer of the sheet toward the opposite side of the bed
	• Tuck the bottom sheet securely under the head of the mattress (approximately 20–30 cm)
	• Make a mitered corner:
	  – Pick up the selvage edge with your hand nearest to the hand of the bed
	  – Lay a triangle over the side of the bed
	  – Tuck the hanging part of the sheet under the mattress
	  – Drop the triangle over the side of the bed
	  – Tuck the sheet under the entire side of bed
	• Repeat the same procedure at the end of the corner of the bed
	• Tuck the remainder in along the side
		Unfolding the sheet in this manner allows you to make the bed on one side
		A mitered corner has a neat appearance and keeps the sheet securely under the mattress
		Tucking the bottom sheet will be done by turning the corner of top first and the corner of the bottom later
		To secure the bottom sheet on one side of the bed

8.	Mackintosh and draw sheet: • Place a mackintosh at the middle of the bed (if used), folded half, with the fold in the center of the bed • Lift the right half and spread it forward to the near side • Tuck the mackintosh under the mattress • Place the draw sheet on the mackintosh • Spread and tuck as same as procedure 1–3 • Move to the left side of the bed	Mackintosh and draw sheet are additional protection for the bed, and serves as a lifting or turning sheet for an immobile client

Contd...

Contd...

SI No	Care action	Rationale
9.	Bottom sheet, mackintosh and draw sheet: • Fold and tuck the bottom sheet as in the above procedure 7 • Fold and tuck both the mackintosh and the draw sheet under the mattress, as given in the above procedure 8 • Return to the right side	Secure the bottom sheet, mackintosh; and draw the bottom sheet, mackintosh and draw sheet
10.	Top sheet and blanket: • Place the top sheet evenly on the bed, centering it in the below 20–30 cm from the top of the mattress • Spread it downward • Cover the top sheet with blanket in the below 1 foot from the top of the mattress and spread downward • Fold the cuff (approximately 1 foot) in the neck • Tuck all these together under the bottom of mattress; miter the corner • Tuck the remainder in along the side	A blanket provides warmth Making the cuff at the neck part prevents irritation from blanket edge Tucking all these pieces together saves time and provides a neat appearance To save time in this manner
11.	Repeat the same as in procedure 10 for the left side Return to the right side	
12.	Pillow and pillow cover: • Put a clean pillow cover on the pillow • Place a pillow at the top of the bed in the center with the open end away from the door	A pillow is a comfortable measure Pillow cover keeps cleanliness of the pillow and neat The open end may collect dust or organisms The open end away from the door is also maintained neat
13.	Return the bed, chair and bedside table to their proper place	Bedside necessities will be within easy reach for the client
14.	Replace all equipments in proper place	It makes well-setting for the next procedure
15.	Discard lines appropriately	Proper linen disposal prevents the spread of infection
16.	Perform hand hygiene	To prevent the spread of infection

Nursing Alert

1. Do not let your uniform touch the bed and the floor not to contaminate yourself.
2. Never throw soiled linens on the floor not to contaminate the floor.
3. Staying one side of the bed until one step is completed, save steps and time to do effectively.

CHANGING AN OCCUPIED BED

Definition

The procedure of changing used linens of a hospitalized patient is an occupied bed.

Purposes

1. To provide clean and comfortable bed for the patient.
2. To reduce the risk of infection by maintaining a clean environment.
3. To prevent bed sores by ensuring that there are no wrinkles to cause pressure points.

Equipments Required

- Bed sheets: 2
  - Bottom sheet (or bed cover): 1
  - Top sheet: 1.
- Draw sheet: 1
- Mackintosh: 1 (if contaminated or needed to change)
- Blanket: 1 (if contaminated or needed to change)
- Pillow cover: 1
- Savlon water or Dettol water in bucket
- Sponge cloth: 2
  - To wipe with solution: 1
  - To dry: 1
  - When the procedure is done by two nurses, sponge cloth is needed two each.
- Kidney tray or paper bag: 1
- Laundry bag or bucket:1
- Trolley: 1.

Procedure

Procedure for changing an occupied bed is detailed in Table 1.2.

Table 1.2: Procedure for changing an occupied bed

Sl No	Care action	Rationale
1.	Check the client's identification and condition	To assess necessity and sufficient condition
2.	Explain the purpose and procedure to the client	Providing information fosters cooperation
3.	Perform hand hygiene	To prevent the spread of infection
4.	Prepare all required equipments and bring the articles to the bedside	Organization facilitates accurate skill performance
5.	Close the curtain or door of the room; put screen	To maintain the client's privacy
6.	Remove the client's personal belongings from bedside and put them into the bedside locker or in safe place	To prevent personal belongings from damage and loss
7.	Lift the client's head and move pillow from center to the left side	Pillow is a comfortable measure for the client
8.	Assist the client to turn toward left side of the bed; adjust the pillow and leave top sheet in place	Moving the client as close to the other side of the bed as possible, which give more room to make the bed

Contd...

Contd...

Sl No	Care action	Rationale
		Top sheet keeps the client warm and protect his/her privacy
9.	Stand in right side; loose bottom bed linen and fanfold (or roll) soiled linens from the side of the bed and wedge them close to the client	Placing folded (or rolled) soiled linen close to the client allows more space to place the clean bottom sheets
10.	Wipe the surface of mattress by sponge cloth with wet and dry	To prevent the spread of infection
11.	Bottom sheet, mackintosh and draw sheet: • Place the clean bottom sheet evenly on the bed, folded lengthwise with the center fold as close to the client's back as possible • Adjust and tuck the sheet tightly under the head of the mattress, making mitered the upper corner • Tighten the sheet under the end of the mattress making mitered the lower corner • Tuck in alongside • Place the mackintosh and the draw sheet on the bottom sheet and tuck in them together	Soiled linens can easily be removed and clean linens are positioned to make the other side of the bed
12.	Assist the client to roll over the folded (rolled) linen to right side of the bed; readjust the pillow and top sheet	Moving the client to the bed's other side allows to make the bed on that side
13.	Move to left side; discard the soiled linens appropriately; hold them away from the uniform and place them in the laundry bag (or bucket)	Soiled linens can contaminate the uniform, which may come into contact with other clients
14.	Wipe the surface of the mattress by sponge cloth with wet and dry	To prevent the spread of infection
15.	Bottom sheet, mackintosh and draw sheet: • Grasp clean linens and gently pull them out from under the client • Spread them over the bed's unmade side; pull the linens taut • Tuck the bottom sheet tightly under the head of the mattress and miter the corner • Tighten the sheet under the end of the mattress and make mitered the lower corner • Tuck in alongside • Tuck the mackintosh and the draw sheet under the mattress	Wrinkled linens can cause skin irritation
16.	Assist the client back to the center of the bed; adjust the pillow	Pillow is a comfort measure for the client
17.	Return to right side: • Clean the top sheet, blanket • Place the clean top sheet at the top side of the soiled top sheet	Tucking these pieces together saves time and provides neat, tight corners

Contd...

Contd...

SI No	Care action	Rationale
	• Ask the client to hold the upper edge of the clean top sheet • Hold both the top of the soiled sheet and the end of the clean sheet with right hand and withdraw to downward; remove the soiled top sheet and put it into a laundry bag (or a bucket) • Place the blanket over the top sheet; fold top sheet back over the blanket over the client • Tuck the lower ends securely under the mattress; miter corners • After finishing the right side, repeat for the left side	
18.	Remove the pillow, replace the pillow cover with clean one and reposition the pillow to the bed under the client's head	Pillow is a comfortable measure for the client
19.	Replace personal belongings back; return the bedside locker and the bed as usual	To prevent personal belongings from loss and provide safe surroundings
20.	Return all equipments to proper place	To prepare for the next procedure
21.	Discard linens appropriately; perform hand hygiene	To prevent the spread of infection

MAKING A POSTOPERATIVE BED

Definition

Postoperative bed is a special bed prepared to receive and take care of a patient returning from surgery.

Purposes

1. To receive the postoperative client from surgery and transfer him/her from a stretcher to a bed.
2. To arrange client's convenience and safety.

Equipments Required

- Bed sheets:
  - Bottom sheet: 1
  - Top sheet: 1.
- Draw sheet: 1–2
- Mackintosh or rubber sheet: 1–2 (according to the type of operation, the number required of mackintosh and draw sheet is different)
- Blanket: 1
- Hot water bag with hot water (104°F–140°F): 1 (if needed)
- Tray: 1
- Thermometer, stethoscope, sphygmomanometer: 1 each

- Spirit swab
- Artery forceps: 1
- Gauze pieces
- Adhesive tape: 1
- Kidney tray: 1
- Trolley: 1
- Intravenous (IV) stand
- Client's chart
- According to doctor's orders:
  - Oxygen cylinder with flow meter
  - Oxygen cannula or simple mask
  - Suction machine with suction tube
  - Airway, tongue depressor
  - Electrocardiogram (ECG), SpO_2 (peripheral O_2 saturation) monitor.

Procedure

Procedure for making a postoperative bed is detailed in Table 1.3.

Table 1.3: Procedure for making postoperative bed

Sl No	Care action	Rationale
1.	Perform hand hygiene	To prevent the spread of infection
2.	Assemble equipments and bring to bedside	Organization facilitates accurate skill performance
3.	Strip bed; make foundation bed as usual with a large mackintosh and cotton draw sheet	Mackintosh prevents bottom sheet from wetting or soiled by sweat, drain or excrement Place mackintosh according to operative technique Cotton draw sheet makes the client feel dry or comfortable without touching the mackintosh directly
4.	Place top bedding as for closed bed, but do not tuck at foot	Tuck at foot may hamper the client to enter the bed from a stretcher
5.	Fold back top bedding at the foot of bed	To make the client's transfer smooth
6.	Tuck the top bedding on one side only	Tucking the top bedding on one side stops the bed linens from slipping out of place
7.	On the other side, do not tuck the top sheet: • Bring head and foot corners of it at the center of bed and form right angles • Fold back suspending portion in one third and repeat folding top bedding twice to opposite side of bed	The open side of bed is more convenient for receiving client than the (other) closed side
8.	Remove the pillow	To maintain the airway
9.	Place a kidney tray on bedside	To receive secretion
10.	Place intravenous (IV) stand near the bed	To prepare it to hang IV soon

Contd...

Contd...

Sl No	Care action	Rationale
11.	Check locked wheel of the bed	To prevent moving the bed accidentally, when the client is shifted from a stretcher to the bed
12.	Place hot water bags (or hot bottles) in the middle of the bed and cover with fan-folded top, if needed	Hot water bags (or hot bottles) prevent the client from taking hypothermia
13.	When the patient comes, remove hot water bags if put before	To prepare enough space for receiving the client
14.	Transfer the client: • Help lifting the client on to the bed • Cover the client by the top sheet and blanket immediately • Tuck top bedding and miter a corner in the end of the bed	To prevent the client from chilling and/or having hypothermia

Checking Vital Signs

CHECKING ORAL AND AXILLARY TEMPERATURE

Definition

The temperature is defined as the expression of heat or coldness in terms of a specific scale; a measure of the average kinetic energy due to thermal disturbance of the particles in a system.

Purposes

1. To assess the progress and recovery of the patient from illness.
2. To diagnose significant conditions.
3. To ensure fitness of patient prior to procedures/surgeries.
4. To assess the patient response to medication and treatment.

Equipments

- A tray containing a bottle of disinfectant and a bottle of water (if glass thermometer)
- Thermometer (mercury in glass thermometer, electronic thermometer, tympanic thermometer)
- Clean cotton balls
- Towel/tissue paper.

Procedure

The procedure for checking axillary temperature and oral temperature are detailed in Tables 2.1 and 2.2.

Table 2.1: Procedure for checking axillary temperature

Sl No	Care action	Rationale
1.	Explain the procedure to the patient	To ensure that the patient understands the procedure and give consent
2.	Carry out handwashing	To prevent cross infection
3.	Place the patient in a comfortable position	To reduce uneasiness

Contd...

Contd...

SI No	Care action	Rationale
4.	Read mercury level, while gently rotating thermometer at eye level; grasp thermometer with thumb and forefinger, and shake gently by snapping the wrist in a downward motion to move mercury to a level until reading lowers mercury level to 35.6°C (96°F)	To get the accurate value, as the brisk shaking lowers mercury level in the glass tube
5.	Clean and dry axilla with towel	To get the exact value; moisture may also alter the temperature
6.	Place the thermometer in axilla, the bulb of thermometer is well in contact with the skin, while the patient's hand is held across chest	Ensures correct contact with the blood vessels in the axilla
7.	Wait for 5 minutes	To trace the temperature correctly
8.	Remove the thermometer, clean from stem to bulb and read at eye level	Reduces transmission of microorganisms to the bulb
9.	Shake gently the thermometer so that the mercury level falls below 35°C (95°F)	Keeps it set for use again
10.	Place the thermometer in disinfectant solution	To reduce cross infection
11.	Discard used tissue paper/cotton balls	Reduce transmission of microorganisms
12.	Record temperature on the graph sheet of temperature, pulse, respiration (TPR) record	Provides proper data for clinical data analysis

Points to Note

- Collect the history from the patient/relatives about the bathing time; the bath just before taking axillary temperature can alter the reading.

Table 2.2: Procedure for checking oral temperature

SI No	Care action	Rationale
1.	Explain the procedure to the patient	To ensure that the patient understand the procedure and to reduce the anxiety
2.	Wash the hands	To prevent cross infection
3.	Place the patient in a comfortable position (sitting or lying down)	To relieve anxiety
4.	Read mercury level, while gently rotating thermometer at eye level; shake it until reading lowers mercury level to 35.6°C (96°F)	To get the accurate readings
5.	Ask the patient to open the mouth and gently place thermometer under tongue in posterior sublingual pocket lateral to center of lower jaw	Ensures proper contact with the blood vessels in the mouth
6.	Wait for 3 minutes	To record the temperature accurately
7.	Remove the thermometer, clean from stem to bulb and read at eye level	Reduces transmission of microorganisms to the bulb

Contd...

Contd...

SI No	Care action	Rationale
8.	Shake gently so that mercury level falls below 35°C (95°F)	Keeps it set for use again
9.	Place the thermometer in disinfectant solution	To reduce cross infection
10.	Discard used tissue paper/cotton balls	Reduce transmission of microbes
11.	Record temperature on the graph sheet of temperature, pulse, respiration (TPR) record	Provides proper data for clinical data analysis

Points to Note

✦ Collect the details from the patient or relative about if he/she has taken any cold or hot food or fluids, or has smoked. If yes, the nurse is supposed to wait for 30 minutes to prevent the false reading.

OBSERVATION OF PULSE

Definition

Pulse is the rhythmic expansion and contraction of an artery caused by the impact of blood pumped by the heart. The pulse can be felt with the fingers at different pulse pressure points throughout the body.

Purposes

1. To ensure an accurate and effective assessment of the rate, rhythm and amplitude (strength) of the pulse.
2. To identify any trends/discrepancies and/or to detect early signs of alteration of cardiovascular function.

Equipments

* A watch
* A stethoscope.

Procedure

The procedure for observation of pulse is detailed in Table 2.3.

Table 2.3: Procedure for observation of pulse

SI No	Care action	Rationale
1.	Explain the procedure to the patient	To get the consent and cooperation
2.	Wash and dry hands thoroughly	To prevent cross infection
3.	Encourage the patient to relaxed	To provide consistent readings
4.	Explain and discuss the procedure with the patient	To ensure that the patient understands the procedure and gives his/her valid consent

Contd...

Contd...

SI No	Care action	Rationale
5.	If supine, place patient's forearm straight or across lower chest or abdomen with wrist extended straight If sitting, bend patient's elbow 90° and support lower arm on chair; slightly flex the wrist with palm down	Relaxed position of lower arm and flexion of wrist permits full exposure of radial artery for palpation
6.	Place second and/or third finger tips over radial artery and press gently until the pulse is felt	Fingertip is the most sensitive part of hand to palpate pulse
7.	Determine pulse amplitude and rhythm	Strength reflects volume of blood ejected against arterial wall with each heart contraction
8.	When pulse has been detected, look at watch's and count pulse rate for 60 seconds	Adequate time is essential to detect irregularities or any other defect
9.	Document any abnormalities in amplitude and rhythm	To maintain accurate records, and allow for monitoring and detection of trends
10.	Use disinfectant hand rub, once the procedure is over	To minimize cross infection risks between patients
11.	Document any relevant evaluation or changes in patient's record	To provide ongoing evaluation
12.	For the assessment of apical pulse, give details to the patient that expose sternum and left side of chest and position the diaphragm of the stethoscope over the point of maximal impulse (PMI) at the left fifth intercostal space, medial to the midclavicular line; if the heart beat is regular, count for 30 seconds and multiply by 2; if irregular, auscultate for one full minute	It provides a more accurate assessment

Points to Note

- Collect the details from the patient/relative, if he/she has been mobilized or done any such motion within the previous 15 minutes. Activity and anxiety can elevate heart rate. These activities may alter pulse rate.
- Thumb and forefinger are not equal, as they have their own pulse.
- Pulse is more accurately assessed with moderate pressure. Too much pressure can occlude pulse and impairs blood flow.

Pulse Sites

Sites of pulse is detailed in Table 2.4.

Table 2.4: Sites of pulse

Site	Location	Assessment criteria
Temporal	Above temporal bone of head, above and lateral to the eye	Easily accessible site to assess pulse in children
Carotid	Along medial edge of sternocleidomastoid muscle in neck	Easily accessible, used during physiological shock or cardiac arrest when other sites are not palpable
Brachial	Groove between biceps and triceps muscles at antecubital fossa	Site used to assess pulse rate; site used to auscultate blood pressure
Radial (commonly used)	Radial or thumb side of forearm at wrist	Common site used to assess character of pulse peripherally and assess status of circulation to hand
Femoral	Below inguinal ligament; midway between symphysis pubis and anterior superior iliac spine	Site used to assess character of pulse during physiological shock or cardiac arrest when other pulses are not palpable
Popliteal	Behind knee in popliteal fossa	Site used to auscultate lower extremity blood pressure
Posterior tibial	Inner side of ankle, below medial malleolus	Site used to assess circulation to foot
Dorsalis pedis	Along top of foot, between extension tendons of great and first toe	Site used to assess circulation to foot

OBSERVATION OF RESPIRATION

Definition

Monitoring the exchange of oxygen and carbon dioxide between the atmosphere and the body cells, including ventilation (inhalation and exhalation).

Purposes

1. To reveal the deviation from the normal body function.
2. To identify any changes in the condition of the patient.
3. To obtain specific information, which will help in the diagnosis of disease, the result of treatment, medications and nursing care.

Equipment

- A watch that has a second's hand.

Procedure

The procedure for observation of respiration is detailed in Table 2.5.

Table 2.5: Procedure for observation of respiration

SI No	Care action	Rationale
1.	Explain the procedure to the patient	To gain consent and cooperation
2.	Patient shall be in sitting or supine position in a quiet environment	Optimum position for recording respiration
3.	Allow the patient to rest for at least 5 minutes before the reading is taken	To gain an accurate reading; respiratory rate settles on rest
4.	Instruct the patient to stop talking during the procedure	Activity, including talking will cause an inaccurate respiratory rate
5.	Promote the patient to place his/her hand over the abdomen or chest, or place nurse's hand directly over patient's upper abdomen	Sufficient time is required to detect irregularities or other defects
6.	Watch complete respiratory cycle (inspiration and one expiration)	Rate is correctly determined only after the nurse had viewed respiratory cycle
7.	Count the respirations for 60 seconds	To observe the abnormality of rate, quality or rhythm
8.	Observe abnormal breathing patterns	To observe any deterioration in patient's respiratory pattern
9.	Observe for regularity of chest movement	To observe for abnormalities in chest movement
10.	Record the respirations on the observation chart as soon as possible	Do not rely on memory; each reading is a vital recording for each patient to maintain accurate records, and allow for monitoring and detection of trends

MEASUREMENT OF BLOOD PRESSURE

Definition

Arterial blood pressure is the force exerted by the blood on the wall of a blood vessel as the heart pumps (contracts) and relaxes. Systolic blood pressure is the degree of force when the heart is pumping (contracting). The diastolic blood pressure is the degree of force when the heart is relaxed.

Indications

1. To determine the patient's blood pressure at initial assessment as a base for subsequent evaluation.
2. To monitor fluctuations in blood pressure.
3. To assess the cardiac status.
4. To identify and monitor changes resulting from a disease process and medical/surgical therapy.
5. To determine patient's hemodynamic status.

Equipments

- Sphygmomanometer
- Stethoscope

- A bowl with spirit cotton swab
- Kidney tray.

Procedure

The procedure for measurement of blood pressure is detailed in Table 2.6.

Table 2.6: Procedure for measurement of blood pressure

Sl No	Care action	Rationale
1.	Wash and dry the hands	To prevent cross infection
2.	Explain the procedure to the patients	Gain consent and cooperation, and ensure the patient is comfortable
3.	Make the patient preferably in supine position or sitting position, if not contraindicated	Tense muscles can raise diastolic pressure hence the need to support the limbs
4.	Position the sphygmomanometer at the level of the heart with palm facing upwards	To ensure an accurate reading is obtained
5.	The meniscus of mercury should be read at the eye level and more than 3 feet away	To prevent errors in recording values
6.	Remove tight clothing from the limb to be used and support the limb	To obtain correct reading
7.	Apply the correct-sized sphygmomanometer cuff 2.5 cm above the antecubital fossa directly over the patient's skin and in level with the heart	The incorrect position of the cuff can lead to inaccuracy of 0.8 mm Hg/cm above or below heart level (Hill and Grim, 1991); the cuff should be sufficient enough to nearly/completely encircle arm and too smaller cuff raises blood pressure artificially
8.	Ensure the level of mercury in the manometer; it should be within zero	To get correct value
9.	Close the valve of the pump; palpate the radial artery gently with the non-dominant hand and inflate the cuff, and note the point where the pulsations disappear (palpation method)	This recognizes a predictable value of systolic pressure, which helps to reduce errors caused by auscultatory gap (a gap occurring when Korotkoff sounds disappear after K5 and reappear after a gap of 5–40 mm Hg)
10.	Palpate the brachial artery with the fingers and place the stethoscope in the ear, and keep the diaphragm of stethoscope over the brachial artery gently; do not allow the stethoscope to touch the clothing or the cuff	Hearing of the pulsation sound should be clear; the pressure of the inflated cuff will prevent blood flow through the artery and light pressure on the stethoscope maintains full skin contact, but when excessive, it distorts/lengthens Korotkoff sounds
11.	Inflate the cuff until the mercury rises up to 2–3 mm Hg/s; the deflation should not be too fast or too slow	If the deflation is too fast, it gives false low reading; if it is too slow, it causes venous congestion and arm pain can result in false high reading and discomfort to the patient
12.	Note the point at which the sound become clear and louder; read the pressure to the closest even number and continue deflating the cuff, and observe the point	To get the exact value of the patient's blood pressure and the markings on the sphygmomanometer at 2 mm Hg intervals; so, rounding up/down to 5 mm Hg factors leads to errors, which could give rise to inappropriate or inconsistent treatment

Contd...

Contd...

Sl No	Care action	Rationale
13.	Do not show evidence of panic on the face when a considerably low or high reading is obtained	To prevent the anxiety of the patient
14.	To double check the reading, deflate the cuff fully and repeat the steps 9–14 after 30–60 seconds	To avoid patient discomfort To avoid the misconception of the values
15.	Allow the remaining air to escape quickly; remove the cuff and fold and keep it in place	To ensure the patient is comfortable To keep it ready for use again
16.	Record the systolic and diastolic pressures in the nurses' chart and on the vitals record	Documentation is necessary to identify the variances in future recordings

Points to Note

+ Collect the history from the patient or relatives whether he/she ingested caffeine or has smoked within 30 minutes prior to measurement. These activities may alter the blood pressure. Factors such as a recent meal, full bladder and cigarette smoking can affect blood pressure. Ideally they should have rested 5–15 minutes preprocedure.
+ The nurse should instruct the patient to keep their feet flat. Crossing of feet may increase the blood pressure.

Contraindications

- The arm has intravenous line
- The arm has got affected with any injury, e.g. fracture, burns, open wound, etc.
- The arm has a shunt or fistula for renal dialysis
- The side on which a breast or axillary surgery is done.

Performing Hygienic Procedures and Other Basic Procedures

MOUTH CARE

Definition

Mouth care is defined as the scientific care of the teeth and mouth by using antiseptic solutions.

Purposes

1. To keep the mucosa clean, soft, moist and intact.
2. To keep the lips clean, soft, moist and intact.
3. To prevent oral infections.
4. To remove the food debris as well as dental plaque without damaging the gum.
5. To alleviate pain, discomfort and enhance oral intake with appetite.
6. To prevent halitosis or relieve it and freshen the mouth.

Equipments

A clean tray containing:
- Sterile dressing tray
- Mackintosh and towel
- Toothbrush and paste/tooth powder (if needed)
- Mouthwash solution
- Cup of water (needed amount)
- Face towel
- Sponge cloth
- A tongue depressor/spatula
- A pair of gloves
- Gauze pieces
- Emollient
- Kidney tray
- A bowl with clean water (for dentures as applicable).

Procedure

The procedure for mouth care is detailed in Table 3.1.

Table 3.1: Procedure for mouth care

Sl No	Care action	Rationale
1.	Explain the procedure to patient	To reduce the unease and get the cooperation from the patient
2.	Wash hands	To reduce transmission of microorganisms
3.	Gather all equipment near the patient side	To promote efficiency
4.	Discuss procedure with patient	To discover hygiene preferences
5.	Wear clean gloves	To prevent contact with microorganisms or body fluids
6.	Assess oral mucosa, teeth and throat	To determine status of oral cavity and patient's need for care and teaching
7.	Take the patient to the edge of bed and if possible in semi-Fowler, if it is not contraindicated	For no difficulty of doing the procedure and to prevent the aspiration
8.	Put a small mackintosh with a face towel on the patient's chest and tuck it under the chin	To prevent the soil and make the patient comfortable
9.	Place kidney tray against the cheek and directly under the mouth	To dispose the used gauze
10.	Raise the head end of the bed to 45°	To avoid the aspiration
11.	If the patient is unconscious, with help of tongue depressor, gently open the jaw	To prevent injury and bleeding
12.	Examine the patient's oral cavity completely with the help of torch, tongue depressor or spatula and gauze	To identify any changes in moisture, cleanliness, infection or bleeding, ulcers in the oral cavity
13.	Pour antiseptic solution into a cup and soak gauze in solution, and squeeze nicely with help of artery forceps	To prevent the infection and easy to do the procedure
14.	Clean teeth from incisors to molars using up and down movements, from gums to crown	To promote the circulation and proper cleanliness
15.	Use one clamp to pick up gauze and the other to clean (avoid interchanging of clamps)	To avoid cross-contamination
16.	Clean oral cavity from proximal to distal, using one gauze for each stroke with wet gauze	To avoid cross-contamination
17.	For supportive and oriented patients, toothbrush might be used to clean the teeth	This facilitates the patient to involve in self-care
18.	Discard used gauze into K-basin	To help for proper disposal and make the patient comfortable
19.	Provide a tumbler of water and instruct the patient to gargle mouth	Rinsing takes away loosened debris and make the mouth taste and fresher
20.	Position K-basin properly	To prevent the spillage to other area
21.	Clean tongue from inner to outer aspect, folding rag piece in such a way that the tip of clamp is completely protected	To prevent injury and remove the bad taste in the mouth
22.	Provide water to rinse mouth	Rinsing removes loosened debris and make the mouth taste fresher

Contd...

Contd...

SI No	Care action	Rationale
23.	Lubricate lips using swab stick	To prevent dry lips and lip cracks
24.	Wipe face with towel	To make the patient comfortable and promote the positive body image
25.	Rinse used articles and replace equipment	To promote the safe and comfortable environment to the patient

> **Points to Note**
>
> ✦ Common antiseptic solutions (dentifrices) used:
>   - Thymol glycerin.
>   - Sodium bicarbonate (1%).
>   - Borax glycerin.
>   - Vaseline.
> ✦ Pay more attention to lips, buccal mucosa, lateral and ventral surfaces of the tongue, floor of the mouth and soft palate.
> ✦ Ask the patient about taste changes, changes in saliva production and composition, oral discomfort or any problem in swallowing.

HAIR COMBING

Purposes

- To keep the hair clean and healthy
- To appear neat and make the patient comfortable
- Help to observe the scalp
- To promote growth of the hair and reduce hair fall
- To prevent itching and infection of the scalp
- To prevent the accumulation of dirt and dandruff
- To provide the sense of well-being
- To wipe out the pediculi.

Equipments

A clean tray containing:
- Towel
- Clean comb with coarse and fine teeth
- Kidney tray
- Oil in container (if necessary).

Procedure

The procedure for hair combing is described in Table 3.2.

Table 3.2: Procedure for hair combing

SI No	Care action	Rationale
1.	Explain the procedure to the patient	To get the cooperation
2.	Wash your hands	To prevent cross-contamination
3.	If possible, make the patient to sit on a bed/chair/stool	To make the patient comfortable for the procedure
4.	Place a towel across the pillow if the patient is in bed; for the sitting patient, place a towel around shoulders	To prevent hair accumulation on the bed/surrounding area
5.	Ensure each half of the hair is treated separately	To make the patient comfortable and to make the procedure painless
6.	Separate the hair in small strands	To enable too easy comb
7.	Hold the strands above the part to be combed (anchoring)	To enhance the comfort
8.	Comb the tangles out from the ends first and then go up gradually	Easy to remove the tangles and ensure the comfort of the patient
9.	Brush from the scalp toward hair end	To promote the circulation and feel the patient comfortable
10.	If tangles are more, use the fingers to take apart small lock of hair, comb loose end of the hair	Easy to remove the tangles and ensure the comfort of the patient
11.	Comb one side of patient's head and repeat the same for other side	To make the patient neat and comfortable
12.	Discard loose hair into kidney tray	To make the area clean
13.	Secure the plait, it should not be too tight	To avoid the discomfort for the patient
14.	Remove the towel and kidney tray	To promote the patient comfort

Points to Note

◆ For patients who can be assisted with hair care, the nurse should advocate timely combing of hair and make sure that they are presentable.

HAIR WASH

Definition

Giving hair wash, while patient is bedridden.

Purposes

- To improve the scalp condition
- To keep the hair clean and healthy
- To reduce the hair loss
- To prevent dandruff and infection
- To increase the patient cleanliness and neat appearance.

Equipments

A tray containing:
- Shampoo
- Comb
- Small bowl
- Mackintosh
- Bath towel
- Sponge towel
- Rag pieces
- Bucket to collect waste water
- Jugs of hot and tepid water
- Basin
- Mug
- Non-absorbent cotton
- Kidney tray.

Procedure

The procedure for hair wash is detailed in Table 3.3.

Table 3.3: Procedure for hair wash

SI No	Care action	Rationale
1.	Explain the procedure to the patient	To relieve the anxiety and to get the cooperation
2.	Place the mackintosh and towel under the neck, head and shoulder	To prevent the soiling of linen
3.	Consign the patient diagonally across the bed over the mackintosh, so that the head and shoulder are at the edge of the bed; other end of the mackintosh should be placed in the bucket	To make the patient comfortable for the procedure and to prevent the water spill over the floor
4.	Check the temperature of the water before starting the procedure	To prevent the burs and to promote comfort of the patient
5.	Place the small towel over the eyes and plug ears with the cotton balls	To prevent the entry of water into the ears
6.	Wear the personal protective equipment (PPE), i.e. apron, gloves, etc.	To protect the uniforms
7.	Loosen the hair and remove tangles, and wet the hair with warm water; apply the shampoo equally on the scalp	To enable proper washing
8.	Work up foam with both hands and start at hair line and work in the direction of back of neck by massage of all the scalp area	To promote circulation and to ensure that all the areas are cleaned
9.	Immerse the hair into the bucket, shower the water slowly and wash the hair, raise the head to some extent with one hand and rinse the back side of the head and squeeze the water thoroughly	To take away the shampoo comprehensively and prevent the water spill over the floor

Contd...

Contd...

Sl No	Care action	Rationale
10.	Apply the shampoo again, if the hair is found dirty	To ensure the cleanliness of the hair
11.	Drape the hair with towel and remove the water away	To make the patient comfortable and to ensure cleanliness of the area
12.	Fold the mackintosh into the bucket	To prevent the spill of water on the floor
13.	Remove the ear plugs and towel, which has covered the eyes; dry the neck and hair thoroughly	To make the hair waterless of hair and ease
14.	Spread the hair on the pillow for some time	To dry completely
15.	Wipe face with towel thoroughly after the bath; dry the hair	To keep the patient comfortable
16.	Replace the articles; discard dirty water and wash the hands	To maintain a safe environment

> **Points to Note**
>
> • For patients who can be assisted with hair care, the nurse should advocate timely washing of hair and make sure that they are presentable.

EYE CARE

Definition

Eye care is the procedure of assessing, cleaning or irrigating the eye and/or instillation of prescribed ocular preparations.

Purposes

- To relieve pain and discomfort
- To prevent or treat infection
- To prevent or treat injury to the eye
- To detect disease at an early stage
- To detect drug-induced toxicity at an early stage
- To prevent damage to the cornea in sedated or unconscious patients.

Equipments

Sterile tray containing:
- Cotton balls
- Thumb forceps
- Bowl
- Kidney tray
- Towel
- Sterile 0.9% sodium chloride.

Procedure

The procedure for eye care is detailed in Table 3.4.

Table 3.4: Procedure for eye care

SI No	Care action	Rationale
1.	Explain the procedure to the patient	To get consent from the patient
2.	Place the patient head well supported with tilted back	To make the patient comfortable and easy to do the procedure
3.	Wash hands thoroughly using bactericidal soap	To reduce the risk of cross infection
4.	Make sure enough light source is available	For the better observation
5.	For all time, treat uninfected or uninflamed eye first	To reduce the risk of cross infection
6.	Take two cotton balls, dip in sterile 0.9% normal saline and squeeze them nicely; start to clean the eye from inner canthus to outer canthus in a straight single stroke	If the swab is not squeezed properly, the solution will run downward to the patient's cheek; this may induce the risk of cross infection and cause the patient discomfort
7.	Ensure to use new swab each time; repeat the procedure until all the discharge has been removed	To reduce the risk of cross infection
8.	Once both eyelids have been cleaned and dried out, make the patient comfortable	To ensure patient's comfort
9.	Discard the waste according to the hospital policy	To minimize the cross-contamination
10.	Replace the equipment	To arrange and keep for next use
11.	Wash hands	To reduce the cross infection
12.	Record the procedure in the nurse's record	To follow-up any fluctuations and continuity of care

SPONGE BATH

Definition

Sponge bath is the procedure of cleaning the body of the patient, who is in the bed (unable to take bath himself/herself).

Purposes

- To prevent bacteria spreading on skin
- To clean the patient's body
- To stimulate the circulation
- To improve general muscular tone and joint
- To make patient comfort and help to induce sleep
- To observe skin condition and objective symptom.

Equipments

- A pair of gloves
- Apron
- Emollient
- Soap with soap dish
- Jug
- Basin

- Bucket
- Sponge cloth
- Face towel
- Bath towel
- Gauze piece: 2–3
- Mackintosh
- Bottom sheet, top sheet, draw sheets
- Nail cutter.

Procedure

The procedure for sponge bath is detailed in Table 3.5.

Table 3.5: Procedure for sponge bath

Sl No	Care action	Rationale
1.	Explain the purpose and procedure to the patient; if he/she is alert or oriented, question the patient about personal hygiene preferences and ability to assist with the bath	Providing information to get cooperation; encourage the patient to assist with care and to promote independence
2.	Gather all required equipments near the patient bedside	Organization facilitates accurate skill performance
3.	Assess and plan care in action with the patient and family/friend, if needed	To plan care will support participation and independence
4.	Check the room temperature; switch off air cooler (AC)/fan if not needed	To make the patient comfortable, and prevent the chillness and cold
5.	Wash your hands and put on gloves	To prevent the spread of organisms
6.	Provide urinals, bedpan or commode to the patient	To avoid any disturbance during procedure and to prevent any discomfort
7.	Remove the gloves and wash hands, use disposable gloves and apron	To prevent the cross-contamination and to prevent soiling of uniforms
8.	Provide proper privacy to the patient	To maintain the self-esteem and to make patient more comfortable
9.	Assist to remove clothing without exposing the patient	To maintain privacy and dignity, and body temperature
10.	Remove the patient's cloth and cover the patient body with top sheet; if an intravenous (IV) tubing is present on the patient's upper extremity, thread the IV tubing and bag through the sleeve of the soiled cloth and rehang the IV solution; check the IV flow rate	Removing the cloth permits easier access when cleansing the patient body and be sure that IV delivery is uninterrupted and to maintain the sterile setup
11.	Fill two basins about two third full with warm water (43°C–46°C or 110°F–115°F)	Water at proper temperature relaxes the patient and provides warmthness
12.	Assist the patient to move toward the right side of the cot	Easy to do the procedure
13.	Lift the patient's head and shoulder, and put mackintosh and big towel under the patient's body from the head to shoulders; place face towel under the chin, which has also covered the top sheet	To prevent the bottom sheet from becoming wet Soap irritates the eyes

Contd...

Contd...

Sl No	Care action	Rationale
	Make a mitt with the sponge towel and moisten it with plain water Wash the patient's eyes; clean from inner to outer corner; use a different section of the mitt to wash each eye Wash the patient's face, neck and ears; use soap on these areas only if the patient prefers; rinse and dry carefully	Washing from inner to outer corner prevents sweeping debris into the patient's eyes Using a separate portion of the mitt for each eye prevents the spread of infection
14.	Wash, rinse and dry upper half of the body, starting with the side furthest away from your side; care needs to be taken not to wet drains/dressings and IV devices	To promote patient well-being and cleanliness, and reduce the risk of cross infection
15.	Wash, rinse and dry legs, starting with the side furthest away from your side; roll patient, wash back; then using disposable pads, wash sacral area, check pressure points and cover areas that are not being washed Return patient on to their back, ensuring they are covered; apply napkin as required	To prevent and treat pressure ulcer and make the patient comfortable
16.	Clear area of any obstacles, ensure the environment warm and draw curtains, close doors to guarantee privacy and dignity	To maintain comfort, a safe environment, and promote privacy and dignity
17.	Change the water and wash the genital area with patient's verbal consent, (if patient is willing to wash this area themself, provide enough water to wipe); using a separate wipe, wash around the area and then dry it	To decrease risk of infection
18.	If patient is on urinary catheter, wear the gloves and wash the tubing away from the genital area; avoid using soap in genital area	To avoid the irritancy and to reduce risk of infection
19.	Turn the patient one side and remove the soiled sheet, and advance the new bottom sheet and draw sheet, if they are to remain in bed; ensure that a minimum of two nurses are present during this procedure	To reduce unnecessary activity and ensure the safe of the patient
20.	Dry and comb patient's hair as desired	To improve patient's comfort and promote self-esteem
21.	Cover the patient with top sheet; position the patient comfortably	To improve the patient's comfort and reduce the risk of pressure ulcers
22.	Take away all used articles and linen from the patient side	To maintain a safe environment and promote patient independence
23.	Remove the aprons and gloves, and dispose it according to hospital policy and wash the hands thoroughly	To prevent cross infection

Points to Note

- Remember, when washing genital area of female patients, wash from perineum to rectum.
- For male patients, retract the foreskin if uncircumcised when washing the penis.

NAIL CARE

Definition

Nail care is one of the nursing cares for maintaining the personal hygiene and to prevent the infections.

Purposes

- To keep nails clean
- To make the nails look neat
- To prevent the patient's skin from scratching
- To avoid infection caused by dirty nail.

Equipments

- Nail cutter
- Bowl with water
- Cotton
- Kidney tray
- Sponge cloth
- Middle towel
- Mackintosh
- Plastic bowl of small size
- Soap with soapdish
- Warm water
- Body lotion
- Clean gloves
- Face towel.

Procedure

The procedure for nail care is detailed in Table 3.6.

Table 3.6: Procedure for nail care

Sl No	Care action	Rationale
1.	Explain the procedure to the patient	To reduce the anxiety and to get the cooperation
2.	Arrange all the articles near to the patient	To minimize the time
3.	Wash your hands and wear gloves	To prevent the infection
4.	If patient is in bed, raise the backrest and place a towel under the hand; if the patient is in a chair, place a table in front and place a towel on the table	To make the patient comfortable till end of the procedure
5.	By using cotton with remover, remove nail polish from the nail	To prevent the infection
6.	Fill up the wash basin with warm water; immerse hands into a bowl of warm water	Warm water shall soften the nails and thicken the epithelial cells; to decrease the inflammation of skin and promote the local circulation

Contd...

Contd...

SI No	Care action	Rationale
7.	Soak the fingers in the warm water for 5–10 minutes; soak one hand at a time or soak both at the same time	Soaking helps to cleanse the nails and make it easy to remove dirt and debris
8.	Place towel under patient's dried hands; gently remove dirt around and under each fingernails	To reduce the infections
9.	Cut short the finger nails by using nail clipper; shape and smooth the nails with nail file; wipe each fingertip with cotton dipped in antiseptic solution	Cutting straight prevents splitting of nail margins To prevent the irregularity of the nail and formation of sharp that can irritate lateral margins
10.	Dry the hands with towel	To make comfortable
11.	Remove and replace the articles from the patient care area	To make the patient comfortable with safety

Points to Note

* Before starting the nail care, examine the exterior part of fingers, toes, feet and nails, to give particular attention to areas of dryness, inflammation and cracking; also inspect areas between toes, heels and soles of feet.
* The integrity of feet and nails determines frequency and level of hygiene required.
* Heels, soles and sides of the feet are prone to irritation from ill-fitting shoes.

BACK CARE

Definition

Back care means cleaning and massaging the back, paying special attention to pressure points. Especially back massage provides comfort and relaxes the patient; thereby it facilitates the physical stimulation to the skin and the emotional relaxation.

Purposes

* To improve circulation to the back
* To refresh the mode and feeling
* To relieve from fatigue, pain and stress
* To induce sleep.

Equipments

* A clean gown
* Clean gloves
* Towels (face towels and bath towel)
* Basin with warm water

- Kidney tray
- Soap
- Oil/White paraffin/Emollient
- Mackintosh.

Procedure

The procedure for back care is detailed in Table 3.7.

Table 3.7: Procedure for back care

Sl No	Care action	Rationale
1.	Perform hand hygiene	To prevent spread of infection
2.	Assemble all equipments required	Organization facilitates accurate skill and performance
3.	Identify the patient, and his/her identification status and condition	To evaluate sufficient condition of the patient
4.	Explain the patient about the purpose of the procedure	Providing information and to get cooperation
5.	Put all required equipments to the bedside	Appropriate setting can make the time of the procedure minimum and effective
6.	Close all windows and doors, and put the screen or/and utilize the curtain, if it is there	To ensure that the room is warm; to maintain the privacy
7.	Expose the patient's back fully and observe whether there are any abnormalities	To find any abnormalities soon is important to prevent more complication and/or provide proper medication as soon as possible If you find out some redness, heat or sores, you cannot massage that place If the patient has already some red sore or broken down area, you need to report the senior staff and/or doctor
8.	Lather soap by sponge towel; wipe with soap and rinse with plain warm water	To maintain the self-esteem and to make patient more comfortable
9.	Provide a gentle massage over the patient's back by using emollients; the pattern for massage includes: • Using your palm, begin in sacral area with smooth, circular strokes • Move your hands up the center of the back and then over the both scapula • Massage in a circular motion over scapula • Move your hands down the sides of the back • Massage the areas over right and left iliac crest • Apply firm, continuous pressure without breaking contact with the patient's skin • Repeat the above steps for 3–5 minutes using more lotion as necessary • Pat dry excess lotion with the towel	To improve circulation and to provide sense of comfort for the patient

Contd...

Contd...

Sl No	Care action	Rationale
10.	Help the patient to put on the clothes and in returning the patient to comfortable position	To keep the patient warm and comfortable
11.	Replace all equipments to their proper place	To prepare for the next procedure
12.	Perform hand hygiene	To prevent the spread of infection
13.	Document on the chart with your signature, including date, time and the skin condition; report any findings to senior staff	Documentation provides coordination of care; giving signature maintains professional accountability

Points to Note

- Back care must be provided during every shift for patients, who are admitted in the intensive care unit (ICU). For patient with pressure ulcers, back massage need to be provided every 2nd hourly.

Steps of Back Massage

Steps of back massage is given in Table 3.8.

Table 3.8: Steps of back massage

Sl No	Steps	Rationale
1.	Effleurage/Stroking: Start with long gliding strokes; use your entire hand or thumb pad. Start from sacral region to scapular region and the shoulder (do not apply pressure on the spinal cord)	To improve the blood flow. To prevent injury
2.	Petrissage: Use gentle pressure to knead or squeeze the muscles; use thumb and distal phalanges	To relieve the deeper muscle tension and clear out toxins
3.	Friction: Use fingertips or thumb pads and do circulatory motion	To breakdown knots and to achieve muscles flexibility
4.	Cupping: Use cupped hands to strike either side of the back/spinal cord	To percuss the area
5.	Tapotement: Use edge of the palm and strike briskly on either side of the back	To stimulate circulation

FOOT CARE

Definition

Foot care involves all aspects of preventive and corrective care of the foot and ankle.

Purposes

1. To make the patient comfortable.
2. To prevent ingrown nails.

3. Help to reduce developing of foot ulcer in diabetes mellitus (DM) patients.
4. To assess the foot problems including foot pain, joint inflammation, plantar warts, fungal infections (e.g. athlete's foot), nerve disorders, torn ligaments, broken bones, bacterial infections and tissue injuries such as frostbite.

Equipments

- Nail cutter
- Kidney tray
- Sponge cloth
- Middle towel
- Mackintosh
- A basin with warm water
- Soap with soapdish, if needed
- Cream or lotion
- Clean gloves.

Procedure

The procedure for foot care is detailed in Table 3.9.

Table 3.9: Procedure for foot care

Sl No	Care action	Rationale
1.	Explain the procedure to the patient	To reduce the anxiety and to get the cooperation
2.	Arrange all the articles near the patient	To easily access and to minimize the time
3.	Wash your hands and wear gloves	To prevent the infection
4.	If patient is in bed, raise the backrest; if not contraindicated, make the patient to sit in the chair comfortably	Make the patient comfortable till the end of the procedure
5.	Inspect the feet, observe for redness, edema, ulceration, callus formation or ingrown toenails and report promptly	To identify the early stage of infections and helping to teach the patient, the signs and symptoms of infection
6.	By using cotton with remover, remove nail polish from the nail	To prevent the infection
7.	Fill up the washbasin with warm water; immerse foot into a bowl of warm water	Warm water softens the hard skin, and calluses and thickens the epithelial cells to decrease the inflammation of skin and promote the local circulation
8.	Soak the foot in the warm water for 5–10 minutes; soak one foot at a time or soak both at the same time	Prolonged positioning may cause discomfort

Contd...

Contd...

Sl No	Care action	Rationale
9.	Wash feet and legs with soap, unless their medical condition hinders access to the feet/legs	To avoid other complication
10.	Dry your feet and toes thoroughly after washing them, and apply a moisturizing foot cream	To remove the dirt and prevent the infection
11.	Gently remove hard skin and calluses with a pumice stone or foot file thoroughly	To prevent infection and complications, and promote the comfort
12.	Trim your toenails straight across, never at an angle or down the edges	To prevent ingrown toenails and inflammations
13.	Apply lotion generously to all areas below the knee; avoid putting lotion on broken skin, in between the toes or on nail beds	To prevent the dryness and cracks
14.	Position the patient on cot, if needed	To make the patient comfortable
15.	Remove and replace the articles from the patient care area and replace it	Remove and replace the articles from the patient care area and replace it
16.	Document the procedure in the nurse's record; if any signs and symptoms of infection report these signs promptly to the physician	To prevent the progress to worsen and to do the comparison study of the patient condition from present to future

Points to Note

♦ Educate the patient to wear footwear (non-skid socks included) at all times. Stress the importance of not going bare foot.
♦ Instruct the patient to not go to bed without washing the feet. If they leave dirt on the skin's surface, it can become irritated and infected. Wash the feet every evening with soap and water.

PERINEAL CARE

Definition

Perineal care is a aseptic procedure, which involves cleaning of the genitalia and surrounding area by using antiseptic solution. Proper assessment and care of the perineal area will need professional clinical judgment.

Purposes

• To keep the perineal area clean
• To prevent infection
• To make the patient comfortable.

Equipments

• Sterile perineal care pack containing cup with cotton balls
• Artery clamp and thumb forceps

- Antiseptic solution (Betadine)
- Extra cotton balls
- Mackintosh
- A pair of clean gloves.

Procedure

The procedure for perineal care is detailed in Table 3.10.

Table 3.10: Procedure for perineal care

Sl No	Care action	Rationale
1.	Explain the procedure to the patient	To make sure that the patient understands the procedure
2.	Gather all the equipment near the bedside	To save time
3.	Provide privacy	To make the patient sense comfortable and treat patient with self-esteem
4.	Wash hands thoroughly	To minimize risk of cross infection
5.	Help out patient to lie down in dorsal recumbent position	Easy to do the procedure and make the patient comfortable
6.	Put the mackintosh; cover the patient with a draw sheet or sheet that is folded double	To prevent the staining of antiseptic solution in the top sheet
7.	Open the sterile perineal pack and pour antiseptic solution	To minimize risk of cross infection
8.	Wash hands again; wear a pair of clean gloves	To minimize risk of cross infection
9.	Clean thighs by using the cotton ball from the center to the peripheral area; use a separate cotton ball for each stroke	To minimize risk of cross infection
10.	Use non-dominant hand too gently and clean labia majora; retract labia from thigh with dominant hand, clean from perineum to rectum; give more attention in skin folds	Wiping from perineum to rectum reduces chance of transmitting fecal organisms to urinary meatus; skin folds may contain microorganisms
11.	Separate labia minora with non-dominant hand to expose urethral meatus and vaginal orifice; with dominant hand, clean downward from pubic area toward rectum in one smooth stroke	Reduces chance of transmitting microorganisms to urinary meatus
12.	Follow the front to back method, dry perineal area thoroughly (perineum to rectum)	To prevent the cross-contamination
13.	Position the patient as he/she desire	To make the patient comfortable
14.	Replace articles and wash hands	To arrange and keep it ready for next use, and minimize risk of cross infection
15.	Document procedure in the nurses record; if there is any foul-smelling discharge or any other abnormalities, inform the doctor	Help to identify the infection in early stage

> **Points to Note**
>
> For male catheter care:
> + Gently grasp the patient's penis.
> + In an uncircumcised male, carefully retract the foreskin prior to washing the penis.
> + Cleanse in a circular motion, moving from the tip of the penis backwards toward the pubic area.
> + Return the foreskin to its former position.
> + Wash, rinse and dry the scrotum carefully.

PERFORMING PHYSICAL EXAMINATION

Definition

Physical examination is an important tool in assessing the client's health status. Approximately, 15% of the information used in the assessment, comes from the physical examination. It is performed to collect objective data and to correlate it with subjective data.

Purposes

- To collect objective data from the client
- To detect the abnormalities with systematic technique early
- To diagnose diseases
- To determine the status of present health in health checkup and refer the client for consultation, if needed.

Principles of Physical Examination

A systematic approach should be used, while doing physical examination. This helps avoiding any duplication or omission. Generally, a cephalocaudal approach (head to toe) is used, but in the case of infant, examination of heart and lung function should be done before the examination of other body parts, because when the infant starts crying, his/her breath and heart rate may change.

Methods of Physical Examination

- Inspection
- Palpation
- Percussion
- Auscultation.

Inspection

Inspection means looking at the client carefully to discover any signs of illness. Inspection gives more information than other method and is therefore the most useful method of physical examination.

Palpation

Palpation means using hands to touch and feel. Different parts of hands are used for different sensations such as temperature, texture of skin, vibration, tenderness, etc. For example, fingertips are used for fine tactile surfaces, the back of fingers for feeling temperature, and the flat of the palm and fingers for feeling vibrations.

Percussion

Percussion determines the density of various parts of the body from the sound produced by them, when they are tapped with fingers. Percussion helps to find out abnormal solid masses, fluid and gas in the body, and to map out the size and borders of certain organ like the heart.

Methods of percussion are:
1. Put the middle fingers of the patient's left hand against the body part to be percussed.
2. Tap the end joint of this finger with the middle finger of the right hand.
3. Give two or three taps at each area to be percussed.
4. Compare the sound produced at different areas.

Auscultation

Auscultation means listening the sounds transmitted by a stethoscope, which is used to listen to the heart, lungs and bowel sounds.

Equipments

- Tray: 1
- Watch with a seconds hand: 1
- Height scale: 1
- Weight scale: 1
- Thermometer: 1
- Stethoscope: 1
- Sphygmomanometer: 1
- Measuring tape: 1
- Scale: 1
- Torchlight or penlight: 1
- Spatula: 1
- Reflex hammer: 1
- Otoscope if available: 1 set
- Disposable gloves: 1 pair
- Cotton swabs and cotton gauze pad
- Examination table
- Record form
- Ballpoint pen, pencils.

Procedure

The procedure for performing physical examination is detailed in Table 3.11.

Table 3.11: Procedure for performing physical examination

SI No	Action/Rationale	Normal finding	Abnormal finding
1.	**Explain the purpose and procedure** Providing information fosters patient's cooperation and allays anxiety	Preparation of the patient for physical examination	
2.	**Close doors and put screen** To provide privacy		
3.	**Encourage the client to empty bladder** A full bladder makes the patient uncomfortable		
4.	**Perform physical examination** ***General examination*** Assess overall body appearance and mental status ***Inspection*** a. Observe the client's ability to respond to verbal commands (responses indicate the client's speech and cognitive function) b. Observe the client's level of consciousness (LOC) and orientation; ask the client to state his/her own name, current location and approximate day, month or year (responses indicate the client's brain function; LOC is the degree of awareness of environmental stimuli; it varies from full wakefulness and alertness to coma; orientation is a measure of cognitive function or the ability to think and reason)	Client responds appropriately to commands The client is fully awake and alert; eyes are open and follow people or objects; the client is attentive to questions and responds promptly and accurately to commands If the patient is sleeping, he/she responds readily to verbal or physical stimuli and demonstrates wakefulness and alertness; the client is aware of who he/she is (orientation to person), where he/she is (orientation to place) and when it is (orientation to time)	Client has confused, disoriented or inappropriate responses Client has a lowered LOC and shows irritability, short attention span or dulled perceptions Client is uncooperative or unable to follow simple commands or answer simple questions At a lowered LOC, the client may respond to physical stimuli only; the lowest extreme is coma, when the eyes are closed and the client fails to respond to verbal or physical stimuli with no voluntary movement If LOC is between full awareness and coma, objectively note the client's eye movements; voluntary, withdrawal to stimuli or withdrawal to noxious stimuli (pain) only

Contd...

Contd...

SI No	Action/Rationale	Normal finding	Abnormal finding
	c. Observe the client's ability to think, remember, process information and communicate (these processes indicate cognitive functioning) Inspect articulation on speech, style and contents of speaking	The client is able to follow commands, repeat and remember information Smooth, appropriate native language	Dysphasia, dysarthria, memory loss, disorientation, hallucination Not clear/not smooth/inappropriate contents
	d. Observe the client's ability to see, hear, smell and distinguish tactile sensations	The client can hear even though the speaker turns away He/She can identify objects or reads a clock in the room and distinguish between sharp and soft objects	The client cannot hear tones and must look directly at the speaker He/She cannot read a clock or distinguish sharp from soft
	e. Observe signs of distress (alert the examiner to immediate concerns; if distress is noted, the client may require healthcare interventions before continuing the examination)		The client shows labored breathing, wheezing, coughing, wincing, sweating, guarding of body part (suggests pain), anxious facial expression or fidgety movements Posture is stopped or twisted Limb movements are uneven or unilateral
	f. Observe for facial expression and mood (these could be effected by disease or ill condition)	Eyes are alert and in contact with examiner The client is relaxed, smiles or frowns appropriately and has a calm demeanor	Eyes are closed or averted The client is frowning or grimacing and is unable to answer questions
	g. Observe general appearance: Posture, gait and movement (to identify obvious changes)	Posture is upright, gait is smooth and equal for the client's age and development; limb movements are bilateral	Posture is stopped or twisted; limb movements are uneven or unilateral
	h. Observe grooming, personal hygiene and dress (personal appearance can indicate self-comfort; grooming suggests his/her ability to perform self-care)	Clothing reflects gender, age, climate; hair, skin and clothing are clean, well-groomed and appropriate for the occasion	The client wears unusual clothing for gender, age or climate Hair is poor groomed, lack of cleanliness Excessive oil on the skin Body odor is present
5.	**Measurement** a. Height: i. Ask the client to remove shoes and stand with his/her back and heels touching the wall		

Contd...

Contd...

SI No	Action/Rationale	Normal finding	Abnormal finding
	ii. Place a pencil flat on client's head, so that it makes a mark on the wall iii. This shows his/her height measured with centimeter tape from the floor to the mark on the wall (or if available, measure the height with measuring scale) b. Weight:	> 140 cm (or 145 cm) in female	< 140 cm (or 145 cm) in female
	i. Weigh client without shoes and much clothing	Body mass index (BMI) is used to assess the status of nutrition using weight and height in the world Formula for BMI = weight (kg)/ height (m²) Normal BMI = 18.5–24.5	**Classification** **BMI** • Under weight < 18.5 • Healthy weight 18.5–24.5 • Over weight 25–29.9 • Obesity > 30
6.	**Take vital signs** Vital signs provide baseline data a. Temperature	36.5°C–37°C	• Hypothermia < 35°C • Pyrexia 38°C–40°C • Hyperpyrexia > 40°C
	b. Pulse (rate/minute) Take the pulse rate and check the beats	In adult, 60–80/min, regular and steady	• Bradycardia • Tachycardia • Pulse deficit, arrhythmia
	c. Respiration Count the breaths without giving notice	Breaths per minute: 16–20/min Clear sound of breaths, regular and steady	• Bradypnea < 10/min • Tachypnea > 20/min • Cheyne-Stokes • Kussmaul's respiration, wheeze, stridor
	d. Blood pressure Take blood pressure under quiet and war	120/80 mm Hg	• Hypotension: In normal adults, blood pressure (BP) < 95/60 mm Hg • Hypertension: BP > 140/90 mm Hg
7.	**Integumentary assessment** Assess integumentary structures (skin, hair, nails) and function ***Skin*** *Inspection and palpation* a. Inspect the back and palms of the client's hands for skin color; compare the right and	The color varies from black brown or fair, depending upon the genetic factors	Erythema, loss of pigmentation, cyanosis, pallor, jaundice

Contd...

Contd...

Sl No	Action/Rationale	Normal finding	Abnormal finding
	left sides make a similar inspection of the feet and toes	Color variations on dark pigmented skin may be best seen in the mucous membranes, nail beds, sclera or lips	
	b. Palpate the skin on the back and palms of the client's hands for moisture, texture: • Moisture • Texture	Slightly moist, no excessive moisture or dryness—firm, smooth, soft, elastic skin	Excessive dryness indicates hypothyroidism Oiliness in acne Roughness in hypothyroidism Velvety texture in hyperthyroidism
	c. Palpate the skin's temperature with the back of your hand	Warmth	Generalized warmth in fever and local warmth, coolness in hypothyroidism
	d. Pinch and release the skin on the back (this palpation indicates the skin's degree of hydration and turgor)	Pinched skin that promptly or gently returns to its previous state, when released signifies normal turgor	Pinched skin is very slow to return to normal position of the client's hand
	e. Press suspected edematous areas with the edge of fingers for 10 seconds and observe for the depression	Depression recovers quickly	Depression recovers slowly or remains Edema indicates fluid retention, a sign of circulatory disorders
	f. Inspect the skin for lesions; note the appearance, size, location, presence and appearance of drainage	Skin is intact, without reddened areas, but with variations in pigmentation and texture, depending on the area's location and its exposure to light and pressure; moles, warts are normal	Erythema, ecchymosis, lesions include rashes, macules, papules, vesicles, wheals, nodules, pustules, tumors or ulcers Wounds include incisions, abrasions, lacerations, pressure ulcers
	Nail a. Inspect the color, shape and lesions of the nails	Pink color and longitudinal bands may be seen in the nails of some people	Koilonychia (spoon-shaped nails) seen in protein deficiency anemia

Contd...

Contd...

Sl No	Action/Rationale	Normal finding	Abnormal finding
	b. Check capillary refill by pressing the nail to blanch; then quickly release pressure, note the return of color	Normally the color returns to pink within 3 seconds; absence of discoloration, cyanosis, clubbing, separation from the edge, etc.	Cyanosis and clubbing is present if there is poor oxygen saturation in the blood Sluggish color return indicates respiratory or cardiovascular dysfunction
	Hair and scalp Inspect the hair for color, distribution, growth and texture	Color may differ from gray to complete black Texture varies from straight to curly The scalp should be clean and absence of scales, lesions, etc.	Alopecia (excessive hair loss is seen in cancer patients) Pediculosis Dandruff Redness and scaling
8.	**Head and neck assessment** ***Face*** Inspect the client's facial expression, symmetry, movement, etc.	Relaxed facial expression without having any deviation and involuntary movement	Blunt expression indicates Parkinson disease Moon face, i.e. Cushing's syndrome Edema around the eyes—glomerulonephritis
	Eyes a. Eyebrows: Observe the eyebrow for color and distribution	Normal black- or brown-colored lashes with normal distribution	Scaliness in seborrheic dermatitis
	b. Eyelids: Inspect the eyelids for edema, lesions, distribution and direction of eyelashes	Eyelashes grow in a downward direction	Ptosis Sty Ectropion Entropion Failure of the eyelids to close
	c. Conjunctiva and sclera: Inspect the color of the sclera and conjunctiva	Transparent white color of the sclera and dark pink conjunctiva	A yellow sclera indicates jaundice and pale conjunctiva indicates anemia
	d. Cornea and lens: Inspect the cornea under good lighting; note any opacities of the lens	Transparent	Opacities in the lens due to cataract
	e. Pupils: Inspect the papillary size, shape, symmetry and reaction	Pupils are equal, round, symmetrical and equally reacting to light	Unequal pupils Miosis—constriction of the pupils Mydriasis—dilation of the pupils
	• Pupillary response to light: – Ask the client to look straight and focus the torchlight from the periphery to the center of the eye	The pupils constrict when the torch approaches the center and it dilates as it is removed	Unresponsive to light otitis media or otitis externa

Contd...

Contd...

SI No	Action/Rationale	Normal finding	Abnormal finding
	– Remove it to the other side and observe how the pupils react f. Coordination of eye movements: • Ask the client to keep the head still and follow the object in the examiner's hand with the eyes only • Move the object toward right, left, up and down	Both eyes move together to follow the direction of the object without moving his head	Eyes do not move together when the object moves indicates paralysis of cranial nerves
	g. Visual acuity test: • Use Snellen chart to check the visual acuity • Make the patient to sit 20 feet away from the Snellen chart and ask to read the letters /numbers by closing one eye • Repeat the same in the other eye • Compare visual acuity of the client with normal vision	20/20 is normal	Myopia (near sightedness) Hypermetropia (far sightedness)
	Ears a. Inspect the shape, location of ears and measure the size	Equal size bilaterally The top of the pinnae meet the eye-occiput line	Microtica or macrotica The top of the pinnae do not meet the eye-occiput line; commonly seen in mentally retarded children
	b. External auditory meatus: Inspect the external auditory meatus using torchlight or otoscope to assess redness, foreign body, swelling, discharge and cerumen		Clear blood from the ear indicates brain hemorrhage Impacted cerumen causes conductive hearing loss A sticky yellow discharge indicates otitis media or otitis externa
	c. Hearing test: i. Whisper test: Stay 30–60 cm away from client's ear and whisper slowly some two syllable words	Normally client repeats the word correctly	If the client does not repeat the words, it indicates hearing loss

Contd...

Contd...

SI No	Action/Rationale	Normal finding	Abnormal finding
ii.	Rinne test: This test is performed by placing a high-frequency (512 Hz) vibrating tuning fork against the patient's mastoid bone and asking the patient to tell you, when the sound is no longer heard; once the client signal that cannot hear it, quickly position the still vibrating tuning fork 1–2 cm from the auditory canal and again ask the patient to tell you if they are able to hear the tuning fork	Air conduction should be greater than bone conduction and so the patient should be able to hear the tuning fork next to the pinna after they can no longer hear it, when held against the mastoid	If they are not able to hear the tuning fork after mastoid test, it means that their bone conduction is more than air conduction; this indicates conductive hearing loss Sensorineural hearing loss—patients usually can hear better on the mastoid process than air process, but indicate the sound has stopped much earlier than conductive loss patients
iii.	Weber test: Keep the vibrated tuning fork in the vertex of the head	The client will hear the sound equally in both the ears	If the client hears more sound in left ear than the right, it means the client has conductive hearing loss in left ear because the sound gets lateralized to the deafer ear
	Nose		
a.	Inspect the shape, size, symmetry of the nose	Nostrils are uniform in size, no flare, no deviation and no obstruction in both vestibule	Asymmetrical in size Deviated nasal septum Flaring nostrils Obstruction in the nose by polyps
b.	Inspect the interior aspect of the nose using pen/torchlight or rhinoscope	No polyps, inflammation, bleeding and foreign body	Nasal mucosa is red and swollen (rhinitis) Deviation of the lower septum is common
c.	Palpate for frontal and maxillary sinus tenderness	No tenderness and pain	Local pain, tenderness, nasal discharge and tenderness suggest acute sinusitis
	Mouth		
a.	Observe the color, moisture and cracking of the lips	No bluish discoloration, cracks and ulcers	Lips bluish (cyanosis) and pallor Cracks, ulcer
b.	Inspect the gums, teeth and tongue	No inflammation and infection in gums, tongue and teeth	Gingivitis Loose teeth Dental caries Coated tongue in typhoid
	Pharynx Ask the client to open the mouth and say 'aah', which helps to see	Pink throat No difficulty in swallowing	Tonsillitis Adenoiditis

Contd...

Contd...

SI No	Action/Rationale	Normal finding	Abnormal finding
	the pharynx well; if not, use spatula to press the tongue; inspect soft palate, tonsils, pharynx and uvula to detect symmetry, swelling or tonsillar enlargement	Pink and small tonsils	Difficulty in swallowing In cranial nerve X paralysis, the soft palate fails to rise and the uvula deviates to the opposite side
	Neck		
	a. Inspect the neck for its symmetry, enlargement of lymph nodes; observe the range of motion of the neck	Head positions centered in the midline and head should be held erect	Rigid neck occurs with arthritis
	b. Lymph nodes: Palpate the lymph nodes by using the pads of your index and middle fingers to detect any palpable nodes with size, shape, mobility, consistency and tenderness	Lymph nodes are neither visible nor becomes red Normal nodes feel movable, discrete, soft, nontender	Enlargement of lymph nodes Lymph adenopathy (> 1 cm) due to infection, allergy or neoplasm Diffuse lymphadenopathy may be seen in human immunodeficiency virus/ acquired immunodeficiency syndrome (HIV/AIDS)
	c. Trachea: • Inspect the trachea to find out any deviation from its normal • Palpate for any tracheal shift; place the index finger on the trachea in the sternal notch and slip it off to each side	Normally trachea is in midline No deviation from the midline	Tracheal push toward one side suggests mass in the neck Tracheal deviation suggests mediastinal mass, atelectasis, etc.
	d. Thyroid gland i. Inspect the thyroid gland and confirm that it rise with swallowing and then fall to their resting position	Normally thyroid gland cannot be palpable; no enlargement, presence of nodules and tenderness	Diffuse enlargement suggests goiter Firm suggests malignancy Soft in Graves' disease Tenderness in thyroiditis
	ii. Palpate the thyroid gland • Stand behind the client • Ask the client to flex the neck slightly forward • Place the fingers of both hands on the client's neck and ask him/her to swallow water; feel for the thyroidisthmus rising up under your finger pads		

Contd...

Contd...

Sl No	Action/Rationale	Normal finding	Abnormal finding
9.	**Chest and lungs** a. Inspection: Make the patient in supine or sitting or semi-Fowler's position to examine the chest; observe the shape and movement of anterior and posterior chest	Anteroposterior (AP) diameter may increase with age Shoulders are even, spine is midline and straight Posterior chest slightly rises and falls on respiration	Barrel chest; AP diameter may increase in chronic obstructive pulmonary disease Structural deformities Scoliosis (lateral curvature) Lordosis (pronounced lumbar curvature) Kyphosis (abnormal spinal curvature and vertebral rotation deform the chest)
	b. Palpation: Palpate the posterior wall over areas to detect any tender masses, swelling or painful area	No tenderness, superficial lumps or masses, normal skin mobility and turgor	Tender pectoral muscles or costal cartilage Pain Masses
	c. Percussion: Percuss the posterior chest to identify any area with an abnormal percussion	Resonance is normal lung sound	Hyperresonance is found in chronic obstructive pulmonary disease (COPD) and asthma Dullness is found in pneumonia, pleural effusion and atelectasis
	d. Auscultation: Listen to the breath posteriorly with mouth open and more deeply than the normal, to note intensity; identify any variation and any adventitious sounds; repeat auscultation in the posterior chest	Breath sounds are usually louder in upper anterior lung fields Bronchial, bronchovesicular, vesicular sounds are the normal breath sounds	Decreased or absent breath sounds suggest atelectasis, pleural effusion, pneumothorax and COPD Increased breath sound suggests pneumonia
10.	**Heart/Pericardium** Make the patient to be in supine position with the head elevated 30°: a. Inspection: Inspect the anterior chest for apical pulsation	Normally seen in children and those with thinner chest	A heave or lift suggests ventricular hypertrophy
	b. Palpation: Palpate the apical pulse by using finger pad to detect some abnormal condition; ask the client to exhale and then hold it; aids the examiner in locating the pulsation in the fourth or fifth intercostal space	The apical pulse is palpable in about half of adult But not palpable in obese clients with thick chest walls	Not palpable in pulmonary emphysema due to overriding lungs

Contd...

Contd...

Sl No	Action/Rationale	Normal finding	Abnormal finding
	c. Percussion: It is done to outline the heart's borders and detect cardiac enlargement: • Place your non-dominant hand's fingers on the client's fifth intercostal space over the left side of the chest near the anterior axillary line • Slide your non-dominant hand's finger toward yourself, percussing as you go • Note the change of sound from resonance over the lung to dull over the heart d. Auscultation: • Place the stethoscope on the chest and hear the sound in second right (aortic valve area) and left (pulmonic area) intercostal space • Then auscultate left lower sternal border (tricuspid valve area) and fifth intercostal space at left midclavicular line (mitral valve area) • Listen S1 and S2; note the rate and rhythm • Listen for murmurs	Percussion sound does not increase Rate ranges from 60 to 100 beats per minute S1 is loudest at the apex and S2, at the base; the rhythm should be regular	Cardiac enlargement is due to increased ventricular wall thickness Irregular rhythm suggests cardiac diseases Both heart sounds are diminished in emphysema, obesity and pericardial effusion Diastolic murmur suggests heart diseases
11.	**Breasts and axillae** a. Inspection: Observe for the size, shape and symmetry of the breasts; inspect color, dimpling, edema or skin lesions and discharge in the breast and nipple; and observe the axillary and subclavicular regions for lymphatic drainage; note any bulging, edema and discoloration	Symmetrical in shape Often the left breast is slightly larger than the right No edema and discoloration normally But fine blue vascular network is visible during pregnancy	Sudden enlargement of breast suggests inflammation or new growth Edema, hyperpigmentation, redness and heat with inflammation, unilateral superficial veins in a non-pregnant woman; recent nipple retraction signifies acquired disease

Contd...

Contd...

Sl No	Action/Rationale	Normal finding	Abnormal finding
	b. Palpation: • Help her to be in a supine position • Place a small pad or towel under the side to be palpated and raise her arm over the head • Use the pads of your three fingers and make a gentle rotary motion on the breast; start at the nipple and palpate out to the periphery • Move in a clockwise direction • Apply gentle pressure on the nipple from outside the areola toward the center and observe any discharge appears; note its color and consistency	In nulliparous woman, normal breast tissue feels firm, smooth and elastic Premenstrual enlargement is normal During lactation, milk secretion is normal	Heat, redness and swelling in non-lactating woman suggests inflammation
12.	**Abdomen** Make the client to lie down in supine position after emptying the bladder: a. Inspection: • Observe the contour and symmetry of the abdomen • Inspect symmetry of the abdomen • Observe the location, contour and bulges of umbilicus • Observe for peristalsis movement and aortic pulsation in the epigastric region b. Auscultation: • Listen to the abdomen before performing percussion or palpation	Normally ranges from flat to round The abdomen should be symmetric bilaterally Normally it is in midline and inverted with no signs of inflammation Normally, peristalsis waves are visible in very thin persons and aortic pulsation is visible in epigastrium Normal sound consists of clicks and gurgles	Abdominal distension Scaphoid abdomen Hernia Enlarged and everted with umbilical hernia Increased peristalsis with the abdominal distension, suggests intestinal obstruction Marked pulsation of the aorta occurs with widened pulse pressure Hyperactive sound will be loud, rushing and high pitched, which suggests increased motility in gastrointestinal infections

Contd...

Contd...

SI No	Action/Rationale	Normal finding	Abnormal finding
	• Listen for the bowel sounds using stethoscope		Hypoactive or absence of sound indicates paralytic ileus or peritonitis
	• Listen for the vascular sounds or bruit with the stethoscope	Normally no sound will be heard	Systolic bruit occurs with stenosis or occlusion of an artery
	c. Percussion: It is done to assess the presence of gas in the abdomen and to identify possible masses:		
	• Percuss the abdomen lightly in all four quadrants	Tympany should dominate because of the presence of gas in the gastrointestinal tract	Absence of tympany
	• Note any large areas of dullness	Normal dullness in the liver and spleen	
	d. Palpation: It is done to screen for organomegaly, mass or tenderness:		
	• Place the client in supine position; keeping your finger pads on the abdominal surface, gently depress the surface about 1–5 cm	No abdominal mass Normally, liver edge, full bladder and right kidney can be palpable	Mass, tenderness, rigidity
	• Move clockwise and explore the entire abdomen		
	Liver		
	• Stand on the client's right side	Liver is normally not palpable	If the liver is palpable more than 1–2 cm below the right costal margin, it indicates enlargement
	• Place your left hand under the client's back parallel to the 11th and 12th ribs		
	• Lift up to support the abdominal contents		
	• Place your right hand on the right upper quadrant with fingers parallel to the midline		
	• Push deeply down when the client takes deep breath		
	• Feel for liver sliding over the fingers, as the client inspires		
	• Note any enlargement or tenderness		

Contd...

Contd...

SI No	Action/Rationale	Normal finding	Abnormal finding
	Spleen Make the patient to lie in supine position: • Stand on the client's right side • Place your left hand over the abdomen and behind the left side at the 11th and 12th ribs • Lift up, to support the abdominal contents • Place your right hand on the left upper quadrant with fingers pointing toward the left axilla • Push deeply down and under the left costal margin, when the client takes deep breath • Note any enlargement or tenderness	Normally spleen is not palpable No enlargement and tenderness	The enlarged spleen is palpable about 2 cm below the left costal margin on inspiration
	Kidneys • Place the client in supine position • Place your left hand between the client's lowest rib and pelvic bone • Place your right hand on the client's right flank region • As the client takes deep inspiration, press your right hand deeply just below the costal margin • Try to capture the kidney between two hands • Note the enlargement or tenderness	Normally both kidneys are not palpable	Enlarged kidney Tenderness Kidney mass Bilateral enlargement suggests polycystic kidney disease
	Percussion in the kidney It is performed to assess the tenderness in the kidney: • Place the ball of one hand in the costovertebral angle • Strike it with the ulnar surface of your fist	Normally painless	Pain with fist percussion suggests pyelonephritis Sometimes it may be due to musculoskeletal cause

Contd...

Contd...

Sl No	Action/Rationale	Normal finding	Abnormal finding
13.	**Genitalia and excretory system** *Female genitalia* • Place the patient in dorsal recumbent position; observe the skin color, hair distribution, labia majora, any lesions • Look for any discharge or bleeding from the vagina, prolapsed, etc.	No redness or swelling in labia Usually no discharge from the vagina No prolapsed and bleeding from the vagina, except during menstruation	Foul smelling; white, yellow discharge from the vagina Bleeding per vagina
	Male genitalia • Inspect the skin, glans and urethral meatus • Observe for urethral discharge • Inspect and palpate the scrotum and penis; palpate gently each scrotal half between thumb and first two fingers	The glans looks smooth without lesions and the foreskin easily retractable Asymmetry is normal, with the left scrotal half, lower than the right No lump, no tenderness Testes are equal in size	Phimosis—unable to retract the foreskin Purulent discharge from the urethra suggests urethritis Abnormalities in scrotum are varicocele, hydrocele, tumor, orchitis, hernia
	Anus Inspect the anal region for any irritation, cracks, fissure and dilated vessels using torchlight or proctoscope	No irritation, fissure, cracks No dilated vessels in anus	Hemorrhoids Fissures
14.	**Musculoskeletal system** • Ask the client to stand and then inspect neck, shoulder, arms, hands, hips, knees, legs, ankle and feet; compare the symmetry of both sides	No bone or joint deformities No swelling or redness of joints No muscle wasting	Presence of bone and joint deformities Redness or swelling suggests joint inflammation Muscle wasting suggests degenerative diseases
	• Check the range of motion and watch for signs of pain	Able to move joints freely and no signs of pain, while moving	Signs of pain, while moving the joint indicates dislocation or subluxation
15.	**Peripheral vascular examination** • Inspect the arms and legs for color, size, any lesion and skin changes • Palpate peripheral pulses	Symmetrical in shape No edema, no changes in skin color and normal pulse rate	Edema of upper extremities Varicose vein in lower extremities

Contd...

Contd...

Sl No	Action/Rationale	Normal finding	Abnormal finding
	• Press the skin gently and firmly at the tibia, ankles and feet for 5 seconds and then release; note whether the fingers leave an impression on the skin • Ask the client to stand and assess the venous system for dilated and tortuous veins	No impression left on the skin, when pressed Edema during pregnancy is common due to weight bearing	Pallor with vasoconstriction Cyanosis Bilateral pitting edema occurs with heart failure, diabetic neuropathy or hepatic cirrhosis
16.	**Nervous system** ***Assessing sensation*** • Ask the client to close the eyes • Select areas on face arms, hands, legs and feet • Give a superficial pain, light touch and vibration to each site by turn • Note the client's ability of sensation on each site	Feels pain sensation, light touch and vibration Equally in both sides	Decreased pain or touch sensation suggests paralysis or paresthesia; it is commonly seen in patients with hemiparesis
	Assessing motor function Ask the client to stand and walk across the room in his/her regular walk backward and turn toward you	Straight and balanced walk	Unbalanced walk, limping Uncoordinated or unsteady walk suggests cerebellar dysfunction
	Checking reflexes It is done to detect the intactness of the arc at specific spinal canal *Deep tendon reflexes* a. Biceps reflex (C5–C6): • **Support the client's forearm** • **Place your thumb on the** biceps tendon and strike a blow on your thumb with the knee hammer • **Observe the response**	Normal response is contraction of the biceps muscle and flexion of the forearm	Hyperreflexia Hyporeflexia
	b. Triceps reflex (C7–C8): • **Tell the client to flex the** arm toward the chest and keep it in a relaxed manner • **Strike the triceps tendon** directly just above the elbow • **Observe the response**	Normal response is extension of the forearm	

Contd...

Contd...

SI No	Action/Rationale	Normal finding	Abnormal finding
	c. Brachioradialis reflex (C5–C6): • Hold the client's thumb to suspend the forearms in relaxation • Strike the forearm directly, about 2–3 cm above the radial styloid process • Observe the response	Normal response is flexion and supination of the forearm	
	d. Quadriceps reflex or 'knee jerk' (L2–L4): • Let the lower legs dangle freely to flex the knee and stretch the tendons • Strike the tendon directly just below the patella • Observe the response and palpate contraction of the quadriceps	Normal response is extension of the lower leg	
	e. Achilles reflex or 'ankle jerk' (L5 to S2): • Position the client with the knee flexed • Hold the foot in dorsiflexion • Strike the Achilles tendon directly • Feel the response	Normal response is the foot plantar flexion against your hand	
	Superficial reflex a. Plantar reflex (L4 to S2) • Position the thigh in slight external rotation • With the reflex hammer, draw a light stroke up the lateral side of the sole of the foot and inward across the ball of the foot • Observe the response	Normal response is plantar flexion of all the toes, extension of big toe and inversion, and flexion of the forefoot	Fanning of toes indicates upper motor neuron disease

NASOGASTRIC TUBE INSERTION

Definition

Nasogastric intubation refers to the process of placing a soft plastic nasogastric (NG) tube through a patient's nostril, past the pharynx and down the esophagus into a patient's stomach.

Purposes

1. To remove substances from the stomach or as a means of testing stomach function or contents.
2. To deliver tube feedings to a patient when they are unable to eat.
3. Other substances that are delivered through a NG tube may include ice water to stop bleeding in the stomach or medications to neutralize swallowed poisons.
4. To remove air that accumulates in the stomach during cardiopulmonary resuscitation (CPR).
5. To remove stomach contents after major trauma or surgery, to prevent aspiration of the stomach contents.
6. To prevent nausea and vomiting by removing stomach contents and preventing distention of the stomach when a patient has a bleeding ulcer, bowel obstruction or other gastrointestinal diseases.
7. For laboratory studies.

Equipments

- Sterile gloves
- Appropriate size of Ryle's tube
- Xylocaine jelly (2%)
- Stethoscope
- Disposable syringe
- A cup of water
- Adhesive plaster
- Appropriate size suction catheter (if needed)
- Laryngoscope (if needed)
- Mask.

Procedure

The procedure for nasogastric tube insertion is detailed in Table 3.12.

Table 3.12: Procedure for nasogastric tube insertion

Sl No	Care action	Rationale
1.	Explain the procedure to the patient/patient relatives	To get valid consent from the patient/patient relatives
2.	Arrange needed articles near the bedside	Easy to perform the procedure and to prevent unnecessary contamination
3.	Place the mackintosh and draw sheet under the head and neck	To prevent the soiling of the linen
4.	Position the patient; if possible, make the patient to sit in upright for optimal neck/stomach alignment	Easy to insert the tube into the gastrointestinal (GI) tract

Contd...

Contd...

Sl No	Care action	Rationale
5.	Examine nostrils for deformity/obstructions to determine the best side for insertion	To prevent bleeding, while doing the procedure
6.	Measure tubing from bridge of nose to earlobe, then to the point halfway between the end of the sternum and the navel; mark measured length with a marker or note the distance	To insert the appropriate size to prevent coiling of the tube inside the GI tract
7.	Lubricate 2–4 inches of tube with lubricant (preferably 2% Xylocaine); this procedure is very uncomfortable for many patients, so a squirt of Xylocaine jelly in the nostril not and a spray of Xylocaine to the back of the throat, will help alleviate the discomfort	For easy insertion of tube into the stomach
8.	• Pass tube via either nare posteriorly, past the pharynx into the esophagus and then the stomach • Instruct the patient to swallow (may offer ice chips/water) and advance the tube as the patient swallows; swallowing of small sips of water may enhance passage of tube into esophagus • If resistance is met, rotate tube slowly downward advancement toward ear; do not force	To ensure the cleanliness of the hair
9.	Withdraw tube immediately if changes occur in patient's respiratory status, if tube coils in mouth; if the patient begins to cough or turns pretty colors	To prevent the complication
10.	Advance tube until mark is reached	To place the tube into the stomach accurately
11.	Check for placement by attaching syringe to free end of the tube, aspirate sample of gastric contents; obtain an X-ray to verify placement before instilling any feedings/medications or if you have concerns about the placement of the tube	To prevent the misplacement of the tube
12.	Secure tube with tape or commercially prepared tube holder	To prevent the misplacement of the tube
13.	Monitor the vital signs of the patient	To identify the abnormalities immediately
14.	Remove the mackintosh form the patient side	To make the patient comfortable
15.	Wash and replace the equipments	To make it arrange for next use
16.	Document the procedure and patient's parameters (during and after the procedure) in the nurse's record	To follow-up care for the patient

NASOGASTRIC TUBE FEEDING

Definition

Ryle's tube feeding or nasogastric feeding is nourishing through the tube to stomach, when the patient is unable to eat or drink by mouth. It is called nasogastric tube because it passes through the nose, down the throat and into the stomach. It is also called NG tube.

Purposes

1. To provide sufficient nourishment and hydration support to the patient.
2. For therapeutic purposes.
3. Help to drain out the stomach content in case of gastric problem or postoperative, etc.
4. To assess acceptance level of feeds in postoperative patients who undergo surgery and have NG tube in situ.

Equipments

A tray containing:
- A 20 cc syringe
- Measured amount of feed
- Stethoscope
- Bowl with water
- Kidney tray
- Water
- Towel
- Adhesives and scissors, if needed.

Procedure

The procedure for nasogastric tube feeding is detailed in Table 3.13.

Table 3.13: Procedure for nasogastric tube feeding

SI No	Care action	Rationale
1.	Explain procedure to patient	To get the cooperation from the patient
2.	Assist the patient to a Fowler's position in bed or sitting position on chair; if the sitting position is contraindicated, a slightly elevated right side lying position is acceptable	To enhance the gravitational flow of the solution and to prevent the aspiration
3.	Wash the hands with soap and water	To prevent cross infection
4.	Place towel around the neck	To prevent soiling of the patient cloth
5.	Assess the tube placement by attaching the syringe to open end of the tube and aspirate gastric secretion	To check the position of the tube as well as to assess the absorption of the last feeding

Contd...

Contd...

SI No	Care action	Rationale
6.	Before administering the feeding , check the temperature and texture of the feed	The excessive cold feeding may cause cramps and minimize the risk of contamination
7.	Pinch the loop and remove the syringe from the tube and rinse it	To prevent air entry into the stomach
8.	Connect the barrel of the syringe to a pinched or clamped nasogastric tube	To make sure the gravity flow of the fluid
9.	Allow the feeding to flow slowly at the prescribed rate and pinch or clamp the tube, stop the feed if the patient feels discomfort	Quickly administering the feed can cause the flatus, pain and reflex vomiting
10.	At the end of the feed, flush the tube with a measured amount of water	To keep the tube clean
11.	Pinch the loop of the tube and remove the syringe, and close the tube with plunger	To prevent air entry into the stomach
12.	Allow the patient in semi-Fowler's position for 5–10 minutes	To enhance the patient comfortable and prevent aspiration of the fluid
13.	Document in the nurse's record, and in intake and output chart	To maintain the accurate record
14.	Replace all the articles	To keep it ready for next use

ADMINISTRATION OF OXYGEN THERAPY

Definition

Method by which oxygen is supplemented at higher percentages than what is available in atmospheric air.

Purposes

- To relieve dyspnea
- To reduce or prevent hypoxemia and hypoxia
- To alleviate the struggle associated with breathing.

Sources of Oxygen

Therapeutic oxygen is available from two sources:
- Wall outlets (central supply)
- Oxygen cylinders.

Nursing Alert

1. Explain the client the dangers of lighting matches or smoking cigarettes, cigars, pipes, etc. Be sure the client has no matches, cigarettes or smoking materials on the bedside table.
2. Make sure that warning signs (Oxygen—No Smoking) are posted on the client's door and above the client's bed.

Contd...

Sl No	Care action	Rationale
4.	Assemble equipments	Organization facilitates accurate skill performance
5.	Prepare the oxygen equipment: • Attach the flowmeter into the wall outlet or oxygen cylinder • Fill humidifier about one third with sterile water or boiled water • Blowout dusts from the oxygen cylinder • Attach the cannula with the connecting tubing to the adapter, on the humidifier	Humidification prevents drying of the nasal mucosa To prevent entering dust from exit of cylinder to the nostril
6.	Test flow by setting flowmeter at 2–3 L/min and check the flow on the hand	Testing flow before use is needed to provide prescribed oxygen to the client
7.	Adjust the flowmeter's setting to the ordered flow rate	The flow rate via the cannula should not exceed 6 L/min Higher rates may cause excess drying of nasal mucosa
8.	Insert the nasal cannula into client's nostrils, adjust the tubing behind the client's ears and slide the plastic adapter under the client's chin, until he/she is comfortable	Proper position allows unobstructed oxygen flow and eases the client's respirations
9.	Maintain sufficient slack in oxygen tubing	To prevent the tubing from getting out of place accidentally
10.	Encourage the client to breathe through the nose rather than the mouth and expire from the mouth	Breathing through the nose inhales more oxygen into the trachea, which is less likely to be exhaled through the mouth
11.	Initiate oxygen flow	To maintain doctor's prescription and avoid oxygen toxicity
12.	Assess the patient's response to oxygen and comfort level	Anxiety increases the demand for oxygen
13.	Dispose of gloves if worn and perform hand hygiene	To prevent the spread of infection
14.	Place 'No Smoking' signboard at entry into the room	The sign warns the client and visitors that smoking is prohibited because oxygen is combustible
15.	Document the following: Date, time, method, flow rate, respiratory condition and response to oxygen	Documentation provides coordination of care Sometimes oxygen inhalation can bring oxygen intoxication
16.	Sign the chart	To maintain professional accountability
17.	Check the oxygen setup including the water level in the humidifier; clean the cannula and assess the client's nares at least every 8 hours	Sterile water needs to be added when the level falls below the line on the humidification container Nares may become dry and irritated, and require the use of a water-soluble lubricant In long use cases, evaluate for pressure sores over ears, cheeks and nares

Simple Face Mask Method

The procedure of simple face mask method is detailed in Table 3.16.

Table 3.16: Procedure of simple face mask method

SI No	Care action	Rationale
1.	Perform hands hygiene and put on gloves if available	To prevent the spread of infection
2.	Explain the procedure and the need for oxygen to the client	The client has a right to know what is happening and why Providing explanations allay client's anxiety
3.	Prepare the oxygen equipment: • Attach the humidifier to the threaded outlet of the flowmeter or regulator • Connect the tubing from the simple mask to the nipple outlet on the humidifier • Set the oxygen at the prescribed flow rate	To maintain the proper setting The oxygen must be flowing before the mask is applied to the client
4.	To apply the mask, guide the elastic strap over the top of the client's head; bring the strap down to just below the client's ears	This position will hold the mask most firmly
5.	Gently, but firmly pull the strap extensions to center the mask on the client's face with a tight seal	The seal prevents leaks as much as possible
6.	Make sure that the client is comfortable	Comfort helps relieve apprehension and lowers oxygen need
7.	Remove and properly dispose gloves; wash your hands	Respiratory secretions are considered contaminated
8.	Document the procedure and record the client's reactions	Documentation provides for coordination of care
9.	Sign the chart and report the senior staffs	To maintain professional accountability
10.	Check periodically for depressed respirations or increased pulse	To assess the respiratory condition and find out any abnormalities as soon as possible
11.	Check for reddened pressure areas under the straps	The straps, when snug, place pressure on the underlying skin areas

Nursing alert: The simple mask is a low-flow device that provides an oxygen concentration in the 40%–60% range, with a liter flow of 6–10 L/min. But, the simple mask requires a minimum oxygen flow rate of 6 L/min to prevent carbon dioxide build up.

SURGICAL DRESSING

Definition

Surgical dressing is a sterile procedure, which is a loosely woven cotton dressing for incisions made during surgery.

Purposes

- To prevent the infection
- To prevent further tissue damage
- To promote wound healing
- To absorb inflammatory exudates and to promote drainage
- To change the contaminated wound into a clean wound
- To absorb fluid and provide a dry environment
- To immobilize and support wound.

Equipments

- Sterile dressing tray
- Cleaning solution prescribed, Betadine/Normal saline
- Sterile gloves
- Adhesives/Bandages/Tegaderm
- Scissors
- Extra sterile packs of cotton balls and gauze
- A pair of clean gloves
- Mackintosh and draw sheet
- Disposable mask and apron
- Medication as per doctors order (if needed)
- Labeled specimen container (if needed)
- Roller bandage (if needed)
- Kidney tray.

Procedure

The procedure for surgical dressing is detailed in Table 3.17.

Table 3.17: Procedure for surgical dressing

Sl No	Care action	Rationale
1.	Explain the procedure to the patient	Make sure the patient and the relatives understand importance of the dressing and to give valid consent
2.	Before starting the procedure, ensure that the sweeping and the mopping of the ward is completed	To allow dust and airborne organisms to settle, before the insertion site and sterile fields are exposed
3.	Arrange and keep the needed articles near the bedside	To minimize unnecessary contamination and to perform the procedure easily
4.	Wash the hands	To reduce the risk of cross-contamination
5.	Make sure that foot-controlled dustbins are present at the bedside with appropriate covers	To minimize airborne contamination
6.	Provide privacy to the patient	To ensure the patient's comfortableness

Contd...

Contd...

Sl No	Care action	Rationale
7.	Position the patient comfortably and drape the patient appropriately	To make the patient feel comfortable and to perform the procedure easily
8.	Wear gloves, remove the adhesive tape and old dressing, and remove the glove and wash the hands	To minimize the infection and contamination
9.	Wash the hands and wear sterile gloves	To minimize the infection and contamination
10.	Open the tray and pour the normal saline into the bowl	To clean the wound
11.	Using thumb forceps, pick up cotton ball, wet with saline and using artery clamp, soak adherent gauze	To remove the adherent gauze without causing trauma to the wound
12.	Using the same artery clamp, remove gauze and cotton ball, and discard in appropriate waste bin	To prevent cross-contamination
13.	Clean the wound from less contaminated area to more contaminated area	To reduce the risk of transfer of microorganism from contaminated to non-contaminated area
14.	Use separate cotton ball for each stroke	To minimize the risk of contamination
15.	Move in progressive strokes away from the incision line to wound edge	To enable disinfection process to be completed; to prevent skin reaction in response to the application of a transparent dressing to moist skin
16.	Use dry gauze to clean the incision	To promote healing
17.	Apply antiseptic as prescribed, using the same technique as for cleaning; include drainage site	To prevent sepsis
18.	Apply the sterile dressing to incision/ wound/ drain site	Avoids infection
19.	If drain is present, use sterile gauze and wrap around drain incision site	To prevent infection at the drain site
20.	Avoid the application of bulky dressing that may disturb the patient's mobility; ensure proper coverage of entire wound If using a commercially available dressing such as Tegaderm with pad, make sure that the size is appropriate; when fixing the commercially available dressing, mold it into place so that there are no creases or folds	Provides esthetic sense
21.	Secure dressing with bandage or adhesive, if needed	To prevent dislodgement
22.	Remove the gloves and wash the hands	To minimize the cross-contamination
23.	Make the patient to sit in a comfortable position and wash, replace the articles	To make it ready for next usage
24.	Document the procedure in the nurse's record	Helps to do the continuous assessment for the patient

---

Points to Note

- Observe character and amount of drainage, and assess condition of wound using the REEDA assessment scale:
  - R: Redness.
  - E: Ecchymosis.
  - E: Edema.
  - D: Drainage.
  - A: Approximation of the skin.
- Removal of old dressing:
  - Clean and dry wound: Remove with gloved hand by pinching the pad.
  - Dry dressing, adherent to the wound: Soak with normal saline. After a while, remove with gloved hand. Remove the gloves.
  - Wet or infected dressing : Remove with gloved hand. Remove the gloves.
- Wound care:
  - Clean wound: Clean the wound from inside or from the center toward outside with each stroke.
  - Infected wound: Clean the wound from outside toward inside with each stroke.
  - Transverse or horizontal incision: Clean the wound from the center toward outside on either side with each stroke.
  - Vertical incision: Clean the wound from top to downwards with one stroke and toward outside on either side in the same vertical direction.
  - Circular wound: Clean from center toward outside with a circular stroke.

Specimen Collection

COLLECTION OF BLOOD SPECIMEN

Performing Venipuncture

Definition

Venipuncture is using a needle to withdraw blood from a vein, often from the inside surface of the forearm near the elbow.

Purposes

1. To examine the condition of client and assess the present treatment.
2. To diagnose disease.

Equipments

- Laboratory form
- Sterilized syringe
- Sterilized needles
- Tourniquet: 1
- Blood collection tubes or specimen vials as ordered
- Spirit swabs
- Dry gauze
- Disposable gloves if available: 1
- Adhesive tape or bandages
- Sharps disposal container: 1
- Steel tray: 1
- Ballpoint pen: 1.

Procedure

The procedure of venipuncture is given in Table 4.1.

Table 4.1: Procedure of venipuncture

Sl No	Care action	Rationale
1.	Identify the patient: • Outpatient are called into the phlebotomy area and asked their name and date of birth • Inpatient are identified by asking their name and date of birth	This information must match the requisition

Contd...

Contd...

Sl No	Care action	Rationale
2.	Reassure the client that the minimum amount of blood required for testing will be drawn	To perform once properly without any unnecessary venipuncture
3.	Assemble the necessary equipment appropriate to the client's physical characteristics	Organization facilitates accurate skill performance
4.	Explain to the client about the purpose and the procedure	Providing explanation fosters his/her cooperation and allays anxiety
5.	Perform hand hygiene and put on gloves if available	To prevent the infection of spreading
6.	Positioning: • Make the client to be seated comfortably or supine position • Assist the client with the arm extended to form a straight-line from shoulder to wrist • Place a protective sheet under the arm	To make the position safe and comfortable is helpful to success venipuncture at one try To prevent the spread of blood
7.	Check the client's requisition form, blood collection tubes or vials and make the syringe-needle ready	To assure the doctor's order with the correct client and to make the procedure smooth
8.	Select the appropriate vein for venipuncture	The larger median cubital, basilica and cephalic veins are most frequently used, but other may be necessary and will become more prominent if the client closes his/her fist tightly
9.	Applying the tourniquet: • Apply the tourniquet 3–4 inches (8–10 cm) above the collection site; never leave the tourniquet on for over 1 minute • If a tourniquet is used for preliminary vein selection, release it and reapply after 2 minutes	To prevent the venipuncture site from touching the tourniquet and keep clear vision Tightening of more than 1 minute may bring erroneous result due to the change of some blood composition
10.	Selection of the vein: • Feel the vein using the tip of the finger and detect the direction, depth and size of vein • Massage the arm from wrist to elbow; if the vein is not prominent, try the other arm	To assure venipuncture at one try
11.	Disinfect the selected site: • Clean the puncture site by making a smooth circular pass over the site with the spirit swab, moving in an outward spiral from the zone of penetration • Allow the skin to dry before proceeding • Do not touch the puncture site after cleaning • After blood is drawn the desired amount, release the tourniquet and ask the client to open his/her fist • Place a dry gauze over the puncture site and remove the needle • Immediately apply slight pressure; ask the client to apply pressure for at least 2 minutes	To prevent the infection from venipuncture site Disinfectant has the effect on drying To prevent the site from contaminating To avoid making ecchymoma The normal coagulation time is 2–5 minutes

Contd...

Contd...

Sl No	Care action	Rationale
	• When bleeding stops, apply a fresh bandage or gauze with tape	Rinsing removes loosened debris and make the mouth taste fresher
12.	• Transfer blood drawn into appropriate blood specimen bottles or tubes as soon as possible using a needless syringe • The container or tube containing an additive should be gently inverted five to eight times or shaking the specimen container by making figure of 8	• A delay could cause improper coagulation • Do not shake or mix vigorously
13.	Dispose of the syringe and needle as a unit into an appropriate sharps container	To prevent the spread of infection
14.	Label all tubes or specimen bottle with client name, age, sex, inpatient number, date and time	To prevent the blood tubes or bottles from misdealing
15.	Send the blood specimen to the laboratory immediately along with the laboratory order form	To avoid misdealing and taking erroneous results
16.	Replace equipments and disinfects materials if needed	To prepare for the next procedure and prevent the spread of infection
17.	Put off gloves and perform hand hygiene	To prevent the spread of infection

Collection of Blood for Culture

Definition

A blood culture is a collection and inoculation of blood into culture medium with the aim of growing pathogenic bacteria or fungi for diagnostic purposes.

Purposes

1. To identify the type of bacteria/fungi present and specific type of antibiotics to use to eradicate the microorganism.
2. To determine whether microorganisms have invaded the patient's bloodstream.

Equipments

A tray containing:
• A pair of sterile gloves
• Alcohol swabs
• Blood culture bottles (two bottles per set)
• Disposable syringe
• Tourniquet
• Sterile gauze pad
• Adhesive strip or tape.

Procedure

The procedure of blood collection for culture is given in Table 4.2.

Table 4.2: Procedure of blood collection for culture

Sl No	Care action	Rationale
1.	Explain procedure to the patient	To get cooperation from the patient
2.	Arrange and keep the entire article near the patient side	To minimize the unnecessary contamination
3.	Position the patient comfortably	To do the procedure easily
4.	Select and keep the appropriate sample collection container and stick patient profile	To get accurate results and to avoid the specimen does not get missed
5.	Wash hands with soap and water with friction for 15 seconds or use alcohol based hand rub	To prevent infections
6.	Clean the rubber cap of the blood culture bottles with an alcohol pad in a circular motion; allow the alcohol to dry	To prepare the specimen container ready to receive the sample and to prevent the cross contamination
7.	Apply tourniquet 3–4 inches above intended site; palpate for a vein and select site, preferably in the antecubital fossa	To assess the patency of the vein, to get the adequate blood sample and to increase the venous pressure
8.	Wear sterile gloves	To minimize the contamination
9.	Site preparation to be done by: • Vigorously clean the venipuncture site with alcohol swabs and allow drying • Starting at the center of the site, swab concentrically with alcohol swab for 1 minute • Allow the site to dry • Do not touch the venipuncture site after preparation and prior to puncture	To minimize the contamination
10.	Hold the syringe with the bevel of needle facing upwards	To ensure the correct position of the needle
11.	Advance the needle into the patient vein, with patient's arm in a downward position and tube stopper uppermost	This reduces the risk of backflow of any anticoagulant into the patient's circulation
12.	As blood come into view in syringe, withdraw the plunger of syringe softly with steady suction until the required sample is obtained	To get accurate report; in sufficient sample may cause again repuncture for the patient
13.	Remove the tourniquet	To release the pressure
14.	Take out the needle from the punctured area and place the dry sterile cotton and apply gentle pressure	To prevent bleeding
15.	Do not recap the needle and remove the needle from the syringe, discard into sharps container as per institutional policy	To prevent the needle stick injury
16.	Distribute blood equally into aerobic and anaerobic labeled sample container	For investigation process

Contd...

Contd...

SI No	Care action	Rationale
17.	Gently rotate the bottles to mix the blood and the broth (do not shake vigorously) and send specimen to respective laboratories	To enhance the blood to mix with the liquid
18.	Make the patient comfortable; replace the equipment and wash hands	To make the patient feel comfortable and prevent cross infection
19.	Record the procedure with details and investigation as well as collection	Helps to assess the continuity of care

Arterial Blood Collection

Definition

Arterial blood gases (ABGs) are diagnostic tests performed on blood taken from an artery.

Purposes

1. Arterial blood gases or ABGs are done to evaluate oxygenation and acid-base balance in the body.
2. An ABG test measures the acidity (pH) and the levels of oxygen and carbon dioxide in the blood from an artery.
3. This test is used to check how well your lungs are able to move oxygen into the blood and remove carbon dioxide from the blood.

Equipments

A tray containing:
- A pair of gloves
- Dry cotton/gauze pieces
- Adhesive plaster
- Heparinized syringe and needle
- Alcohol swab
- Injection Xylocaine 2%.

Procedure

The procedure of arterial blood collection is given in Table 4.3.

Table 4.3: Procedure of arterial blood collection

SI No	Care action	Rationale
1.	Explain the procedure to the patient	To reduce the anxiety and to get the cooperation
2.	Prepare all the articles near the patient bedside	To ease to do the procedure

Contd...

Sl No	Care action	Rationale
3.	Check the patient coagulation factors and platelet count before starting the procedure	To prevent bleeding
4.	Feel for radial pulses on both wrists to determine which will be the better site, from which to draw	To avoid to perform an arterial puncture on an extremity; it may cause an inadequate blood supply
5.	Perform the Allen's test on the hand, which has been selected for the puncture	To determine adequate collateral flow
6.	Prepare the puncture site aseptically	To prevent infection
7.	Put sterile gloves and anesthetize the puncture area with 2% Xylocaine, according to the physician order	The use of a local anesthetic is not required, but may relieve uneasiness or be useful in reducing arterial spasm, if any case with difficulty in obtaining an arterial sample
8.	The heparinized syringe should be used to withdraw the blood sample	To prevent clotting of blood
9.	Puncture the skin about 5–10 mm distal to the finger directly over the artery; the puncture angle should be approximately 45° toward the direction of the blood flow	To obtain the blood easily
10.	Slowly advance the needle and syringe with one hand, while continuing to palpate the artery with the other hand; when a flash of arterial blood is observed in the hub of the needle, do not advance the needle further	To prevent deep injury
11.	While holding the syringe and needle motionless with one hand, gently pull back on the plunger of the syringe with the other hand to allow the syringe to fill	To prevent damage of the artery
12.	If the needed amount of blood has been obtained, should remove the needle and syringe rapidly, and press down on the puncture site with sterile gauze	To prevent the bleeding
13.	If any air bubbles present in the syringe, it is to be removed immediately and recap the needle	To prevent the inaccuracy in results
14.	Send the specimen to the blood gas analyzer	To do the analysis
15.	The needle is advanced just slightly under the skin; once the needle is in the artery the syringe will readily fill Arterial blood will pulsate whereas blood from a vein will not; arterial blood is also brighter red (if oxygenation is adequate) than blood from a vein When the needle is withdrawn, a gauze should be placed over the punctured site and pressure applied for about 5 minutes (longer if the patient has bleeding tendencies), if any bleeding occurs at the end of this time, pressure should be maintained until no further bleeding occurs	To obtain the sample

Contd...

Contd...

Sl No	Care action	Rationale
16.	Once the sample is obtained, remove the visible gas bubbles; label the syringe with patient profile	Air bubbles can dissolve into the sample and cause inaccurate results
17.	The sealed syringe is taken to a blood gas analyzer	The sample cannot be immediately analyzed; it is chilled in an ice bath in a glass syringe to slow metabolic processes, which can cause inaccuracy Samples drawn in plastic syringes are not iced and are analyzed within 30 minutes
18.	Document the procedure; collect the arterial blood gas (ABG) report and paste it in the appropriate place in the clinical chart	To monitor differences and detect trends; any irregularities should be brought to the attention of the appropriate senior nursing and medical teams

Points to Note

+ Allen test is used to test blood supply to the hand, specifically, the patency of the radial and ulnar arteries. It is performed prior to radial arterial blood sampling or cannulation.

Allen test procedure
1. The hand is elevated and the patient is asked to make a fist for about 30 seconds.
2. Pressure is applied over the ulnar and the radial arteries so as to occlude both of them.
3. Still elevated, the hand is then opened. It should appear blanched (pallor can be observed at the finger nails).
4. Ulnar pressure is released and the color should return in 7 seconds.
5. Inference: Ulnar artery supply to the hand is sufficient and it is safe to cannulate/prick the radial.
6. If color does not return or returns after 7–10 seconds, the test is considered negative and the ulnar artery supply to the hand is not sufficient. The radial artery therefore cannot be safely pricked/cannulated.

Measurement of Capillary Blood Glucose

Definition

The collection of capillary blood from a fingertip quickly evolved as the standard sampling methodology. It is performed in homes and in hospitals for monitoring purposes that require relatively small samples of blood. It is more cost-effective, less traumatic and more convenient to obtain a blood sample by lancing the skin capillaries than it is by using healthcare practitioners to draw a tube of venous blood.

Purposes

1. Helps to observe immediate and daily levels of blood glucose control and dose adjustments.
2. Helps to identify the value variation of the patient in continuous insulin infusion.
3. To identify hypoglycemia and hyperglycemia.
4. Help out in the safe management of hyperglycemia and hypoglycemia.
5. Determines the effect of daily activities such as physical activity and meals on blood glucose.

Equipments

- Blood glucose meter
- Test strips
- Control solution
- Single use lancets
- Cotton swabs
- Disposable gloves.

Procedure

The procedure of capillary blood glucose measurement is given in Table 4.4.

Table 4.4: Procedure of capillary blood glucose measurement

Sl No	Care action	Rationale
1.	Explain the procedure to the patient	The patient should be attentive of the procedure in order to relieve some of his/her anxiety and to be able to cooperate in the procedure
2.	Ask the patient to sit down or lie down	To ensure the patient's safety
3.	Wash your hands and put on gloves	To decrease the risk of cross infection and risk of contamination
4.	Clean the fingertip with the alcohol swab where has to prick	To minimize the risk of contamination
5.	Allow the area to dry and prick the fingertip with the help of single use lancet	To minimize the risk of cross infection and accidental needle stick injury
6.	Take a blood sample from the pricking side of the finger, ensuring the side of the piercing is rotated; avoid frequent use of the index finger and thumb The finger may bleed without assistance or may need assistance by 'exploiting' to form a droplet of blood, which is large enough to cover the test pad	The side of the finger is used as it is less painful and easier to obtain a hanging droplet of blood; the site is rotated to reduce the risk of infection from multiple stabbing, and to prevent the areas from becoming toughened and to reduce pain

Contd...

Contd...

SI No	Care action	Rationale
7.	Apply the blood to the testing strip; some test strips are hydrophilic and are dosed/filled from the side and are not dropped directly onto the strip	The window on the test strip allows verification of a correctly dosed strip
8.	Dispose of lancet into a puncture proof sharps container	To reduce the risk of needle stick injury
9.	Record value immediately after the test has been done	To ensure the accuracy of the result
10.	Dispose all the waste according to the hospital policy	To reduce the risk of cross infection
11.	Ensure the patient comfortable and watch for bleeding in the puncture side; if bleed, apply pressure with dry cotton balls	To ensure the patient's comfort and safety To minimize the complication
12.	Wash and dry hands	To prevent cross infection
13.	Record the result in the nurses' notes and in appropriate record (diabetic chart); if any variations in the value are found, it should be intimated immediately to the medical team by the nurses	To prevent complications

Points to Note

Before taking the device to the patient, the monitor needs to be checked for the following:
- Opening date of the strip box.
- The test strip should not be left in the open environment.
- It should be kept in the strip box with closed lids.

Collection of Blood Sample from Arterial Cannula

Definition

Arterial blood sampling blood can be drawn from an indwelling arterial cannula.

Purposes

1. To evaluate the adequacy of ventilatory ($PaCO_2$) acid-base (pH and $PaCO_2$) and oxygenation (PaO_2 and SaO_2) status, and the oxygen-carrying capacity of blood (PaO_2, HbO_2, Hb total and dyshemoglobins).
2. To quantitate the patient's response to therapeutic intervention and/or diagnostic evaluation (e.g. oxygen therapy, exercise testing).
3. To monitor severity and progression of a documented disease process.

Equipments

- A pair of gloves
- Disposable syringe (5 mL, 10 mL)
- Heparinized syringe (5 mL, 10 mL)
- Labeled specimen container
- Gauze pieces
- Alcohol swab.

Procedure

The procedure of blood sampling from arterial cannula is detailed in Table 4.5.

Table 4.5: Procedure of blood sampling from arterial cannula

SI No	Care action	Rationale
1.	Explain the procedure to the patient	To ensure that the patient understands the procedure
2.	Arrange and keep all the articles near the patient side	To minimize unnecessary contamination
3.	Wash hands with bactericidal soap and water or bactericidal alcohol hand rub	To minimize the risk of cross infection
4.	Turn stopcock off to patient	To prevent the blood backflow from the line
5.	Remove the bung from stopcock; wipe with alcohol swab and attach sterile syringe to stopcock	To obtain the first sample from the line and prevent the entry of microorganism
6.	Open stopcock to syringe and intra-arterial catheter; aspirate 3 mL of blood and discard it	To get the accurate report
7.	Turn stopcock to the half-closed position, quickly remove syringe and replace with heparinized syringe	To obtain blood sample
8.	Open stopcock to syringe and intra-arterial catheter and obtain arterial blood gas sample	To do the analysis
9.	Close stopcock to the syringe and remove syringe containing blood sample and gently rotate syringe, cover the syringe with an arterial blood gas (ABG) cap to prevent contamination with air	Send for analysis and ensure that the blood and heparin in the syringe are mixed
10.	Activate flush device to clear arterial line	To prevent the clotting of the tube
11.	Turn stopcock off to the patient and flush side port of stopcock into sterile syringe until all blood is cleared from stopcock	To prevent infection and clotting of the tube
12.	Close stopcock, clean with alcohol and replace sterile protective cap	To prevent entry of the microorganisms and direct contamination of the cannula
13.	Check whether pressure infuser cuff is inflated to 300 mm Hg	To prevent back flow of blood into circuit
14.	Analyze or send to nearest blood gas analyzer and document result	To obtain accurate results as soon as possible
15.	Document the procedure in the nurse's record	To perform the follow-up care for the patient

---

Points to Note

→ Before taking blood sample from arterial line, ensure that arterial line is patent, i.e. the pressure bag is pumped up to 300 mm Hg, the tubing from the arterial site to the 3-way tap is clear and the line flushes easily.

Collection of Blood Sample from Central Venous Catheter

Definition

Blood can be drawn from a central venous access device, where the catheter is threaded into the central vasculature.

Purposes

1. To provide fluid resuscitation.
2. To provide parenteral feeding.
3. To measure the central venous pressure.
4. To administer the irritant drugs.
5. To collect the blood sample.
6. To provide long-term access like transfusion of blood or blood products, administration of drugs such as cytotoxic and antibiotic therapy.

Equipments

- Sterile dressing pack
- Alcohol swab
- A pair of gloves
- Labeled specimen container
- Disposable syringe (5 mL, 10 mL)
- Sterile disposable syringes 10 mL
- Injection: Normal saline 0.9%
- Water for injection.

Procedure

The procedure of blood sampling from central venous catheter is given in Table 4.6.

Table 4.6: Procedure of blood sampling from central venous catheter

Sl No	Care action	Rationale
1.	Explain the procedure to the patient	To get the cooperation and reduce the anxiety of the patient
2.	Arrange the articles near the bedside	To minimize unnecessary contamination
3.	Assess all medications and infusions before selecting a port for sampling	To avoid the dilated sample and to get the accurate results

Contd...

Contd...

SI No	Care action	Rationale
4.	Wash hands with soap and water or bactericidal hand rub	To reduce the risk of infection
5.	If intravenous (IV) fluid is on flow, switch it off	To get the accurate results
6.	Before removing bung from stopcock, check the clamp or adaptor of the CVP line whether it is locked or not	To prevent bleeding
7.	Remove the bung from the stopcock and clean the catheter with alcohol swab	To minimize the entry of microorganism into the catheter
8.	Connect 10 mL syringe to the stopcock Open the stopcock Release the clamp and withdraw 5–10 mL of blood, close the clamp and discard the blood sample	To prevent contamination and to prevent the mixing
9.	Connect another disposable syringe in the stopcock and release the clamp, and withdraw the required amount of blood	To do the analysis
10.	Once the blood is withdrawn, close the clamp and transfer the blood to labeled specimen container; flush the line with 0.9% normal saline (NS) or sterile water	To prevent blood clotting in the lines
11.	When required, disconnect the administration set from the catheter and cover the end of the set with sterile cap	To reduce the risk of contaminating the end of the administration set
12.	Reconnect the IV fluids or medication as per physician order	To continue the treatment of the patient
13.	Document the procedure in the nurse's record	To perform the follow-up care of the patient

COLLECTION OF URINE SPECIMEN

Definition

Urinalysis in which the components of urine are identified, is part of every client assessment at the beginning and during an illness.

Purposes

1. To diagnose illness.
2. To monitor the disease process.
3. To evaluate the efficacy of treatment.

Nursing Alert

1. Label specimen containers or bottles before the client voids.
   Rationale: Reduce handling after the container or bottle is contaminated.

2. Note on the specimen label if the female client is menstruating at that time.
   Rationale: One of the tests routinely performed is a test for blood in the urine. If the female client is menstruating at the time a urine specimen is taken, a false-positive reading for blood will be obtained.
3. To avoid contamination and necessity of collecting another specimen, soap and water cleansing of the genitals immediately preceding the collection of the specimen is supported.
   Rationale: Bacteria are normally present on the labia or penis and the perineum and in the anal area.
4. Maintain body substances precautions, when collecting all types of urine specimen.
   Rationale: To maintain safety.
5. Wake a client in the morning to obtain a routine specimen.
   Rationale: If all specimen are collected at the same time, the laboratory can establish a baseline. And also this voided specimen usually represents that was collecting in the bladder all night.
6. Be sure to document the procedure in the designated place and mark it off on the Kardex.
   Rationale: To avoid duplication.

Collection of Single-voided Specimen

Equipments

1. Laboratory form.
2. Clean container with lid or cover: 1 (wide-mouthed container is recommended).
3. Bedpan or urinal: 1 (as required).
4. Disposable gloves: 1 (if available).
5. Toilet paper as required.

Procedure

The procedure for collection of urine sample is given in Table 4.7.

Table 4.7: Procedure for collection of urine sample

Sl No	Care action	Rationale
1.	Explain the procedure	Providing information fosters his/her cooperation
2.	Assemble equipments and check the specimen form with client's name, date and content of urinalysis	Organization facilitates accurate skill performance Ensure that the specimen collecting is correct
3.	Label the bottle or container with the date, client's name, department identification and doctor's name	Ensure correct identification and avoid mistakes

Contd...

Contd...

Sl No	Care action	Rationale
4.	Perform hand hygiene and put on gloves	To prevent the spread of infection
5.	Instruct the client to void in a clean receptacle	To prevent cross contamination
6.	Remove the specimen immediately after the client has voided	Substances in urine decompose when exposed to air; decomposition may alter the test results
7.	Pour about 10–20 mL of urine into the labeled specimen bottle or container and cover the bottle or container	Ensure the client voids enough amount of urine for the required tests Covering the bottle retards decomposition and it prevents added contamination
8.	Dispose of used equipment or clean them; remove gloves and perform hand hygiene	To prevent the spread of infection
9.	Send the specimen bottle or container to the laboratory immediately with the specimen form	Organisms grow quickly at room temperature
10.	Document the procedure in the designated place and mark it off on the Kardex	To avoid duplication Documentation provides coordination of care

Collection of 24-hour Urine Specimen

Definition

Collection of 24-hour urine specimen is defined as the collection of all the urine voided in 24 hours without any spillage of wastage.

Purposes

1. To detect kidney and cardiac diseases or conditions.
2. To measure total urine component.

Equipments

- Laboratory form
- Bedpan or urinal: 1
- A 24 hours collection bottle with lid or cover
- Clean measuring jar: 1
- Disposable gloves: 1 (if available)
- Tissue paper (if available)
- Ballpoint pen: 1.

Procedure

The procedure for collection of 24-hour urine sample is given in Table 4.8.

Table 4.8: Procedure for collection of 24-hour urine sample

Sl No	Care action	Rationale
1.	Explain the procedure	Providing information fosters his/her cooperation
2.	Assemble equipments and check the specimen form with client's name, date and content of urinalysis	Organization facilitates accurate skill performance Ensure that the specimen collecting is correct
3.	Label the bottle or container with the date, client's name, department identification and doctor's name	Ensure correct identification and avoid mistakes
4.	Instruct the client: • Before beginning 24-hour urine collection, ask the client to void completely • Document the starting time of 24-hour urine collection on the specimen form and nursing record • Instruct the client to collect all the urine into a large container for the next 24 hours • In the exact 24 hours later, ask the client to void and pour into the large container • Measure total amount of urine and record it on the specimen form and nursing record • Document the time when finished the collection	To measure urinal component and assess the function of kidney and cardiac function accuracy The entire collected urine should be stored in a covered container in a cool place
5.	Sending the specimen: • Perform hand hygiene and put on gloves if available • Mix the urine thoroughly • Collect some urine as required or all the urine in a clean bottle with lid • Transfer it to the laboratory with the specimen form immediately	To prevent contamination Ensure the client voids enough amount of the urine for the required tests Covering the bottle retards decomposition and it prevents added contamination. Substances in urine decompose, when exposed to air; decomposition may alter the test results
6.	Dispose of used equipment or clean them; remove gloves and perform hand hygiene	To prevent the spread of infection
7.	Document the procedure in the designated place and mark it off on the Kardex	To avoid duplication Documentation provides coordination of care

Collection of Urine for Culture

Definition

Collecting a urine culture is a process that it obtains specimen urine with sterile technique.

Purposes

1. To collect uncontaminated urine specimen for culture and sensitivity test.
2. To detect the microorganisms cause urinary tract infection (UTI).
3. To diagnose and treat with specific antibiotic.

Equipments

- Laboratory form
- Sterile gloves: 1
- Sterile culture bottle with label as required
- Sterile kidney tray or sterile container with wide mouthed if needed
- Bedpan (if needed): 1
- Tissue paper (if needed)
- Ballpoint pen: 1.

Procedure

The procedure of urine culture is given in Table 4.9.

Table 4.9: Procedure of urine culture

Sl No	Care action	Rationale
1.	Assemble equipments and check the specimen form with client's name, date and content of urinalysis	Organization facilitates accurate skill performance Ensure that the specimen collecting is correct
2.	Label the bottle or container with the date, client's name, department identification and doctor's name	Ensure correct identification and avoid mistakes
3.	Explain the procedure to the client	Providing information fosters his/her cooperation
4.	Instruct the client: • Instruct the client to clean perineum with soap and water • Open sterilized container and leave the cover facing inside up • Instruct the client to void into sterile kidney tray or sterilized container with wide mouth • If the client needs bedrest and needs to pass urine more, place bedpan after you collect sufficient amount of sterile specimen	To prevent the contamination of specimen from perineum area The cover should be kept the sterilized state To secure the specimen kept in sterilized container surely
5.	Remove the specimen immediately after the client has voided; obtain 30–50 mL at midstream point of voiding	Substances in urine decompose when exposed to air; decomposition may alter the test results Ensure the client voids enough amount of the urine for the required tests Emphasize first and last portions of voiding to be discarded
6.	Close the container securely without touching inside of cover or cap	Covering the bottle retards decomposition and it prevents added contamination
7.	Dispose of used equipment or clean them Remove gloves and perform hand hygiene	To prevent the spread of infection
8.	Send the specimen bottle or container to the laboratory immediately with the specimen form	Organisms grow quickly at room temperature
9.	Document the procedure in the designated place and mark it off on the Kardex	To avoid duplication Documentation provides coordination of care

Collection of Urine Specimen from Retention Catheter

Equipments

- Laboratory form
- Disposable gloves: 1 (if available)
- Container with label as required
- Spirit swabs or disinfectant swabs
- A 10–20 mL syringe with 21–25-gauge needle
- Clamp or rubber band: 1
- Ballpoint pen: 1.

Procedure

The procedure of urine specimen collection from retention catheter is given in Table 4.10.

Table 4.10: Procedure of urine specimen collection from retention catheter

Sl No	Care action	Rationale
1.	Assemble equipments; label the container	Organization facilitates accurate skill performance
2.	Explain the procedure to the client	Providing information fosters his/her cooperation
3.	Perform hand hygiene and put on gloves if available	To prevent the spread of infection
4.	Clamp the tubing: • Clamp the drainage tubing or bend the tubing • Allow adequate time for urine collection *Nursing alert:* You should not clamp longer than 15 minutes	Collecting urine from the tubing guarantees a fresh urine Long-time clamp can lead back flow of urine and is able to cause urinary tract infection
5.	Cleanse the aspiration port with a spirit swab or another disinfectant swab (e.g. Betadine swab)	Disinfecting the port prevent organisms from entering the catheter
6.	Withdrawing the urine: • Insert the needle into the aspiration port • Withdraw sufficient amount of urine gently into the syringe	This technique for uncontaminated urine specimen, preventing contamination of the client's bladder
7.	Transfer the urine to the labeled specimen container *Nursing alert:* The container should be clean for a routine urinalysis and be sterile for a culture	Careful labeling and transfer prevents contamination or confusion of the urine specimen Appropriate container brings accurate results of urinalysis
8.	Unclamp the catheter	The catheter must be unclamped to allow free urinary flow and to prevent urinary stasis
9.	Prepare and pour urine to the container for transport	Proper packaging ensures that the specimen is not an infection risk
10.	Dispose of used equipments and disinfect if needed; remove gloves and perform hand hygiene	To prevent the spread of infection

Contd...

Contd...

SI No	Care action	Rationale
11.	Send the container to the laboratory immediately	Organisms grow quickly at room temperature
12.	Document the procedure in the designated place and mark it off on the Kardex	To avoid duplication Documentation provides coordination of care

COLLECTION OF SPUTUM SPECIMEN

Sputum for Routine Test

Definition

Sputum specimen collection is a procedure to collect expectorated secretions from a patient's respiratory tract.

Purposes

1. To identify the type of pathogenic microorganism present in the respiratory tract.
2. To monitor the response to treatment.
3. Identification of antibiotics to which cultured organism is sensitive.
4. Suspected pulmonary tuberculosis.

Equipments

A clean tray containing:
- Specimen container
- Gloves
- Mask
- Kidney tray.

Procedure

The procedure of routine test for sputum is given in Table 4.11.

Table 4.11: Procedure of routine test for sputum

SI No	Care action	Rationale
1.	Explain the procedure to the patient	To understand the importance of the investigation
2.	Provide privacy to the patient	To make comfortable to the patient
3.	Wash the hands with soap and water, wear gloves	To reduce the infection
4.	Make the patient to sit straightly, if not contraindicated	To obtain the sample easily
5.	Gargle with water immediately prior to obtaining a sputum specimen	To reduce the number of oral bacteria; do not use a mouthwash or any other gargle

Contd...

Contd...

Sl No	Care action	Rationale
6.	Educate the patient to take two or three deep breaths and cough deeply	Help to bring out the sputum easily
7.	If sputum is raised should be expectorated directly into the labeled sputum container	To obtain sterile specimen
8.	Close the lid securely and send the specimen to the laboratory	To do the analysis
9.	Document the procedure in the nurse's record	Help to follow continuity of care

Points to Note

If the patient is unable to produce the desired amount of sputum:
* Instruct the patient to drink two glasses of water.
* Position the patient for postural drainage.
* Provide support for effective coughing by placing the hands or a pillow over the diaphragmatic area and apply mild pressure.
* Perform chest percussion.

Collection of Sputum for Culture

Definition

Collection of coughed out sputum for culture is a process to identify respiratory pathogens.

Purposes

1. To detect abnormalities.
2. To diagnose disease condition.
3. To detect the microorganism causes respiratory tract infections.
4. To treat with specific antibiotics.

Equipments

* Laboratory form
* Disposable gloves: 1 (if available)
* Sterile covered sputum container: 1
* Label as required
* Kidney tray or plastic bag for dirt: 1
* Tissue paper as required
* Ballpoint pen: 1.

Nursing Alert

Nurse should give proper and understandable explanation to the client:

1. Give specimen container on the previous evening with instruction how to treat.
2. Instruct to raise sputum from lungs by coughing, not to collect only saliva.
3. Instruct the client to collect the sputum in the morning.
4. Instruct the client not to use any antiseptic mouthwashes to rinse his/her mouth before collecting specimen.

Procedure

The procedure of sputum collection for culture is given in Table 4.12.

Table 4.12: Procedure of sputum collection for culture

SI No	Care action	Rationale
1.	Assemble equipments; label the container	Organization facilitates accurate skill performance Careful labeling ensures accuracy of the report and alerts the laboratory personnel to the presence of a contaminated specimen
2.	Explain the procedure to the client	Providing information fosters his/her cooperation
3.	Perform hand hygiene and put on gloves if available	To prevent the spread of infection; the sputum specimen is considered highly contaminated, so you should treat it with caution
4.	Instruct the client: • Instruct the client to collect specimen early morning before brushing teeth • Instruct the client to remove and place lid facing upward • Instruct the client to cough deeply and expectorate directly into specimen container • Instruct the client to expectorate until you collect at least 10 mL of sputum • Close the container immediately when sputum is collected • Instruct the client to wipe around mouth if needed; discard it properly	To obtain overnight accumulated secretions To maintain the inside of lid as well as inside of container A sputum specimen should be from the lungs and bronchi; it should be sputum rather than mucous To obtain accurate results To prevent contamination Tissue papers used by any client are considered contaminated
5.	Remove and discard gloves; perform hand hygiene	To prevent contamination of other objects, including the label
6.	Send specimen to the laboratory immediately	To prevent the increase of organisms
7.	Document the procedure in the designated place and mark it off on the Kardex	To avoid duplication Documentation provides coordination of care

Collection of Throat Swab

Purpose

• To identify the type of pathogenic microorganism present in the throat.

Equipments

A clean tray containing:
- Throat swab culture container
- A pair of gloves
- Towel
- Mackintosh
- Torch/Spotlight
- Wooden spatula/tongue depressor
- Gauze pieces
- Kidney tray.

Procedure

The procedure of sample collection from throat swab is given in Table 4.13.

Table 4.13: Procedure of sample collection from throat swab

Sl No	Care action	Rationale
1.	Explain the procedure to the patient	To get the cooperation
2.	Provide privacy to the patient	To make comfortable to the patient
3.	Make the patient to sit straight in the bed or raise the head end of the bed, if not contraindicated	To obtain the sample correctly
4.	Put the Mackintosh and towel around the neck or below the chin	To prevent the soil
5.	Ask the patient to tilt head backward and open mouth, stretch the tongue out	To ease to take the sample
6.	Visualize the tongue and throat by using the spotlight or torch	To assess any problems like ulceration, bleeding, etc.
7.	Use tongue spatula to press the tongue downward to the floor of the mouth	To ease to take the sample
8.	Use sterile cotton swab to wipe down both of the tonsillar arches and the posterior nasopharynx, without touching the sides of the mouth	To prevent the contamination
9.	Place the swab in labeled culture tube and close the tube	To prevent misusage
10.	Remove the Mackintosh and towel, and place the patient in comfort position	To make the patient comfortable
11.	Send the specimen to the laboratory	To do the analysis
12.	Document the procedure in the nurse's record	Help to follow continuity of care
13.	Document the procedure in the nurse's record in details	To follow-up the continuity of care

Points to Note

- If the patient is unconscious, use tongue depressor to access the peritonsillary region.

STOOL SAMPLE COLLECTION

Definition

Stool specimen collection is the process of obtaining a sample of a patient's feces for diagnostic purposes.

Purposes

1. The purpose of a stool culture (STC) is either to identify the causative agent of diarrhea or to detect the bacterial carrier state in a patient.
2. To identify the abnormal elements in the stool.

Equipments

A clean tray containing:
- Specimen container
- A pair of gloves
- Wooden tongue depressor
- Clean bedpan if needed.

Procedure

The stool sample collection procedure is given in Table 4.14.

Table 4.14: Procedure of stool sample collection

Sl No	Care action	Rationale
1.	Explain the procedure to the patient	To understand about the importance of the test
2.	Provide privacy to the patient	To make patient feel comfortable
3.	Urinate before collecting the stool, so that you do not get any urine in the stool sample; do not urinate while passing the stool	To get the accurate results
4.	If the patient collect the specimen himself/herself, the following steps need to be explained to the patient: • Clean the genitalia with water • Pass the motion in the clean bedpan • Avoid contaminating the stool specimen with urine or water during collection • A small amount of stool is removed with stick and placed in the labeled container	To obtain the stool specimen completely
5.	To collect a stool specimen from a child in diapers, line the diaper with plastic wrap and transfer a portion of the stool to the collection specimen container	To prevent the contamination and to get the accurate result
6.	Wash the hands with soap and water	Wash the hands with soap and water

Contd...

Contd...

Sl No	Care action	Rationale
7.	Send the specimen container to the laboratory	To do the analysis
8.	Document the procedure in the nurse's record	To do the follow-up care for the patient

Points to Note
* Avoid using antacids, barium, bismuth, antibiotics, antiamebics, antidiarrheal medication or oily laxative 1 week prior to collection of the specimen.
* Do not refrigerate the specimen containers.

VAGINAL SWAB COLLECTION

Purpose

The vaginal swab test is done to identify the infections in vaginal area, as well as other abnormalities of vaginal wall and cervical cells.

Equipments

A clean tray containing:
* Specimen container with swab stick
* A pair of gloves
* A gauze pieces
* Kidney tray.

Procedure

The procedure of vaginal swab collection is given in Table 4.15.

Table 4.15: Procedure of vaginal swab collection

Sl No	Care action	Rationale
1.	Explain the procedure to the patient	To get the valid consent
2.	Provide privacy to the patient	To make patient feel comfortable
3.	Arrange all the articles near the bedside	To minimize the unnecessary contamination
4.	Wash the hands with soap and water	To prevent infection
5.	Make the patient in lithotomy position in the bed and tell the patient to be relaxed	To make the patient comfortable and easy to perform the procedure
6.	Wear gloves	To avoid the infection
7.	Remove the swab stick from the collection kit or the tube and do not touch the soft tip or lay the swab down	To avoid the infection

Contd...

Contd...

Sl No	Care action	Rationale
8.	Insert the swab into the vagina about 2 inches; gently rotate the swab for 10–30 seconds and withdraw the swab without touching the skin	To prevent the contamination
9.	Place the swab into the labeled test tube and the tip of the swab is visible below the tube label; recap the container	For the easy visualization of the sample and to identify any abnormalities
10.	Clean the genital area with clean gauze pieces	To feel the patient comfortable
11.	Remove the gloves and discard as per the hospital policy and perform handwashing	To prevent cross infection
12.	Send the sample to laboratory	To do the analysis
13.	Document the procedure in the nurses record	To perform the follow-up care for the patient

WOUND SWAB COLLECTION

Purpose

The wound swab test is to help identify microorganisms causing wound infection.

Equipments

A clean tray containing:
- Dressing tray
- Adhesive plaster
- Specimen container with swab stick
- A pair of gloves
- Gauze pieces
- Kidney tray.

Procedure

The procedure of wound swab collection is given in Table 4.16.

Table 4.16: Procedure of wound swab collection

Sl No	Care action	Rationale
1.	Explain the procedure to the patient	To get the valid consent
2.	Provide privacy to the patient	To make patient feel comfortable
3.	Arrange all the articles near the bedside	To minimize the unnecessary contamination
4.	Wash hands with soap and water	To prevent infection
5.	Make the patient in comfortable position according to the wound site	To make the patient comfortable and easy to perform the procedure

Contd...

Contd...

Sl No	Care action	Rationale
6.	Wear the gloves	To avoid the infection
7.	Remove the solid dressing materials with artery forceps	To prevent the contamination
8.	Wash the hands and wear another pair of gloves	To minimize the contamination
9.	Remove the swab stick from the collection kit or the tube and do not touch the soft tip or lay the swab down	To avoid the infection
10.	Take the swab before cleaning the wound	To collect the maximum number of organisms
11.	Use a 'zig-zag' motion whilst simultaneously rotating between the fingers	Ensure all the swab will contain sufficient amounts of bacteria
12.	Place the swab into the labeled test tube and the tip of the swab is visible below the tube label; recap the container	Easy to visualize the sample and to identify any abnormalities
13.	Perform the dressing in an aseptic manner according to the physician order	To prevent the infection
14.	Remove the gloves, discard as per hospital policy and perform handwashing	To prevent cross infection
15.	Wash the articles and replace it	To keep it ready for next usage
16.	Send the sample to laboratory	To do the analysis
17.	Document the procedure in the nurse's record	To perform the follow-up care for the patient

Administration of Medications

ADMINISTRATION OF ORAL DRUGS

Definition

Oral medication is administration of drugs by mouth via the alimentary tract.

Purpose

Drugs are taken by this route because of convenience, absorption of drug, ease of use and cost containment. It is the most common method used.

Equipments

- Clean tray to keep all the equipments needed
- Medication container to keep the opened tablets to be administered
- Ounce glass
- Clean bowl with gauze piece
- Scissors
- Small kidney basin
- Spoon.

Procedure

The procedure of administration of oral drugs is given in Table 5.1.

Table 5.1: Procedure of administration of oral drugs

SI No	Care action	Rationale
1.	Wash hands	To prevent cross infection
2.	Identify the patient	To prevent error
3.	Check for the physician's order; follow the six rights of the medication administration	To prevent medication error
4.	Empty the required dose into the medicine container; avoid touching the preparation	To minimize the cross infection and contamination of the drug
5.	Explain the action, dose and expected adverse effect of the drug to the patient	Patient has the rights to know the treatment
6.	Administer the drug as prescribed orally through mouth with a spoon	No self-administration of drug according to policy

Contd...

Contd...

SI No	Care action	Rationale
7.	Offer a glass of water	To swallow the medication
8.	Documentation to be done in medication administration record (MAR)	To ensure that patient has received the treatment properly

PREPARATION OF INJECTIONS

Definition

The parenteral route refers to medications that are given by injection or infusion ('para' meaning besides, 'enteron' meaning intestine). It is the forcing of drug in the form of fluid into cavity, a blood vessel or intestine.

Purposes

1. To get a rapid and systematic effect of the drug.
2. To provide the needed effect even when the patient is unconscious or unable to swallow.
3. Assures that the total dosage will be administered and the same will be absorbed for the systematic actions of the drug.
4. Provides the only means of administration for medications that cannot be given orally.
5. To obtain a local effect at the site of injection.
6. To restore blood volume by replacing the fluid (in cases of bolus).
7. To give nourishment when it cannot be taken by mouth (in case of total parenteral nutrition).

Equipments

- Clean tray or receiver in which to place drug and equipment
- Use 21 G needle(s) to ease reconstitution and drawing up; 23 G if from a glass ampule
- Use 21, 23 or 25 G needle, size dependent on route of administration
- Syringe(s) of appropriate size for amount of drug to be given
- Swabs saturated with 70% isopropyl alcohol
- Sterile topical swab, if drug is presented in ampule form
- Drug(s) to be administered
- Patient's prescription chart, to check dose, route, etc.
- Recording sheet or book as required by law or hospital policy
- Any protective clothing required by hospital policy for specified drugs such as antibiotics or cytotoxic drugs.

Procedure

Single-dose Ampule

Solution preparation: Single-dose ampule solution preparation is detailed in Table 5.2.

Table 5.2: Protocol for single-dose ampule solution preparation

SI No	Care action	Rationale
1.	Inspect the solution for cloudiness or particulate matter; if this is present, discard and follow hospital guidelines on what action to take, e.g. return drug to pharmacy	To prevent the patient from receiving an unstable or contaminated drug
2.	Tap the neck of the ampule gently	To ensure that all the solution is in the bottom of the ampule
3.	Cover the neck of the ampule with a sterile topical swab and snap it open; if there is any difficulty a file may be required	To minimize the risk of contamination To prevent aerosol formation or contact with the drug, this could lead to a sensitivity reaction To reduce the risk of injury to the nurse
4.	Inspect the solution for glass fragments; if present, discard	To minimize the risk of injection of foreign matter into the patient
5.	Withdraw the required amount of solution, tilting the ampule if necessary	To avoid drawing in any air
6.	Replace the sheath on the needle and tap the syringe to dislodge any air bubbles; expel air	To prevent aerosol formation To ensure that the correct amount of drug is in the syringe

Powder preparation: Single-dose ampule powder preparation is detailed in the Table 5.3.

Table 5.3: Single-dose ampule powder preparation for injection

SI No	Care action	Rationale
1.	Tap the neck of the ampule	To ensure that any powder lodged here falls to the bottom of the ampule
2.	Cover the neck of the ampule with a sterile topical swab and snap it open; if there is any difficulty a file may be required	To minimize the risk of contamination To prevent contact with the drug this could cause a sensitivity reaction To prevent injury to the nurse
3.	Inject the correct diluents slowly into the powder within the ampule	To ensure that the powder is thoroughly wet before agitation and is not released into the atmosphere
4.	Agitate the ampule	To dissolve the drug
5.	Inspect the contents	To detect any glass fragments or any other particulate matter; if present, continue agitation or discard as appropriate

Contd...

Contd...

SI No	Care action	Rationale
6.	When the solution is clear withdraw the prescribed amount, tilting the ampule if necessary	To ensure the powder is dissolved and has formed a solution with the diluents To avoid drawing in air
7.	Replace the sheath on the needle and tap the syringe to dislodge any air bubbles; expel air	To prevent aerosol formation To ensure that the correct amount of drug is in the syringe
8.	Attach a new needle if required (and discard used needle into appropriate sharps container) or attach a plastic end cap	To reduce the risk of infection To avoid tracking medications though superficial tissues To ensure that the correct size of needle is used for the injection To reduce the risk of injury to the nurse

Multidose Vial

Powder preparation: The procedure is described in the Table 5.4.

Table 5.4: Powder preparation from multidose vial

SI No	Care action	Rationale
1.	Remove the tamper evident seal and clean the rubber septum with the chosen antiseptic and let the air dry for at least 30 seconds	To prevent bacterial contamination of the drug, as the plastic lid prevents damage and does not ensure sterility
2.	**Restitution method** Insert a 21 G needle into the cap to vent the bottle	To prevent pressure differentials, this can cause separation of needle and syringe
3.	Inject the correct diluent slowly into the powder within the vial	To ensure that the powder is thoroughly wet before it is shaken and is not into the atmosphere
4.	Remove the needle and the syringe	To enable adequate mixing of the solution
5.	Place a sterile topical swab over the venting needle and shake to dissolve the powder	To prevent contamination of the drug or the atmosphere To mix the diluents with the powder and dissolve the drug
6.	Inspect the solution for cloudiness or particulate matter, if this is present, discard; follow hospital guidelines on what action to take, e.g. return to pharmacy	To prevent patient from receiving an unstable or contaminated drug
7.	**Reconstitution method** With the needle sheathed draw into the syringe a volume if air equivalent to the required volume of solution to be drawn up	To prevent bacterial contamination of the drug
8.	Remove the needle cover and insert the needle into the vial through the rubber septum	To gain access to the vial
9.	Invert the vial; keep the needle in the solution slowly depress the plunger to push the air into the vial	To create an equilibrium in the vial

Contd...

Contd...

SI No	Care action	Rationale
10.	Release the plunger, so that the solution flows back into the syringe (if a large volume of solution is to be withdrawn use a push pull technique)	To create an equilibrium in the vial
11.	Inject the diluents into the vial; keeping the tip of the needle above the level of the solution in the vial, release the plunger; the syringe will fill with the air, which has been displaced by the solution	This 'equilibrium method' helps to minimize the build up of pressure in the vial
12.	With the needle and syringe in place, gently swirl the vials to dissolve all the powder	To mix the diluents with the powder and dissolve the drug
13.	Inspect the solution for cloudiness or particulate matter; if this is present, discard and follow hospital guidelines on what action to take, e.g. return drug to pharmacy	To prevent patient from receiving an unstable or contaminated drug
14.	**Withdrawal of medication from vial** Withdraw the prescribed amount of solution and inspect for pieces of rubber, which may have 'cored out' of the cap	To ensure that the correct amount of drug is in the syringe To prevent the injection of foreign matter into the patient
15.	Remove air from syringe without spraying into the atmosphere by injecting air back into the vial or replace the sheath on the needle and tap the syringe to dislodge any air bubbles; expel air	To reduce risk of contamination of practitioner To prevent aerosol formation To avoid complication
16.	Attach a new needle if required (and discard used needle into appropriate sharps container) or attach a plastic end cap	To reduce the risk of infection To avoid possible trauma to the patient if the needle has barbed To avoid tracking medications through superficial tissues To ensure that the correct size of needle is used for the injection

Aftercare

- Inspection of the site for bleeding and abscess; if bleeding, apply pressure
- Watch for signs and symptoms of allergic reactions
- If the patient develops numbness or weakness on walking it may be due to nerve injury; ask patient take rest and inform the doctor
- Apply warmth if the patient develops pain redness and induration
- Clean all articles and replace them
- Wash hands.

ADMINISTRATION OF INTRAMUSCULAR INJECTION

Definition

Administration of injection (medication) with an angle of 90° into the muscle.

Purpose

Provides faster medication absorption than the subcutaneous because of a greater muscular vascularity.

Equipments

- Clean tray or receiver in which to place drug and equipment
- Syringe(s) of appropriate size for amount of drug to be given
- Swabs saturated with 70% isopropyl alcohol
- Sterile topical swab, if drug is presented in ampule form
- Drug(s) to be administered
- Patient's prescription chart, to check dose, route, etc.
- Recording sheet or book as required by law or hospital policy
- Any protective clothing required by hospital policy for specified drugs such as antibiotics or cytotoxic drugs.

Sites

- Vastus lateralis
- Ventrogluteal
- Deltoid
- Dorsogluteal.

Procedure

Follow the procedure for administration of intramuscular injection is given in the Table 5.5.

Table 5.5: Procedure for administration of intramuscular injection

Sl No	Care action	Rationale
1.	Cleanse hands with alcoholic hand rub	Hands to be cleansed before and after each patient contact
2.	Explain and discuss the procedure with the patient	To ensure the patient understands the procedure and gives his/her valid consent
3.	Consult the patient's prescription sheet: • Drug • Dose • Date and time of administration • Route and method of administration • Dilute as appropriate • Validity of prescription	To ensure that the patient is given the correct drug in the prescribed dose using the appropriate diluents and by the correct route
4.	Assist the patient into the required position	To access to the injection site and to ensure the designated muscle is flexed and therefore relaxed
5.	Remove the appropriate garment to expose the injection site	To gain access for injection

Contd...

Contd...

Sl No	Care action	Rationale
6.	Assess the injection site for signs of inflammation, edema, infection and skin lesions	To promote effectiveness of administration To reduce the risk of infection To avoid skin lesions and avoid possible trauma to the patient
7.	Clean the injection sites with a swab saturated with 70% isopropyl alcohol for 30 seconds and allow it to dry for 30 seconds	To reduce the number of pathogens introduced into the skin by the needle at the time of insertion, to prevent stinging sensation if alcohol is taken into the tissues upon needle entry
8.	Stretch the skin around the injection site	To facilitate insertion of the needle and to reduce the sensitivity of nerve endings
9.	Holding the needle at an angle of 90°, quickly plunge into the skin	To ensure that the needle penetrates the muscle
10.	Pull back the plunger; if no blood is aspirated, depress the plunger at approximately 1 mL every 10 seconds and inject the drug slowly; if blood appears, withdraw the needle completely, replace it and begin again; explain to the patient what has occurred	To confirm that the needle is in the correct position and not in a vein; this allows time for the muscle fibers to expand and absorb the solution To prevent pain and ensure even distribution of the drug
11.	Wait 10 seconds before withdrawing needle	To allow the medication to spread into the tissue
12.	Withdraw the needle rapidly; apply pressure to any bleeding point	To prevent hematoma
13.	Record the administration on appropriate charts	To maintain accurate records, provide point of reference in the event of any queries and prevent any duplication of treatment
14.	Ensure that all sharps and non-sharp waste are disposed safely and in accordance with locally approved procedures (sharps in the sharps bin and syringes into yellow clinical waste bag)	To ensure safe disposal and to avoid laceration or other injury to staff

ADMINISTRATION OF SUBCUTANEOUS INJECTIONS

Definition

A subcutaneous (SC) injection is a method of drug administration into the subcutaneous tissue. Up to 2 mL of a drug solution can be injected directly beneath the skin. The drug becomes effective within 20 minutes.

Purposes

1. Subcutaneous injection is the method used to administer drugs when a small amount of fluid is to be injected, when the patient is unable to take the drug orally, or the drug is destroyed by intestinal secretions.
2. Administration prevents complication because:

- The skin and underlying tissues are free of abnormalities
- Not over bony prominences
- Free of large blood vessels and nerves.
3. Self-administration is possible.

Equipments

- Clean tray or receiver in which to place drug and equipment
- Use 23 G needle if from a glass ampule
- Use 1–2 mL syringes appropriate for the amount of drugs to be given
- Swabs saturated with 70% isopropyl alcohol
- Sterile topical swabs, if drug is presented in ampule form
- Drugs to be administered
- Patient's prescription chart, to check dose, route, etc.
- Recording sheet (MAR) as required by law policy.

Sites

- Outer aspect of the upper arm
- Posterior chest wall below the scapula
- Anterior abdominal wall from below the breast to the iliac crest
- The anterior and lateral aspect of the thigh.

Procedure

The procedure to be followed in the administration of the subcutaneous injections is explained in the Table 5.6.

Table 5.6: Procedure for administration of subcutaneous injection

Sl No	Care action	Rationale
1.	Explain and discuss the procedure with the patient	To ensure that the patient understands the procedure and gives his/her valid consent
2.	Consult the patient's prescription chart and ascertain the following: • Drug • Dose • Date and time of administration • Route and method of administration • Dilute as appropriate • Validity of prescription • Signature of doctor	To ensure that the patient is given the correct drug in the prescribed dose using the appropriate diluent and the correct route
3.	Assist the patient into the required position	Allow to access to the appropriate injection site
4.	Remove appropriate garments to expose the injection site	To gain access for injection

Contd...

Contd...

SI No	Care action	Rationale
5.	Assess the injection site for signs of inflammation, edema, infection and skin lesions	To promote effectiveness of administration To reduce the risk of infection To avoid skin lesions and avoid possible trauma to the patients
6.	Choose the correct needle size	To minimize the risk of missing the subcutaneous tissue and any ensuing pain
7.	Clean the injection site with a swab saturated with 70% isopropyl alcohol	To reduce the number of pathogens introduced into the skin by the needle at the time of insertion
8.	Gently pinch the skin up into a fold	To elevate the subcutaneous tissue and lift the adipose tissue away from the underlying muscle
9.	Insert the needle into the skin at an angle of 45° and release the grasped skin; inject the drug slowly	Injection mediation into compressed tissue irritated nerve fibers and causes the patient discomfort
10.	Withdraw the needle rapidly; apply pressure to any bleeding point; do not rub	To prevent hematoma formation Interferes with absorption
11.	Ensure that all sharps and non-sharp waste are disposed safely and in accordance with locally approved procedures such as needle into white puncture proof container and syringes into red waste bag	To ensure safe disposal and to avoid laceration or other injury to staff
12.	Record the administration on appropriate sheets	To maintain accurate records, provide a point of reference in the event of any queries and prevent any duplication of treatment

Nursing Alert

With the subcutaneous route, a small thin needle is inserted beneath the skin and the drug injected slowly. The drug moves from the small blood vessels into the bloodstream.

ADMINISTRATION OF INSULIN INJECTIONS

Definition

Insulin is a hormone used to control glycemia. It must be administered by injection because it is a protein and therefore would be broken down and destroyed in the gastrointestinal tract.

Purposes

1. To provide sufficient insulin throughout 24 hours to cover basal requirements.
2. To deliver higher boluses of insulin in an attempt to match the glycemic effect of meals.

3. To control diabetes mellitus.
4. To treat hyperglycemia.

Blood Glucose Monitoring

Blood glucose (BG) levels are often checked qac (30 min before meals), qhs (at bedtime) or prn (as needed):
- Preprandial (fasting or before a meal) 70–130 mg/dL
- Postprandial (1–2 h after the start of a meal) less than 180 mg/dL
- These ranges may vary depending on institution and physician protocols.

Insulin Administration According to the Classification

Rapid Onset-fast Acting Insulin

Rapid onset-fast acting insulin is fast acting. It starts working within1–15 minutes. It is clear in appearance and its peak time is about 1 hour later, and lasts for 3–5 hours. When you inject rapid onset-fast acting type of insulin, patient must eat immediately after the inject. The two rapid onset-fast acting insulin types currently available are:
- NovoRapid (insulin aspart)
- Humalog (Lispro)
- Glulisine (apidra).

Short-acting Insulin

Short-acting insulin looks clear and begins to lower blood glucose levels within 30 minutes, so patient need to take the injection half an hour before eating. Short-acting insulin has peak effect of 4 hours and works for about 6 hours. Short-acting insulin types, currently available include:
- Actrapid
- Humulin
- Hypurin Neutral (highly purified bovine insulin).

Intermediate-acting Insulin

Intermediate-acting insulin looks cloudy. They have either protamine or zinc added to delay their action. This insulin starts to show its effect about 90 minutes after the inject, peak at 4–12 hours and lasts for 16–24 hours.
   Intermediate-acting insulins presently available with protamine:
- Protaphane
- Humulin NPH
- Hypurin Isophane (bovine).

Mixed Insulin

Mixed insulin is cloudy in appearance. It is a combination of either a rapid onset-fast acting or a short-acting insulin and intermediate-acting insulin. Advantage of it is that, two types of insulin can be given in one injection.

When it shows 30/70 then it means 30% of short acting is mixed with 70% of intermediate-acting insulin. The mixed insulins currently available include:
- NovoMix 30
- Humalog Mix 25/75
- Mixtard 30/70
- Mixtard 20/80.

Points to Note

♦ Roll well the vial of insulin in order to mixed them evenly.

Long-acting Insulin

There are two kinds of long-acting insulin available in market, both with clear appearance:
1. Lantus (glargine): It has no peak period as it works constantly when released into your bloodstream at a relatively constant rate (full 24 hour).
2. Levemir (detemir): It has a relatively flat action, can last up to 24 hours and may be given once or twice during the day.

Frequently Used Regimens

1. Two injections daily of a mixture of short- and intermediate-acting insulins (before breakfast and the main evening meal).
2. Three injections daily using a mixture of short- and intermediate-acting insulins before breakfast; short-acting insulin alone before an afternoon snack or main evening meal; intermediate-acting insulin before bed or variations of this:
   - Basal-bolus regimen of short-acting insulin 20–30 minutes before main meals (e.g. breakfast, lunch and the main evening meal); intermediate- or long-acting insulin at bedtime
   - Basal-bolus regimen of rapid-acting insulin analog immediately before main meals (e.g. breakfast, lunch and main evening meal); intermediate- or long-acting insulins at bedtime, probably before breakfast and occasionally at lunchtime
   - Insulin pump regimes are regaining popularity with a fixed or variable basal dose and bolus doses with meal.

None of these regimens can be optimized without frequent assessment by BG monitoring.

Daily Insulin Dosage

Daily insulin dosage varies greatly between individuals and changes over time. It therefore requires regular review and reassessment. Dosage depends on many factors includes the following:
- Age
- Weight

- Stage of puberty
- Duration and phase of diabetes
- State of injection sites
- Nutritional intake and distribution
- Exercise patterns
- Daily routine
- Results of BG monitoring (and glycosylated hemoglobin)
- Concurrent illness.

The 'correct' dose of insulin is that which achieves the best attainable glycemic control for an individual child or adolescent.

> **Points to Note**
>
> ◆ Healthcare professionals have the responsibility to advice patients, other care providers and young people on adjusting insulin therapy safely and effectively. This training requires regular review, reassessment and reinforcement.

Route of Administration

Subcutaneous or Hypodermic (into the Subcutaneous Tissue)

Needles: 25–27 G, 5/8–1/2 inch.

Syringes: Includes the following:
- 1 mL for 100 unit of insulin
- 1 mL for 40 units of insulin.

Position: 45°–90° angle.

Advantages
- Allows slower, more sustained drug administration than IM injection
- Injected into the adipose tissues beneath the skin, a drug moves into the bloodstream more rapidly than if given by mouth
- Minimal tissue risk
- Allows slower absorption
- Minimal risk of hitting blood vessel.

Cautions
- Do not give in scarred areas, in moles, inflamed or edematous areas
- Do not massage after administration
- Outer aspect of the upper arm
- Anterior thigh
- Loose tissue of the lower abdomen
- Upper hips
- Buttock
- Upper back.

Procedure

The procedure for the insulin administration is described in Table 5.7.

Table 5.7: Procedure for insulin injection administration

Sl No	Care action	Rationale
1.	Wash hands	To prevent infection
2.	Check the medicine order and make sure that the solution in the vial matches the ordered solution	Avoids medication error
3.	Obtain an insulin syringe	
4.	Pick up the vial and verify the type of insulin, which is prescribed	Avoids medication error
5.	Check the patient's most recent blood glucose, if in case of doubt or assessment changes always recheck and reassess	To avoid overdosage
6.	If applicable, verify the blood glucose and use sliding scale insulin administration dosage on the patient's medication administration record (MAR)	To avoid overdosage
7.	Wipe the insulin vial with a sterile gauze alcohol pad, if the insulin is cloudy roll between palms of your hands	Rotating the vial between both hands resuspend the modified insulin preparation and help to warm the medication; shaking insulin vial causes bubbles to form, which take up space and alters the dose
8.	Withdraw the appropriate type and amount of insulin	To achieve the therapeutic effect
9.	Pull back on barrel of syringe to draw in a volume of the ordered medication dose; holding the vial between the thumb and fingers of the non-dominant hand, insert the needle through the rubber stopper into the air space, not the solution	Enhances easy withdrawal of medication
10.	Invert the vial and withdraw the ordered dose of medication by pulling back on the plunger; make sure the needle is in the solution to be withdrawn	Prevents the entry of air
11.	Expel air bubbles and adjust dose if necessary	To prevent complication
12.	Remove needle from vial and cover the needle with guard using one hand or scoop method	Avoids needle stick injury
13.	Take medication into patient's room and verify, administer the subcutaneous (SC) injection; remember to never massage the insulin injection site (Figs 5.1A and B)	
14.	Record the administration on appropriate sheets	To maintain accurate records, provide a point of reference in the event of any queries and prevent any duplication of treatment

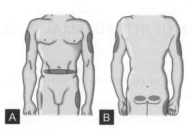

FIGURES 8.1A and B: Insulin injection sites. **A.** Anterior sites; **B.** Posterior sites.

Insulin Pen

Preparation, dosing and rationale of insulin pen is explained in Table 5.8.

Table 5.8: Nursing intervention in insulin pen usage

SI No	Care action	Rationale
1.	Gather supplies; verify insulin type: • Pen device (with cartridge) • Pen needle • Alcohol wipe • Sharps container	To save time
2.	Wash hands	To prevent infection
3.	Choose injection site	To administer medication
4.	Clean injection site	To prevent infection
5.	Screw pen needle firmly onto pen	Ensures the needle from dislodging form the pen
6.	Prime: Dial '2' units	To remove the primary medicine, which is lodged in the pocket of cartridge
7.	Hold upright; remove air by pressing the plunger; repeat 'prime' if no insulin shows at end of needle	To avoid air embolism
8.	Dial number of units to be administered as per order	To avoid medication error
9.	Pinch up the skin	Ensures the correct size of the needle
10.	Push the needle into the skin at 90°	Avoids injury
11.	Release pinched skin	Causes pain
12.	Leave needle in skin and keep pressing the button for 5–10 seconds	To ensure to deliver the required dose completely
13.	Remove and dispose of pen needle	Avoids needle stick injury
14.	Document time, dose, site and blood glucose value	To maintain accurate records, provide a point of reference in the event of any queries and prevent any duplication of treatment

Points to Note

- Check site for leakage, lipoatrophy, lipohypertrophy.
- Check for signs and symptoms of hypoglycemia.
- Meal/Snack dose.
- Timeliness in relation to eating.
- Supervision of food amount.

ADMINISTRATION OF INTRADERMAL INJECTIONS

Definition

Administration of injection (medication) with an angle of 5°–15° into the dermal layer of the skin.

Purpose

Certain medications may be injected intradermally to test the allergy.

Equipments

- Clean tray or receiver in which to place drug and equipment
- Syringe(s) of appropriate size for amount of drug to be given
- Swabs saturated with 70% isopropyl alcohol
- Sterile topical swab, if drug is presented in ampule form
- Drug(s) to be administered
- Patient's prescription chart, to check dose, route, etc.
- Recording sheet or book as required by law or hospital policy
- Any protective clothing required by hospital policy for specified drugs such as antibiotics or cytotoxic drugs.

Site

- Forearm.

Procedure

The procedure for intradermal injection is described in Table 5.9.

Table 5.9: Procedure for administration of intradermal injection

Sl No	Care action	Rationale
1.	Cleanse hands with alcoholic hand rub	Hands to be cleansed before and after each patient contact
2.	Explain and discuss the procedure with the patient	To ensure the patient understands the procedure and gives his/her valid consent
3.	Consult the patient's prescription sheet: • Drug • Dose • Date and time of administration • Route and method of administration • Dilute as appropriate • Validity of prescription	To ensure that the patient is given the correct drug in the prescribed dose using the appropriate diluents and by the correct route
4.	Assist the patient into the required position	Assist the patient into the required position
5.	Remove the appropriate garment to expose the injection site	To gain access for injection
6.	Assess the injection site for signs of inflammation, edema and infection and skin lesions	To promote effectiveness of administration To reduce the risk of infection To avoid skin lesions and avoid possible trauma to the patient
7.	Clean the injection sites with a swab saturated with 70% isopropyl alcohol for 30 seconds and allow it to dry for 30 seconds	To reduce the number of pathogens introduced into the skin by the needle at the time of insertion, to prevent stinging sensation if alcohol is taken into the tissues upon needle entry
8.	Stretch the skin around the injection site	To facilitate insertion of the needle and to reduce the sensitivity of nerve endings

Contd...

Contd...

Sl No	Care action	Rationale
9.	Holding the needle level up at an angle of 5°–15°, slowly plunge into the skin and administer the drug	To ensure that the needle penetrates the dermis
10.	Notice that, while injecting the medication, small bleb approximately 6 mm in diameter appears on the skin surface	Bleb indicates medication is deposited in dermis
11.	Withdraw the needle, while applying alcohol swab or gauze gently over site rapidly	To minimize discomfort
12.	Apply gentle pressure; do not massage site	Massaging damages underlying tissues, it may disperse medication into underlying tissue layers and alter test results
13.	Stay with the patient 3–5 minutes and observe for any allergic reactions	Severe anaphylactic reaction is characterized by dyspnea, wheezing and circulatory collapse
14.	Record the administration on appropriate charts	To maintain accurate records, provide point of reference in the event of any queries and prevent any duplication of treatment
15.	Ensure that all sharps and non-sharp waste are disposed off safely and in accordance with locally approved procedures (sharps in the sharps bin and syringes into yellow clinical waste bag)	To ensure safe disposal and to avoid laceration or other injury to staff

Points to Note

* For intradermal injections, use blue ink pen and draw circle around perimeter of injection site.
* Do not use red ink pen.

ADMINISTRATION OF INTRAVENOUS INJECTIONS

Definition

Intravenous (IV) injection is defined as the parenteral administration of bolus medication directly into the vein through the existing IV line.

Methods of Infusion

In intravenous injection administration there are three methods:
1. Continuous infusion.
2. Intermittent infusion.
3. Direct intermittent injection.

Continuous Infusion

Continuous infusion may be defined as the intravenous delivery of medication or fluid at a constant rate over a prescribed time period, ranging from 24 hours to days, to achieve a controlled therapeutic response.

Intermittent Infusion

Intermittent infusion is the administration of a small volume infusion, i.e. 50–250 mL over a period of between 20 minutes and 2 hours. This may be given as a specified dose at one time or at repeated intervals during 24 hours.

Direct Intermittent Injection

Direct intermittent injection involves the injection of a drug from a syringe into the injection port of the administration set or directly into a vascular access device.

Purposes

1. To administer large volume of fluid.
2. Rapid absorption is achieved.
3. In emergencies, fast-acting medications can be delivered quickly.
4. Establishes continuous fluid infusions.
5. To establish constant therapeutic blood levels.
6. Medications that are highly alkaline and irritating to subcutaneous tissue are given intravenously.
7. Intravenous therapy is used primarily for fluid replacement in patients unable to take oral fluids.

Equipments

- Clean tray or receiver in which to place drug and equipment
- To ease reconstitution 21 G needle(s) and drawing up, 23 G if from a glass ampule
- Needles of 21, 23 or 25 G can be used, size dependent on route of administration
- Syringes of appropriate size for amount of drugs to be given
- Swabs saturated with 70% isopropyl alcohol
- Drugs to be administered
- Patient's prescription chart, to check dose, route, etc.
- Medication administration record (MAR), recording sheets as required by hospital policy
- Any personal protective devices required by hospital policy for specified drugs such as cytotoxic drugs
- Three-way connectors with stopper
- Gloves
- Kidney basin
- Spread sheet to prevent soiling of bedsheet.

Procedure

Procedure for intravenous injection administration is described in the Table 5.10.

Table 5.10: Procedure for administrating intravenous injection

Sl No	Care action	Rationale
1.	Collect and check all equipments	To prevent delays and enable full concentration on the procedure
2.	Check that the packing of all equipment is intact	To ensure sterility, if the seal is damage, discard
3.	Wash hands with bactericidal soap and water or bactericidal alcohol hand rub	To prevent contamination of medication and equipment
4.	Prepare needle(s), syringe(s) and other supplies by placing on a tray or receiver	To contain all items in a clean area
5.	Inspect all equipment	To check that none is damaged; if so, discard or report
6.	Consult the patient's prescription chart and ascertain the following: • Drug • Dose • Date and time of administration • Route and method of administration • Dilute as appropriate • Validity of prescription • Signature of doctor	To ensure that the patient is given the correct drug in the prescribed dose using the appropriate
7.	Check all details with another nurse if required by hospital policy	To minimize any risk of error
8.	Select the drug in the appropriate volume, dilution or dosage and check the expiry date	To reduce wastage; treatment with medication that is outside the expiry is dangerous The expiry date indicates when a particular drug is no longer pharmacologically efficacious
9.	Proceed with the preparation of the drug, using protective clothing if advisable	To protect practitioner during preparation
10.	Take the prepared dose to the patient, whose identity is checked	To prevent error and confirm patient's identity
11.	Evaluate the patient's knowledge of the medication being offered; if this knowledge appears to be faulty or incorrect, offer an explanation of the use, action, dose and potential side-effects of the drug or drugs involved	A patient has a right to know the information about the treatment
12.	Close room door or curtains if appropriate	To ensure patient privacy and dignity
13.	Administer the drug as prescribed	To ensure patient receives treatment
14.	Do not recap; follow biomedical waste management (BWM) policy	To minimize risk of contamination and prevent risk of injury to nurses
15.	Record the administration on appropriate chart; documentation must include date, time, amount, route, name of the drug and reaction of patient; follow-up observation also must be recorded	To maintain accurate records, provide a point of reference in the event of any queries and prevent any duplication of treatment

Points to Note
- The rate and the flow of solution.
- Complications like infection, phlebitis (venous inflammation), thrombophlebitis (clot formation), air embolism, local infiltration and allergic reactions.
- Accuracy of flow is very important.

ADMINISTERING MEDICATIONS BY HEPARIN LOCK

Definition

A heparin lock is an IV catheter that is inserted into a vein and left in place either for intermittent administration of medication or as open line in the case of an emergency.

Administering medications by heparin lock is defined as one of IV therapy, which can allow to be freedom clients while he/she has not received IV therapy.

Purposes

- To provide intermittent administration of medication
- To administer medication under the urgent condition.

Equipments

General

- Client's chart and Kardex
- Prescribed medication
- Spirit swabs
- Disposable gloves, if available: 1
- Kidney tray: 1
- Steel tray: 1.

For Flush

- Saline vial or saline in the syringe: 1
- Heparin flush solution: 1
- Syringe (3–5 mL) with 21–25 gauge needle: 1.

For Intermittent Infusion

- Bottle or IV bag with 50–100 mL solution: 1
- Intravenous tubing set: 1
- Intravenous stand: 1
- Needle of 21–23 gauge: 1
- Adhesive tape.

Nursing Alert

- A heparin lock has an adapter, which is attached to the hub (end) of the catheter
- An anticoagulant, approximately 2 mL heparin, is injected into the heparin lock
- To reduce the possibility of clotting, flush the heparin lock with 2–3 mL of saline 8 hourly (or once a every duty); saline lock
- Choose heparin lock or saline lock to decrease the possibility of making coagulation according to your facility's policy or doctor's order.

Procedure

Procedure for administration of medication by heparin lock is described in Table 5.11.

Table 5.11: Procedure for administration of medication by heparin lock

Sl No	Care action	Rationale
1.	Perform hand hygiene	To prevent the spread of infection
2.	Assemble all equipments	Organization facilities accurate skill performance
3.	Verify the medication order	To reduce the chances of medication errors
4.	Check the medication's expiration date	Out dated medication may be ineffective
5.	**For bolus injection** Prepare the medication; if necessary, withdraw from an ample or a vial	Preparing the medication before entering the client's room facilitates administration
6.	Explain the procedure to the client	Providing information fosters his/her cooperation
7.	Identify the client before giving the medication	Abiding by the 'five rights' prevents medication errors
8.	Put on gloves	Gloves act as a barrier
9.	Cleanse the heparin lock port with a spirit swab	Spirit swab removes surface contaminants and decreases the potential for introducing pathogens into the system
10.	• Steady the heparin lock with your dominant hand • Insert the needle of the syringe containing 1 mL of saline into the center of the port • Aspirate for blood return • Inject the saline • Remove the needle and discard the syringe in the sharps container without recapping it	Blood return on aspiration generally indicates that the catheter is positioned in the vein Saline clears the tubing of any heparin flush or previous medication Most accidental needle-sticks occur during recapping Proper disposal prevents injury

Contd...

Contd...

Sl No	Care action	Rationale
11.	• Cleanse the port again with a spirit swab • Insert the needle of the syringe containing the medication • Inject the medication slowly • Withdraw the syringe and dispose of it properly	Rapid injection of medication can lead to speed shock
12.	• Cleanse the port with a spirit swab • Flush the lock with 1 mL heparin flush solution according to hospital/agency policy	To remove contaminants and prevents infection via the port Flush clears the lock of medication and keeps it open Some agencies recommend only a saline flush to clear the lock
13.	**For intermittent infusion** • Use premixed solution in the bag • Connect the tubing and add the needle or needless component • Prepare the tubing with solution	Preparing the medication before enter the client's room facilitates administration
14.	Follow the former action given in step 6–10	Because the preparation is same like bolus injection
15.	• Cleanse the port again with a spirit swab • Insert the needle or needleless component attached to the intravenous (IV) set up into the port • Attach it to the IV infusion pump or calculate the flow rate • Regulate drip according to the prescribed delivery time • Clamp the tubing and withdraw the needle when all solution has been infused • Discard the equipments used safely according to hospital/agency's policy	To remove contaminants and prevents infection via the port Infusing more than required amount of solution will cause fluid overload Clamping prevents air entry Proper disposal prevents injury
16.	• Cleanse the port with a spirit swab • Flush the lock with 1 mL heparin flush solution according to hospital/agency policy	To remove contaminants and prevents infection via the port Flush clears the lock of medication and keeps it open Some agencies recommend only a saline flush to clear the lock
17.	Remove gloves and perform hand hygiene	To prevent the spread of infection
18.	Record: • Record the IV medication administration on the appropriate form • Record the fluid volume on the client's balance sheet	Documentation provides coordination of care
19.	Check the client's response to the medication within the appropriate time	Drugs administered parenterally have rapid onsets of action

ADMINISTRATION OF EYE MEDICATIONS

Eye Ointment Application

Definition

An eye ointment is a semisolid preparation applied to the eye.

Purpose

Eye ointment is used to treat conditions like, keratitis, scleritis, postexternal and internal ocular surgeries, postglaucoma surgeries, ocular injuries.

Equipments

- Clean tray to keep all the required materials
- Sterile dressing pack
- Sterile water for irrigation
- Sterile swab
- Prescribed eye ointment.

Procedure

The procedure of eye ointment application is listed in Table 5.12.

Table 5.12: Procedure for eye ointment application

Sl No	Care action	Rationale
1.	Explain the procedure to the patient	To get the consent
2.	Follow the six rights of the drug administration	To prevent medication error
3.	Make the patient to lie down in supine position	To ensure the ointment gone into the inferior fornix of the eye
4.	Wash hands	To prevent cross infection
5.	Clean the eyes with sterile water	To remove any discharges
6.	Hold the nozzle of the tube approximately 2.5 cm above the eye; apply a line of ointment to the inner edge of the lower lid from the nasal corner outwards	To reduce the risk of cross infection, contamination of the tube and trauma to the eye
7.	Ask the patient to close the eyes for 1 minute	To ensure the adequate absorption of the drops
8.	Document in medication administration record (MAR); special notes to be documented in the nurse's record	To maintain the accurate record

Instillation of Eyedrops

Definition

Eyedrop instillation is the instillation of sterile ophthalmic medication into the patient eyes.

Purpose

Eyedrops are used to treat the eye disorders like glaucoma, allergies and infections, and it is used to dilate the pupil for ophthalmic examination.

Equipments

- Clean tray to keep all the required materials
- Sterile dressing pack
- Sterile water for irrigation
- Sterile swab
- Prescribed eyedrops.

Procedure

Nursing action and rationale in the instillation of eyedrops is described in the Table 5.13.

Table 5.13: Nursing intervention and rationale in the instillation of eyedrops

Sl No	Care action	Rationale
1.	Explain the procedure to the patient	To get the consent
2.	Follow the six rights of the drug administration	To prevent medication error
3.	Make the patient to lie down in supine position	To ensure the drops instilled into the inferior fornix of the eye
4.	Wash hands	To prevent cross infection
5.	Clean the eyes with sterile water	To remove any discharges
6.	Ask the patient to look up, simultaneously pull down the lower eyelid and instill the prescribed eye drops	To ensure the drops are instilled into the inferior fornix of the eye
7.	Ask the patient to close the eyes for 1 minute	To ensure the adequate absorption of the drops
8.	Document in medication administration record (MAR); special notes to be documented in the nurses record	To maintain the accurate record

INSTILLATION OF EAR MEDICATION

Definition

Administration of medicine into the ear canal.

Purpose

Eardrops is used to treat or prevent ear infections.

Equipments

- Clean tray to keep all the required materials
- Sterile swab
- Prescribed eardrops.

Procedure

Action and rationale related to ear the medicine instillation is listed in the Table 5.14.

Table 5.14: Nursing intervention and rationale in eardrops instillation

SI No	Care action	Rationale
1.	Explain the procedure to the patient	To get the consent and cooperation from the patient
2.	Follow the six rights of the drug administration	To prevent medication error
3.	Make the patient to lie on the lateral position with the affected side uppermost	To ensure the best position for instillation of the drops
4.	Wash hands	To prevent cross infection
5.	Pull the cartilaginous part of the pinna backwards and upwards; instill the drops	To ensure the proper instillation of the ear drops
6.	Advise the patient to be in same position for 1–2 minutes	For the proper absorption of the ear drops
7.	Document in medication administration record (MAR)	To maintain the accurate record

INSTILLATION OF NASAL MEDICATION

Definition

A nasal instillation is a medicine solution prepared for administration into the nasal canal. Nasal medicine is given in the form of nasal drops or nasal sprays.

Purpose

The purpose of a nasal instillation is to deliver medicine directly into the nose and onto the nasal membranes, where it will be absorbed into the body. The most common nasal medicines are decongestant, antihistamine and steroid nasal sprays used to relieve nasal congestion.

Equipments

- Clean tray to keep the equipments needed
- Prescribed nasal drops
- Clean gauze or tissue paper
- Clean kidney basin.

Procedure

Nasal medication instillation procedure is described in Table 5.15.

Table 5.15: Nursing intervention and rationale in nasal medication instillation

Sl No	Care action	Rationale
1.	Wash hands	To prevent cross infection
2.	Explain the procedure to the patient and get the consent	Patient has the rights to know the treatment
3.	Follow the six rights of drug administration	To prevent medication error
4.	Ask the patient to blow the nose (unless clinically contraindicated)	To clear the passage for easy penetration
5.	Extend the patient neck (unless clinically contraindicated), e.g. cervical spondylosis	To get a safe position for instillation of medication
6.	Avoid touching external nostrils and instill the prescribed strength	To prevent cross infection
7.	Instruct the patient to be in the same position for 1–2 minutes	To ensure the absorption of the medicine
8.	Record in medication administration record (MAR)	To maintain the record of treatment

ADMINISTRATION OF RECTAL MEDICATIONS

Definition

Administration of medicine into the rectum.

Purpose

Rectal medicine application method is preferred to administer laxatives, to obtain localized therapeutic effect or for diagnostic purpose. Also it used when the patient has nausea, vomiting, uncooperative patients or before surgeries.

Equipments

- Clean tray to keep all the equipments
- Prescribed medicine
- Clean gloves
- Clean gauze
- Clean kidney tray.

Procedure

Nursing action and rationale in rectal medicine application is listed in Table 5.16.

Table 5.16: Rectal medicine application

Sl No	Care action	Rationale
1.	Explain the procedure to the patient	To get the patient consent and for the cooperation
2.	Make the patient to lie down in left lateral position with right leg flexed	For the proper administration of the medication

Contd...

Contd...

SI No	Care action	Rationale
3.	Wash hands and wear the clean gloves	To prevent cross infection
4.	Ask the patient to relax and to take a deep breath and insert the medicine	For easy administration of the medication and to prevent pain
5.	Advise the patient to lie down for 1 minute	For the good absorption of medication
6.	Document in medication administration record (MAR)	To keep accurate record

ADMINISTRATION OF VAGINAL MEDICATIONS

Definition

Administration of medicine (pessaries) into the vaginal orifice.

Purpose

Pessaries are used to have a therapeutic action.

Equipments

- Clean tray to keep all the equipments
- Prescribed medicine
- Clean glove
- Clean gauze
- Clean kidney tray.

Procedure

Procedure to be followed in the application of vaginal medicine is described in the Table 5.17.

Table 5.17: Nursing intervention and rationale in vaginal medication

SI No	Care action	Rationale
1.	Explain the procedure to the patient	To get the patient consent and for the cooperation
2.	Follow the six rights of drug administration	To prevent medication error
3.	Make the patient to lie down in supine position with knees up	For the correct insertion of the pessaries
4.	Wash hands	To prevent cross infection
5.	Wear gloves and insert the prescribed pessary along the posterior wall of the vagina; ask the patient to lie down on left lateral for 1–2 minutes	To ensure that the pessary should retained
6.	Document in medication administration record (MAR)	To maintain the accurate record

PREPARATION AND ADMINISTRATION OF CHEMOTHERAPY DRUG

Handling, preparation, administration and disposal of cytotoxic agents may constitute an occupational hazard. While it has not been established that handling cytotoxic agents is consistently linked with adverse health risks, handlers must be aware of the possibility. The implementation of suitable safety precautions reduces the possibility of adverse health effects to hospital employees.

Definition

Other medical terms often used to describe cancer chemotherapy are antineoplastic (anticancer) and cytotoxic (cell killing).

Purposes

- To kill cancer cells
- Can be used as a primary form of treatment or as a supplement to other treatments
- Can be used in metastasis
- Can be used as adjuvant therapy
- Can ease the symptoms of cancer (palliative), helping some patients have a better quality life.

Side Effects of Chemotherapy

- Nausea, vomiting
- Myelosuppression
- Mucositis
- Diarrhea
- Constipation
- Cardiotoxicity
- Pulmonary toxicity
- Fever
- Nephrotoxicity
- Bladder toxicity
- Neurotoxicity
- Allergic reactions (i.e. rashes, petechiae, ecchymosis)
- Alopecia
- Hyperpigmentation
- Immunosuppression.

Terminology

Cytotoxic agents: Substances used in the treatment of malignant and other diseases. They are designed to destroys rapidly growing cancer cells. They have been shown to be mutagenic, carcinogenic and/or teratogenic, either in treatment doses or animal and bacterial assays.

Cytotoxic: An agent or process that is toxic to cells.

Chemotherapy: The use of any chemical agents to treat or control disease. Most often used to describe treatment of malignant and other diseases with cytotoxic agent.

Mutagenic: Capable of causing alterations/damage to genes.

Carcinogenic: Capable of causing cancer.

Teratogenic: Capable of causing fetal defects, either anatomic or functional.

Classification of Cytotoxic Drugs

- Cell cycle specific
- Non-cell cycle specific.

Complications of Unsafe Administration of Cytotoxic Drugs

Chemotherapy drugs are divided into several categories based on how they affect specific chemical substances within cancer cells (Table 5.18).

Table 5.18: Different categories of cytotoxic drugs

Vesicants	Irritants	Non-vesicants
Associated with severe local necrosis	May be associated with local necrosis	Uncommonly associated with local necrosis
Amsacrine	Carboplatin	L-asparaginase
Carmustine (BCNU)	Cisplatin	Bleomycin
Dactinomycin	Dacarbazine (DTIC)	Cyclophosphamide
Daunorubicin	Etoposide	Cytarabine
Doxorubicin	Methotrexate	Ifosfamide
Epirubicin	Mitozantrone	Mephalan
Idarubicin	Teniposide	Thiotepa
Vincristin		
Vinblastine		

Types of Drugs

Vesicants: Drugs, which are capable of causing pain, inflammation and blistering of the local skin, underlying flesh and structures, leading to tissue death and necrosis.

Exfoliants: Drugs, which are capable of causing inflammation and shedding of the skin, but less likely to cause tissue death.

Irritants: Drugs, which are capable of causing inflammation, irritation or pain at site of extravasation, but rarely cause tissue breakdown.

Inflammitants: Drugs, which are capable of causing mild to moderate inflammation and flare in local tissues.

Neutrals: Inert or neutral compounds that do not cause inflammation or damage.

Hazardous Cytotoxic Drugs

Drugs that meet one or more of the following criteria should be handled as hazardous:
- Carcinogenicity
- Teratogenicity or developmental toxicity
- Reproductive toxicity
- Organ toxicity at low doses
- Genotoxicity
- Structure or toxicity similar to drugs classified as hazardous using the above criteria.

Routes of Exposure

- Inhalation of aerosolized drug
- Dermal absorption
- Ingestion
- Injection
- Intrathecal.

Responsibilities of Healthcare Worker

- Participating in training before handling hazardous drugs and updating knowledge based on new information
- Referring to guidance documents and hospital policy as necessary for information regarding hazardous drugs
- Pregnant staff or those who are expecting to become pregnant should not handle cytotoxic drugs (Table 5.19)

Table 5.19: Phases of pregnancy and the effects of biohazards

Phase	Duration	Effect
Embryogenesis	Day 0–14	Repair or spontaneous abortion
Organogenesis	Day 15–84	Spontaneous abortion or irreparable malformation
Fetal development	Day 85 to birth	Functional defects

- Utilizing biological safety cabinets (BSCs) in drug preparation or laminar hood
- Follow universal precaution
- Washing hands after drug handling activities
- Disposing of materials contaminated with hazardous drugs separately from other waste in designated containers (black cover)
- Cleaning up hazardous drug spills immediately according to recommended procedures

- Follow institutional procedures for reporting and following up on accidental exposure to hazardous drugs (Table 5.20).

Table 5.20: Guidelines to be followed in the accidental exposure to hazardous drugs

Type of exposure	Immediate care
Skin exposure	Remove contaminated clothing and/or personal protective equipment (PPE) Wash affected area thoroughly with soap and water
Eye exposure	Flush eye(s) with water/isotonic eye wash for 15 minutes; do not rub the eyes
Exposure by inhalation or ingestion	Acute symptoms may require emergency intervention

Section
2

Advanced and Other Nursing Procedures

- ❑ Advanced Nursing Procedures
- ❑ Assisting Procedures
- ❑ Infection Control Procedures

Advanced Nursing Procedures

INTRAVENOUS CANNULATION

Definition

Intravenous (IV) cannulation is the procedure, where the insertion of a cannula into vessels for the purposes of administration of medication and IV fluids, etc.

Purposes

- For fluid and electrolyte replacement
- To administer the medicines
- To administer the blood/blood products
- To administer the total parenteral nutrition
- To assess the hemodynamic levels
- To collect the blood sampling.

Equipments

- Appropriate size of IV cannula
- Alcohol wipe
- A 2 mL syringe
- A 25 G needle
- A 5 mL ampule of 1% lignocaine solution
- Adhesive dressing for fixation of cannula
- Tourniquet
- Sharps container
- Gloves
- Isopropyl alcohol 70% solution (hand rub solution).

Procedure

Procedure for IV cannulation is provided in Table 6.1.

Table 6.1: Nursing intervention and rationale for intravenous cannulation

SI No	Care action	Rationale
1.	Explain the procedure to the patient	To obtain the consent from patient
2.	Assess the condition of the patient	To determine reason for intravenous (IV) cannulation

Contd...

Contd...

Sl No	Care action	Rationale
3.	Position the patient with the arm extended to form a straight line from shoulder to wrist	Easy to perform the procedure and make the patient comfortable
4.	Provide privacy to the patient	To make the patient feel comfortable
5.	Wash the hands with soap and water	To minimize the infection
6.	Select the appropriate vein for IV cannulation; it should be straight and more prominent, e.g. the vein in the forearm or dorsum of the hand	Easy to access the line and to prevent the complication
7.	Palpate the vessel; apply a tourniquet 7–10 cm above site gently and it should not be too tight	To prevent the blood obstruction
8.	Put on gloves and clean skin (selected site) with alcohol wipe	To minimize and prevent the entry of the microorganism
9.	Infiltrate skin over proposed puncture site with 1% lignocaine solution (if the doctor prescribed)	To give anesthetic effect to the patient
10.	Hold patient's hand with your non-dominant hand, using your thumb to keep skin taut and anchor vein	To prevent the rolling of the hand
11.	Remove the protective sleeve from the needle taking care not to touch it at any time	To minimize the contamination
12.	Hold the cannula in your dominant hand, stretch the skin over the vein to anchor the vein with your non-dominant hand (do not repalpate the vein)	To prevent the rolling of the vein and to prevent the contamination
13.	The needle is inserted bevel up; the initial angle of entry should be approximately 15°–30°	Easy to capture and prick the vein correctly
14.	Observe for blood in the flashback chamber	Successful entry into the vessel is indicated by return of blood into the flash chamber
15.	Lower the cannula slightly to ensure the enters of lumen in the vessels and does not	To prevent the puncture of exterior wall of the vessel
16.	Gently advance the cannula over the needle whilst withdrawing the guide, noting secondary flashback along the cannula	To prevent the damage of the vein
17.	Release the tourniquet and apply gentle pressure over the vein (beyond the cannula tip) remove the white cap from the needle	To prevent bleeding
18.	Remove the needle from the cannula; attach the white lock cap and dispose of it into a sharps container	Needle is used only for introducing the cannula into the vein White lock cap prevents leakage of blood from cannula
19.	Secure the cannula with an appropriate dressing and flush the cannula with 2–5 mL of 0.9% sodium chloride or attach an IV giving set and fluid	To prevent the clot
20.	Document the procedure in the nurses record	To provide a point of reference or comparison in the event of later queries

> **Points to Note**
>
> ✦ Do not attempt a venipuncture more than twice. Notify your supervisor or patient's physician if unsuccessful.

INTRAVENOUS INFUSION

Definition

Intravenous infusion is a process that gives insertion of IV catheter for IV therapy.

Purposes

- To give nutrient instead of oral route
- To provide medication by vein continuously.

Equipments

- Prescribed IV solution
- Intravenous infusion set/IV tubing: 1
- Intravenous catheter or butterfly needle in appropriate size: 1
- Spirit swabs
- Adhesive tape
- Disposable gloves, if available: 1
- Intravenous stand: 1
- Arm board, if needed, especially for infant
- Steel tray: 1
- Kidney tray: 1.

Procedure

Procedure for starting an IV infusion is detailed in Table 6.2.

Table 6.2: Procedure for starting an intravenous infusion

Sl No	Care action	Rationale
1.	Assemble all equipments and bring to bedside	To save the time and do the procedure easily
2.	Check intravenous (IV) solution and medication additives with doctor's order	To prevent medication error
3.	Explain procedure to the client	To obtain consent from the patient
4.	Perform hand hygiene	To prevent cross infection
5.	Prepare IV solution and tubing: • Maintain aseptic technique when opening sterile packages and IV solution • Clamp tubing, uncap spike and insert into entry site on bag as manufacturer directs	This prevents spread of microorganisms This punctures the seal in the IV bag Suction effects cause to move into drip chamber also prevents air from moving down the tubing

Contd...

Contd...

SI No	Care action	Rationale
	• Squeeze drip chamber and allow it to fill at least one third to halfway • Remove cap at end of tubing, release clamp, allow fluid to move through tubing; allow fluid to flow until all air bubbles have disappeared • Close clamp and recap end of tubing, maintaining sterility of set up • If an electric device is to be used, follow manufacturer's instructions for inserting tubing and setting infusion rate • Apply label if medication was added to container • Place timetape (or adhesive tape) on container as necessary and hang on IV stand	This removes air from tubing in larger amounts that can act as an air embolus To maintain sterility This ensures correct flow rate and proper use of equipment This provides for administration of correct solution with prescribed medication or additive Pharmacy may have added medication and applied label This permits immediate evaluation of IV according to schedule
6.	Preparation the position: • Have the client in supine position or comfortable position in bed • Place protective pad under the client's arm	Mostly the supine position permits either arm to be used and allows for good body alignment
7.	Selection the site for venipuncture: • Select an appropriate site and palpate accessible veins • Apply a tourniquet 5–6 inches above the venipuncture site to obstruct venous blood flow and distend the vein • Direct the ends of the tourniquet away from the site of injection • Check to be sure that the radial pulse is still present	The selection of an appropriate site decreases discomfort for the client and possible damage to body tissues Interrupting the blood flow to the heart causes the vein to distend Distended veins are easy to see The end of the tourniquet could contaminate the area of injection, if directed toward the site of injection Too much tight the arm makes the client discomfort Interruption of the arterial flow impedes venous filling

8.	Palpation the vein
	• Ask the client to open and close the fist
	• Observe and palpate for a suitable vein
	• If a vein cannot be felt and seen, do the following:
	   – Release the tourniquet and have the client lower his/her arm below the level of the heart to fill the veins; reapply tourniquet and gently over the intended vein to help distend it
	   – Tap the vein gently
	   – Remove tourniquet and place warm, moist compress over the intended vein for 10–15 minutes
		Contraction of the muscle of the forearm forces blood into the veins, thereby distending them further
		To reduce several puncturing
		Lowering the arm below the level of the heart, tapping the vein and applying warmth help distend veins by filling them with blood

9.	Put on clean gloves, if available	Care must be used when handling any blood or body fluids to prevent transmission of human immunodeficiency virus (HIV) and other blood-borne infectious disease

Contd...

Contd...

Sl No	Care action	Rationale
10.	Cleanse the entry site with an antiseptic solution (such as spirit) according to hospital policy: • Use a circular motion to move from the center to outward for several inches • Use several motions with same direction as from the upward to the downward around injection site, approximate 5–6 inches	Cleansing that begins at the site of entry and moves outward in a circular motion carries organisms away from the site of entry Organisms on the skin can be introduced into the tissues or bloodstream with the needle
11.	Holding the arm with non-dominant hand: • Place an non-dominant hand about 1 or 2 inches below entry site to hold the skin taut against the vein • Place an non-dominant hand to support the forearm from the backside *Nursing alert:* Avoid touching the prepared site	Pressure on the vein and surrounding tissues helps prevent movement of the vein as the needle or catheter is being inserted The needle entry site and catheter must remain free of contamination from unsterile hands
12.	Puncturing the vein and withdrawing blood: • Enter the skin gently with the catheter held by the hub in the dominant hand, bevel side up, at a 15°–30° angle • The catheter may be inserted from directly over the vein or the side of the vein • While following the course of the vein, advance the needle or catheter into the vein • A sensation can be felt when the needle enters the vein • When the blood returns through the lumen of the needle or the flashback chamber of the catheter, advance either device 1/8–1/4 inch further into the vein • A catheter needs to be advanced until hub is at the venipuncture site	This technique allows needle or catheter to enter the vein with minimum trauma and deters passage of the needle through the vein The tourniquet causes increased venous pressure resulting in automatic backflow Having the catheter placed well into the vein helps to prevent dislodgement
13.	Connecting to the tube and stabilizing the catheter on the skin: • Release the tourniquet • Quickly remove protective cap from the IV tubing • Attach the tubing to the catheter or needle • Stabilize the catheter or needle with non-dominant hand	The catheter, which immediately is connected to the tube, causes minimum bleeding and patency of the vein is maintained
14.	Starting flow: • Release the clamp on the tubing • Start flow of solution promptly • Examine the drip of solution and the issue around the entry site for sign of infiltration	Blood clots readily if IV flow is not maintained If catheter accidentally slips out of vein, solution will accumulate and infiltrate into surrounding tissue
15.	Fasten the catheter and applying the dressing: • Secure the catheter with narrow non-allergenic tape	Non-allergenic tape is less likely to tear fragile skin

Contd...

Contd...

Sl No	Care action	Rationale
	• Place strictly sided-up under the hub and crossed over the top of the hub • Loop the tubing near the site of entry	The weight of tubing is enough to pull it out of the vein if it is not well anchored There are various ways to anchor the hub You should follow agency/hospital policy To prevent the catheter from removing accidentally
16.	Bring back all equipments and dispose in proper manner	To prepare for the next procedure
17.	Remove gloves and perform hand hygiene	To prevent the spread of infection
18.	If necessary, anchor arm to an arm board for support	An arm board helps to prevent change in the position of the catheter in the vein Site protectors also will be used to protect the IV site
19.	Adjust the rate of IV solution flow according to doctor's order	Doctor prescribed the rate of flow or the amount of solution in day as required to the client's condition Some medications are given very less amount Doctor may use infusion pump to maintain the flow rate
20.	Document the procedure including the time, site, catheter size and the client's response	This ensures continuity of care
21.	Return to check the flow rate and observe for infiltration	To find any abnormalities immediately

Nursing Alert

Nurse should have special consideration for the elderly and infant:

1. To older adults: Avoid vigorous friction at the insertion site and using too much alcohol.

   Rationale: Both can traumatize fragile skin and veins in the elderly.

2. To infant and children: Hand insertion sites should not be the first choice for children.

   Rationale: Nerve endings are more very close to the surface of the skin and it is more painful.

URINARY CATHETERIZATION

Definition

Urinary catheterization or Foley catheterization commonly referred to be an invasive procedure. It involves introducing a plastic or rubber tube into the urethra then advancing the tube into the bladder. Once in the bladder, the catheter provides for a continuous flow of urine.

Indications

Intermittent Catheterization

1. Collection of sterile urine sample.
2. Provide relief from discomfort of bladder distention.
3. Decompression of the bladder.
4. Measure residual urine.
5. Management of patients with spinal cord injury, neuromuscular degeneration or incompetent bladders.

Short-term Indwelling Catheterization

1. Postsurgery and in critically ill patients to monitor urinary output.
2. Surgical procedures involving pelvic or abdominal surgery repair of the bladder, urethra and surrounding structures.
3. Urinary obstruction (e.g. enlarged prostate), acute urinary retention.
4. Prevention of urethral obstruction from blood clots with continuous or intermittent bladder irrigations.
5. Instillation of medication into the bladder.

Long-term Indwelling Catheterization

1. Refractory bladder outlet obstruction and neurogenic bladder with urinary retention.
2. Prolonged and chronic urinary retention.
3. To promote healing of perineal ulcers, where urine may cause further skin breakdown.

Equipments

- Sterile catheterization pack
- Underpad or mackintosh
- Sterile gloves
- Appropriate size of urinary catheters
- Anesthetic lubricating jelly
- Sodium chloride (0.9%) or water for injection
- Adhesive plaster
- Syringe and needle
- Disposable plastic apron
- Sterile drainage bag set.

Procedure

Procedure to set urinary catheterization in females and males is detailed in Tables 6.3 and 6.4.

Table 6.3: Procedure of urinary catheterization in female

Sl No	Care action	Rationale
1.	Explain the procedure to the patient	To obtain the consent from patient
2.	Assess the condition of the patient	To determine reason for catheterization
3.	Collect the history from the patient whether she has any latex allergy	To ensure no latex/coated latex products are used
4.	Provide privacy to the patient	To make the patient feel comfortable
5.	Do not expose the patient and assist into supine position with legs extended and cover patient's genital area	To maintain patient's dignity and comfort
6.	Prior to commencement for procedure, if applicable ensure patient has washed genital area using soap and water and assist, if necessary, wearing non-sterile gloves	To reduce presence of bacteria
7.	Arrange needed equipment near the bedside	To avoid the unnecessary contamination as well as easy to perform the procedure
8.	Place the mackintosh or underpad under the patient's buttocks	To prevent the soiling of the linen
9.	Wash hands using bactericidal soap and water or bactericidal alcohol hand rub	To decrease the risk of infection
10.	Wear sterile gloves (both pairs)	To reduce risk of cross infection
11.	Place sterile towels in patient's thighs and under buttocks in transversely and expose genital area	To create a secondary sterile field
12.	With thumb and one finger of your non-dominant hand, spread labia and identify meatus; be prepared to maintain separation of labia with one hand until urine is flowing well and continuously	Easy to identify and clean the meatus and insert the catheter
13.	Using cotton balls held with forceps, clean around the urethral orifice with 0.9% sodium chloride or an antiseptic solution by using single downward stokes	To reduce the cross-contamination
14.	Instil (3–6 mL) anesthetic gel into urethral meatus; allow sufficient time for 5 minutes (time for anesthetic gel to take effect)	Sufficient lubrication helps to prevent urethral trauma; use of a local anesthetic reduce the discomfort experienced by the patient
15.	Pick up sterile catheter with dominant hand, holding it by its inner wrapper and expose tip of catheter, the remaining length should lie in the container, which should be placed between the patients legs	To maintain sterility
16.	Gently insert the catheter into the meatus and pass along the urethra until urine flows	While inserting the catheter ensures that the balloon is positioned correctly in the bladder
17.	Inflate the balloon with sterile according to the manufacture's direction and ensured that the catheter is draining properly before hand; attach	To prevent urethral trauma

Contd...

Contd...

SI No	Care action	Rationale
	the catheter to the drainage system and tie the bag below and secure the catheter to the thigh	
18.	Make the patient comfortable; ensure the area is dry	To prevent infection and skin irritation
19.	Measure the amount of urine and record drainage	To assess the bladder capacity or to monitor renal capacity/fluid balance It is not necessary to measure the amount of urine if the patient is having routine catheter drainage
20.	Dispose all the used items as per institutional policy	To ensure a safe disposal of biomedical waste
21.	Record the procedure in nurse's record	To be aware of continuity of patient care

Table 6.4: Procedure of urinary catheterization in male

SI No	Care action	Rationale
1.	Explain the procedure to the patient	To obtain the consent from patient
2.	Assess the condition of the patient	To determine reason for catheterization
3.	Collect the history from the patient whether he has any latex allergy	To ensure no latex/coated latex products are used
4.	Provide privacy to the patient	To make the patient feel comfortable
5.	Do not expose the patient and assist into supine position with legs extended and cover patient's genital area	To maintain patient's dignity and comfort
6.	Prior to commencement for procedure, if applicable ensure patient has washed genital area using soap and water and assist, if necessary, wearing non-sterile gloves	To reduce presence of bacteria
7.	Arrange needed equipment near the bedside	To avoid the unnecessary contamination as well as easy to perform the procedure
8.	Place the mackintosh or underpad under the patient's buttocks	To prevent the soiling of the linen
9.	Wash hands using bactericidal soap and water or bactericidal alcohol hand rub	To decrease the risk of infection
10.	Wear sterile gloves (both pairs)	To reduce risk of cross infection
11.	If patient is uncircumcised, it will be necessary to retract the prepuce with non-dominant hand, holding penis with a gauze swab; clean penis with sterile normal saline 0.9% or antiseptic solution with dominant hand	To reduce risk of introducing infection to the urinary tract during the procedure
12.	Instil 11 mL of anesthetic gel into urethral meatus, still holding penis with non-dominant hand gently compress penis behind glans to retain gel and massage gel along urethra; allow 5 minutes for anesthetic gel to take effect	Adequate lubrication helps to prevent urethral trauma Use of a local anesthetic minimizes the discomfort experienced by the patient
13.	Pick up sterile catheter with dominant hand, holding it by its inner wrapper and expose tip of catheter, the remaining	To maintain sterility

Contd...

Contd...

SI No	Care action	Rationale
	length should lie in the container, which should be placed between the patient's legs	
14.	Pick up catheter by holding inner wrapper and expose tip of catheter 1–2 inches (5 cm)	To prevent introduction of infection
15.	Holding penis at angle of 60°–90° to body, gently insert catheter into meatus and pass along urethra maintaining gentle pressure	To get the cooperation and reduce the anxiety
16.	Advance the catheter 6–8 cm and inflate the balloon according to the manufacturer's directions, having ensured that the catheter is draining adequately	Involuntary inflation of the balloon within the urethra is painful and causes urethral trauma
17.	Make the patient comfortable and ensure that the area is dry	If the area is left wet or moist, secondary infection and skin irritation may occur
18.	Record the procedure in details in the nurse's record	To provide a point of reference or comparison in the event of later queries

Points to Note

♦ While inserting the urinary catheter for male patients, if resistance is encountered getting the patient to cough may reduce spasm on the external sphincter and ease the passage of the catheter. Force should not be used and medical advice should be sought if further resistance is felt.

CARE OF URINARY CATHETER

Definition

Catheter care is the sterile procedure, where cleaning of the urinary catheter and perineal area by using the antiseptic solution. A Foley catheter is a tube that is put into the bladder to drain urine out of the body. A Foley catheter can stay in the bladder for hours or weeks.

Purposes

• To prevent infection
• To provide comfort
• To assess the placement of the catheter.

Equipments

A tray containing:
• A sterile dressing tray (thumb forceps and artery forceps, a bowel with sterile gauze and cotton)
• Mackintosh
• A pair of sterile gloves
• Micropore (adhesive tape)
• Mask
• Scissors.

Procedure

Urinary catheter care procedure is given in Table 6.5.

Table 6.5: Procedure of urinary catheter care

Sl No	Care action	Rationale
1.	Explain the procedure to the patient	To get the cooperation and reduce the anxiety
2.	Gather all the equipment, which needed for the catheter care	To save the time and do the procedure easily
3.	Provide privacy	To create the patient comfortable sense and treat patient with self-esteem
4.	Wash hands thoroughly	To minimize risk of cross infection
5.	Place the patient in lying down position	To make the comfortable and ease to perform the work
6.	Place the mackintosh under the perineal region	To prevent soiling of the sheets
7.	Wear mask and sterile gloves	To prevent the infection
8.	Clean the skin near the catheter by using wet cotton or gauze, if possible; gently wash around urinary opening with warm water	To minimize the contamination and prevent the infection
9.	Clean the external meatus for males and introitus for female patients with help of artery forceps by using the antiseptic solutions	To prevent the infection
10.	Hold the end of the catheter and clean around the catheter to remove any blood, crust or mucus; avoid the pulling of catheter	To prevent injury and traction of the tubing
11.	Cover the junction of the penis and the catheter by using sterile gauze, which is soaked with antiseptic solutions	To prevent the infection
12.	Tape the catheter by using the adhesive tape; make sure there is enough tubing left, so the catheter will not be pulled when patient moves his/her leg: • For women tape the catheter to the upper or lateral part of thighs • For men tape the catheter to the lower abdomen, so the catheter does not pull the penis downward	To prevent injury and traction of the tubing
13.	Remove the mackintosh and place the patient as they desire	To feel the comfortable
14.	Replace articles and wash hands	To arrange and keep it ready for next use and minimize risk of cross infection
15.	Document procedure in the nurse's record, if there is any foul smelling discharge or any other abnormalities inform to the concerned doctor	Help to identify the infection in early stage

Points to Note

Clean the skin around the catheter everyday and after every bowel movement:
• For females, always wash from their front to the back.
• For males, always wash from the tip of the penis to down.

BLADDER IRRIGATION

Definition

Bladder irrigation is the procedure in which instillation of a solution into the bladder to provide cleansing or to medication.

Purposes

1. To maintain patency of the retention catheter by removing bladder sediment or blood clots.
2. To instill medications/fluids as ordered.
3. To clean the bladder and maintain the patency of the urinary catheter.
4. To relieve congestion, swelling and pain in the bladder.
5. To arrest hemorrhage and to prevent clot formation after surgery.
6. To prepare the patient for bladder surgeries.
7. To promote healing.

Equipments

- Catheterization set
- Dressing pack
- Pair of sterile gloves
- Irrigation solution
- Asepto syringe
- Double lumen Foley catheter with drainage tubing bag
- Three-way adaptor
- Alcohol swab
- Antiseptic solution
- Kidney tray
- Mackintosh/Underpad
- Adhesive plaster and scissors.

Procedure

Procedure for bladder irrigation is detailed in Table 6.6.

Table 6.6: Procedure for bladder irrigation

Sl No	Care action	Rationale
Closed method		
1.	Explain the procedure to the patient	Explanations make easy to get cooperation and provide comfort for the patient
2.	Arrange all the articles and keep near the patient's bedside	To minimize the unnecessary consultation
3.	Provide privacy for the patient	To feel comfortable

Contd...

Contd...

SI No	Care action	Rationale
4.	Check the physician's order before administering the solution	To know the type and amount of solution to be used
5.	Place the mackintosh/underpad under the patient buttocks	To prevent the soiling of the linen
6.	Position the patient in modified dorsal recumbent position	Easy to perform the position
7.	Drape the patient well	To make the patient comfortable
8.	Wash hands	To prevent the spread of infection
9.	Open the bladder irrigation set and keep additional dressing materials and pour the solution required	To carry out the procedure in an easy way
10.	Wear sterile gloves	To maintain the sterile environment while doing the procedure
11.	Follow the sterile catheterization procedure to insert the catheter	To prevent the infection
12.	If the patient is on urinary catheter, detach the uro sac or uro bag and cover the tip with sterile gauze pieces	To prevent the entry of the microorganisms
13.	Load the bladder wash syringe with solution prescribed and expel the air, attach the tip of the syringe into the catheter	To prevent positive pressure within the asepto syringe
14.	Install the solution slowly into the bladder usually not more than, 80–100 cc at a time	To prevent trauma to the bladder mucosa
15.	Remove the syringe and allow the urine to drain into the kidney tray	
16.	Repeat installing and emptying till the return flow is clean	To ensure proper removal of the block
17.	Connect the catheter to the uro sac and measure the return flow	To drain the urine continuously and follow-up care
18.	Remove the mackintosh and make the patient to lie down comfortably	To make the patient feel comfortable
19.	Remove the gloves; wash all the articles and replace properly	To prevent the cross-contamination and make the articles ready for further usage
20.	Document the procedure in the nurse's record	To assess the condition of the patient and perform the continuity of care
Continuous method		
1.	Prepare the bladder irrigation solution as prepared for intravenous (IV) infusion, hang the solution bottle on irrigation stand at a height of about 6–8 inches above the level of meatus and allow expelling air from the irrigating set	It helps to increase the flow rate of solution Expelling air in the irrigating set prevents air embolism

Contd...

Contd...

Sl No	Care action	Rationale
2.	Place the mackintosh under the patient buttocks	To prevent the soiling of the linen
3.	Place the patient in dorsal recumbent position	To perform the procedure in an easy way
4.	Clean the catheter and uro bag junction with alcohol swab	To minimize the entry of microorganisms
5.	Wear gloves	To prevent the contamination
6.	Connect the tubing to the 3-way urinary catheter and allow about 500–800 mL of fluid at a time	To ensure that proper amount of solution flows into the bladder to wash out the bladder completely
7.	Do not clamp the irrigation tubing	To allow the free flow of fluids
8.	Assess the color of the return flow and measure the return flow for each 500 mL bottle	To assess for any abnormalities
9.	Continue irrigation till the return flow is clear	To ensure proper removal of the block from the bladder
10.	If the patient is post-transurethral resection of the prostate (TURP), the procedure is continued for 24 hours	To wash out the blood clot from the bladder
11.	Remove the mackintosh	To make the patient comfortable
12.	Remove the glove and wash hands	To prevent the cross-contamination
13.	Record time, amount and kind of solution used, character of return flow and response of the patient	To identify any abnormalities and report immediately

Points to Note

+ For continuous irrigation: Unclamp the irrigating tube and adjust the flow rate similar to an IV infusion. The solution along with urine will continuously flow out of catheter into the drainage bag.
+ For intermittent irrigation: Clamp the drainage tubing and unclamp the irrigating tube, adjust the flow rate and allow a specified amount of solution to flow.

EAR IRRIGATION

Definition

The ear irrigation is the procedure to remove the discharge of the ear canal, to soften and remove impacted cerumen or to dislodge a foreign object.

Purposes

- To relieve congestion, inflammation and pain in the ear
- To administer antiseptics
- To remove foreign bodies, earwax or discharges
- To evaluate the vestibular functions.

Equipments

A tray containing the following articles:
- Prescribed irrigating solution warmed to 37°C (98.6°F)
- Irrigation set (container and irrigating or bulb syringe)
- Basin
- Cotton-tipped applicator and cotton balls
- Mackintosh or underpad
- Kidney tray
- Otoscope, if needed.

Procedure

Procedure for ear irrigation is given in Table 6.7.

Table 6.7: Procedure for ear irrigation

Sl No	Care action	Rationale
1.	Explain the procedure to the patient	Explanations make easy to get cooperation and provide comfort for the patient
2.	Arrange and keep the needed articles near the patient bedside	For the planned approach to the work
3.	Provide privacy	To reduces unease of the patient
4.	Wash your hands	To prevent the spread of microorganisms
5.	Spread the mackintosh/underpads under the patient	To protect the linen soiling
6.	Make the patient sit up or lie with the head tilted toward the side of the affected ear and support a basin under the ear to receive the irrigating solution	Gravity causes the irrigating solution to flow from the ear to the basin
7.	Wear the sterile gloves	To keep up sterile technique while doing the procedure
8.	Clean the pinna and the meatus at the auditory canal, as necessary, with the normal saline or the irrigating solution	Materials lodged on the pinna and the meatus may be washed into the ear
9.	Fill the bulb syringe with solution, if an irrigating container is used, check for air bubbles	Air forced into the ear canal is noisy and therefore unpleasant for the patient
10.	Straightening the auditory canal by pulling the pinna down and back for an infant and up and back for an adult patient	Straightening the ear canal aids in allowing solution to reach all areas of the ears easily
11.	Direct a steady, slow stream of solution against the roof of the auditory canal, using only sufficient force to remove secretions; do not occlude the auditory canal with the irrigating nozzle and allow solution to flow out unimpeded	Solution directed at the roof of the canal aids in preventing injury to the tympanic membrane; continuous in- and out-flow of the irrigating solution helps prevent pressure in the canal
12.	Continue to irrigate till the ear is clear of discharge	To ensure that ear is cleaned completely
13.	Dry the ear with sterile cotton applicator	To ensure clean and dry surface

Contd...

Contd...

Sl No	Care action	Rationale
14.	Remove all wet mackintosh/underpad from the patient side	To make the patient comfortable
15.	When the irrigation is completed, place a dry cotton ball loosely in the auditory meatus and have the patient lie on the side of the affected ear on a an towel/underpad	The cotton ball absorbs excess fluid; gravity allows the remaining solution in the canal to escape from the ear
16.	Wash your hands; clean and replace the articles	Keep it ready for next use and to deters the spread of microorganisms
17.	Document the irrigation, the appearance of the drainage and the patient's response	To provide accurate documentation and help to provide follow-up care for the patient

Points to Note

- Avoid dropping or squirting on the eardrum.
- Never use more than 500 mL of solution.
- If the tympanic membrane is ruptured, check with the doctor before irrigation.
- Monitor temperature of solution carefully.
- Forceful instillation of the solution can rupture the tympanic membrane.
- If pain or dizziness occurs, stop the procedure.
- If irrigation is done to dislodge the wax, it is better to soften it by putting soda glycerin or hydrogen peroxide 3–4 days prior to the procedure.
- If syringe is used for irrigation, do not use a large syringe as it is difficult to control and may exert undue pressure in forcing the fluid into the auditory canal.

EYE IRRIGATION

Definition

Eye irrigation is the procedure, where to flush eye(s) with solution to remove secretion and foreign bodies or to dilute chemicals.

Purposes

- Remove secretions from the conjunctival site
- Irrigate following the instillation of certain diagnostic drugs
- To relieve congestion, inflammation and pain in the eye
- To administer medications
- To remove foreign bodies, chemicals or discharge
- To prepare the patient for eye surgery.

Equipments

A tray containing the following articles:
- Sterile irrigating solution warmed to 37°C (98.6°F)
- Disposable gloves

- Sterile irrigating set (sterile container and irrigating or bulb syringe)
- Basin or irrigation basin
- Disposable syringe
- Solution container
- Cotton swabs
- Gauze pieces
- Warm sterile solution in a sterile jug
- Eye medicine, if needed
- Towel
- Kidney tray.

Procedure

The procedure of eye irrigation is detailed in the Table 6.8.

Table 6.8: Procedure for eye irrigation

SI No	Care action	Rationale
1.	Explain the procedure to the patient	Explanations make easy to get cooperation and provide comfort for the patient
2.	Arrange and keep the needed articles near the patient bedside	For a planned approach to the work
3.	Provide privacy	To reduces unease of the patient
4.	Wash your hands	To prevent the spread of microorganisms
5.	Spread the mackintosh/underpads under the patient	To protect the linen soiling
6.	Make the patient sit or lie with the head tilted toward the side of the affected eye; protect the patient and the bed with waterproof pad	Gravity will aid the flow of solution away from the unaffected eye and from the inner canthus of the affected eye toward the outer canthus
7.	Wear disposable gloves, clean the lids and the lashes with a cotton ball moistened with normal saline or the solution ordered for the irrigation; wipe from the inner canthus to the outer canthus and discard the cotton ball after each wipe	Materials lodged on the lids or in the lashes may be washed into the eye This cleansing motion protects the nasolacrimal duct and the other eye
8.	Place the curved basin at the cheek on the side of the affected eye to receive the irrigating solution; if sitting up, ask the patient to support the basin	Gravity will aid the flow of solution
9.	Expose the lower conjunctival sac and hold the upper lid open with your non-dominant hand	The solution is directed on to the lower conjunctival sac because the cornea is very sensitive and easily injured This also prevents reflex blinking
10.	Hold the irrigator about 2.5 cm (1 inch) from the eye; direct the flow of the solution from the inner canthus to the outer canthus along the conjunctival sac	This minimizes the risk of injury to the cornea; solution directed toward the outer canthus helps prevent the spread of contamination from the eye to the lacrimal sac, the lacrimal duct and the nose

Contd...

Contd...

SI No	Care action	Rationale
11.	Irrigate until the solution is clear or all the solution has been used; use only sufficient force gently to remove secretions from the conjunctiva; avoid touching any part of the eye with the irrigating tip	Directing solutions with force may cause injury to the tissues of the eyes as well as to the conjunctiva Touching the eye is uncomfortable for the patient
12.	Make the patient close the eye periodically during the procedure	It helps to move secretions from the upper conjunctival sac to the lower
13.	Dry the area after the irrigation with cotton balls or a gauze sponge; offer a towel to the patient if the face and neck are wet	Leaving the skin moist after irrigation is uncomfortable for the patient
14.	Wash the hands, clean and replace the equipments	To prevent the risk of cross infection and make it ready for next usage
15.	Document the irrigation, the appearance of the eye, drainage and the patient's response	To provide accurate documentation and to provide follow-up care for the patient

> **Points to Note**
>
> + When irrigating both eyes, have the patient tilt his/her head toward the side being irrigated to avoid cross-contamination.
> + For chemical burns, irrigate each eye with at least 1,000 mL of normal saline solutions.
> + In case of chemical burn, irrigation could last 10–15 minutes.

ENDOTRACHEAL/TRACHEAL SUCTIONING

Definition

Oropharyngeal, tracheal and endotracheal suction are methods of clearing secretions by the application of negative pressure via either a Yankauer sucker (oropharyngeal) or an appropriately sized tracheal suction catheter (tracheal/endotracheal).

Indications

- To remove thick mucus secretions from the trachea and lower respiratory tract
- Maintain a patent airway to ensure adequate oxygenation and ventilation
- To prevent or treat pulmonary infection
- To prevent hypoxia.

Equipments

- Appropriate size of suction catheters
- Sterile water for rinsing catheter
- Normal saline (0.9%)
- Suction apparatus (portable or wall suction) with tubing

- A pair of sterile gloves
- Kidney tray
- Disposable face mask
- Goggles
- Clean gloves
- Disposable apron
- Syringe to instill normal saline.

Procedure

Endotracheal/Tracheal suctioning is given in Table 6.9.

Table 6.9: Procedure for endotracheal/tracheal suctioning

Sl No	Care action	Rationale
1.	Confirm the patient's identity, explain the procedure	To identify the patient correctly and gain informed consent
2.	Assess the patient to ensure that suction is necessary (including the effectiveness of their cough)	To reduce potential complications from endotracheal suction and avoid unnecessary interventions
3.	Collect the needed equipments on a trolley and take to the bedside	Easy to perform the procedure
4.	Assist the patient into an upright position (if possible)	To allow optimum lung expansion and effective cough
5.	Check the saturation level (SpO_2) of the patient by using pulse oximeter	To enable evaluation of patient's oxygenation prior to and following the suction procedure to prevent the complication
6.	Wash hands	To reduce the risk of cross infection
7.	Put on disposable apron and protective visor/eyewear, according to institutional policy	To reduce risk of cross infection and to protect yourself from droplets/sputum contamination
8.	Connect suction catheter to suction tubing and turn suction machine on	To allow suction to begin
9.	Use sterile/clean glove	To reduce risk of cross infection
10.	Withdraw suction catheter from sleeve with clean gloved hand and grasp catheter with sterile/clean gloved hand away from catheter tip	To reduce risk of cross infection
11.	Advance catheter gently until a cough is stimulated or resistance is felt; do not apply suction during catheter insertion	To minimize risk of mucosal trauma
12.	When a cough is initiated or resistance is felt, withdraw the catheter approximately 1 cm and apply suction by occluding suction control port on catheter with thumb; withdraw gently and procedure should last not more than 15 seconds	To reduce potential complications from suctioning

Contd...

Contd...

SI No	Care action	Rationale
13.	Rinse the suction tubing by dipping its end into the sterile water bottle and applying suction until the solution has rinsed the tubing through	To ensure sputum is removed from suction tubing
14.	Dispose of suction catheter and gloves in clinical waste disposable bin, as per institutional policy	To reduce risk of cross infection and ensure clinical waste is correctly disposed of
15.	Clear patient's oral secretions, if required	To maintain patient comfort
16.	Wash hands with soap and water	To reduce the risk of cross infection
17.	Record the procedure in the nurse's record	To assess the continuity of care

PERCUTANEOUS ENDOSCOPIC GASTROSTOMY FEEDING

Definition

Percutaneous endoscopic gastrostomy (PEG) is a procedure for placing a feeding tube directly into the stomach through a small incision in the abdominal wall using an instrument known as an endoscope.

Purposes

1. To provide sufficient nourishment and hydration support to the patient.
2. For therapeutic purposes.
3. Help to drain out the stomach content in case of gastric problem or postoperative, etc.
4. To assess acceptance level of feeds in postoperative patients, who undergone surgery and have nasogastric (NG) tube in situ.

Equipments

Clean tray containing:
- A 50 mL syringe
- Tissue paper
- Towel
- Measuring cup
- A cup of feed
- A cup of water
- Gloves (if needed)
- Disposable feeding bag
- Stethoscope
- Intravenous stand
- Administration set
- Infusion pump.

Procedure

Percutaneous endoscopic gastrostomy feeding and jejunostomy feeding are detailed in Table 6.10.

Table 6.10: Procedure of percutaneous endoscopic gastrostomy and jejunostomy feeding

Sl No	Care action	Rationale
1.	Make clear the procedure to the patient	To get the patient's cooperation and consent
2.	Ensure rate, frequency and formula of the feed as per consultant order	To prevent the overload of the feed and complications
3.	Check the dressing site of the percutaneous endoscopic gastrostomy (PEG) tube for any redness, edema or oozing	Help to identify the infection in early stage
4.	Ensure the patient to lie down in Fowler's position or in supine with 30° of head end elevation	To avoid aspiration
5.	Arrange the entire needed article near the right side of the patient	Easy to perform the procedure
6.	Wash hands with soap and water	To prevent cross infection
7.	Check the tube potion by using the syringe, aspirate the gastric secretion or auscultate over the left upper quadrant with stethoscope and push 10–20 mL of air into the tube using syringe	To ensure the write position of tube that is placed in the stomach
8.	Connect the barrel of the syringe in the PEG tube connector	To make sure the gravity flow of the fluid
9.	Pore the measured amount of feed into the feeding tube, in case of 2-way tube, one way has to be used for feeding and another way for water to flush after the use	To keep the feeding tube clean
10.	In case of bag feed method: • Connect the tube to the bag • Fill the bag with feed • Expel the air in the connecting tube • Hang the bag to intravenous (IV) stand • Raise the bag up to 18 inches above the patient's abdomen • Fix the bag to the infusion pump and set the rate • Connect the proximal end of the tube to the feeding bag • Allow the feed to go off into the stomach	To ensure the proper amount and technique of feeding and to prevent complications
11.	Push measured amount of water into the tube after the feed	To prevent the obstruction of feed in the feeding tube and keep the tube clean
12.	Once the feed is over, wash the feeding bag with warm water	To avoid feed steamy over the bag and to ensure the bag is ready for next use
13.	Make the patient to continue the same Fowler's position for 5–10 minutes	To prevent aspiration
14.	Replace the articles and wash hands	To make it ready for next use and to prevent the contamination
15.	Document the procedure in the nurse's chart in detail and maintain the intake and output chart	To continue the perfect record of the patient

JEJUNOSTOMY FEEDING

Definition

The administration of nutritionally balanced liquefied foods or nutrients through a tube inserted into jejunum.

Purposes

To provide adequate nutrition to the patient, who has undergone gastrointestinal tract bypass surgery.

Equipments

- Clean tray to collect all the things
- Disposable feeding bag
- Stethoscope
- Measured amount of feed
- Intravenous stand
- Administration set
- Infusion pump.

Procedure

For jejunostomy procedure refer Table 6.10.

ADMINISTRATION OF TOTAL PARENTERAL NUTRITION

Definition

Total parenteral nutrition (TPN) is a solution, which contains all the required nutrients including protein, fat, calories, vitamins and minerals is injected over the course of several hours through intravenously into the body. TPN provides a complete and balanced source of nutrients for patients, who cannot consume a normal diet.

Purposes

1. Total parenteral nutrition is the intravenous administration of essential nutrients and is initiated when the gastrointestinal (GI) tract does not provide for adequate ingestion, digestion and absorption.
2. A general indication is anticipation of undernutrition (< 50% of metabolic needs) for more than 7 days.
3. Total parenteral nutrition is given before and after treatment to severely undernourished patients, who cannot ingest large volumes of oral feeding and are being prepared for surgery, radiation therapy or chemotherapy.

Equipments

Clean tray containing:
- Total parenteral nutrition solution
- Administration set or IV set
- Hand care gloves
- Alcohol swab
- Kidney tray.

Procedure

Procedure for administration of total parenteral nutrition is given in Table 6.11.

Table 6.11: Procedure for administration of total parenteral nutrition

SI No	Care action	Rationale
1.	Explain the procedure to the patient	To get the consent and cooperation from the patient
2.	Arrange all the articles to keep in the medicine preparation trolley	To reduce the cross-contamination
3.	Wash hands with soap and water and dry the hands thoroughly	To prevent cross infection
4.	Wear hand care gloves	To prevent the infection
5.	Clean the intravenous (IV) port insertion site with alcohol swab for at least 15 seconds	To prevent bacterial growth and contamination
6.	Insert the sterile IV set into the port and let out the air in the set by flushing the set with the solution	To prevent the growth of bacteria and entry of air in the vein
7.	Label the bag with the started date and time or the drug name, which is added in the fluid	To prevent the continuous usage of total parenteral nutrition (TPN)
8.	Connect TPN to the infusion pump; set the pump on prescribed drops	To make sure the accurate flow rate
9.	Check the patency of IV line or central venous pressure (CVP) line before starting the TPN; using aseptic technique, attach tubing to appropriate IV line	To prevent the complication like extravasations and to prevent the entry of the microorganisms
10.	Start the infusion as per consultant prescription	To avoid the over usage of drugs
11.	Document in medication administration record (MAR)	To maintain an accurate record
12.	Record the procedure clearly in the nurse's notes	To assess the patient condition periodically

Points to Note

- In case of continuous infusion, the total parenteral nutrition solution should be changed every 24 hours.
- Before starting the infusion, the pump should be checked thoroughly to prevent hypo- or hyper-glycemia.
- Sugar level shall be checked every 2nd hourly or as per consultant's order.
- Frequent monitoring of the patient is very essential.

BLOOD TRANSFUSION

Definition

Blood transfusion is the process of transferring blood or blood-based products from one person into the circulatory system of another.

Purposes

- To treat a severe anemia or thrombocytopenia
- To raise the blood pressure
- To treat the critically ill patient like massive blood loss, major surgery, trauma, etc.
- To provide selected cellular components as a replacement therapy (e.g. clotting factors, platelets and albumin).

Equipments

- Appropriate blood administration set
- Intravenous stand
- Infusion pump (if needed)
- Equipment for patient's intravenous access requirements (if necessary)
- Blood pressure (BP) apparatus
- Stethoscope
- Intravenous cannulation tray (if needed).

Procedure

Procedure for blood transfusion is detailed in Table 6.12.

Table 6.12: Procedure for blood transfusion

Sl No	Care action	Rationale
1.	Explain the procedure to the patient/patient relatives	To understand importance of the transfusion and get the valid consent from patient/patient relatives
2.	Check the doctor's order for premedication	To prevent the allergic reaction
3.	Confirm the blood grouping and typing and crossmatching details	To prevent incorrect blood component transfused error
4.	Check the patient vital signs [blood pressure (BP), pulse, respiration, temperature]	Help to identify any abnormal reaction immediately
5.	The blood component should be cross-checked by duty medical officer (DMO)/consultant and nursing supervisor/senior staff nurse	To prevent the administration of outdated/expired blood products
6.	The following details to be checked in the blood component: • Blood group and crossmatch • Donor's name, patient's name	To ensure the safe delivery of blood components

Contd...

Contd...

SI No	Care action	Rationale
	• The date of blood drawn • Date of expiry • Consent is obtained from the duty doctor for verification in the record • Checks for any clots or any other abnormality is present, if found the blood/blood product is return to blood bank	
7.	Intravenous (IV) cannula is checked for the patency before staring the transfusion	To prevent the extravasations
8.	Blood infusion started slowly for first 20 minutes; if no allergic reaction the transfusion can be continued by set up infusion via a volumetric infusion pump, if appropriate	To observe for the allergic reaction and to maintain the accurate transfusion rate
9.	Check and record the patient's temperature, pulse, BP and respiratory rate every 15 minutes during the 1st hour, followed by every 30 minutes till the transfusion is completed	Help to identify any abnormalities (allergic reaction) in an early stage itself
10.	As per the doctor's order the infusion rate should be followed; infusion should be finished within 4 hours of started	To prevent the risk of transfusion reaction and complications
11.	Record the procedure in the nurse's record in details	Help to assess the continuous progress of the patient
12.	Once the blood transfusion over, disconnect the blood transfusion set and discard as per institutional policy	To prevent the contamination

Points to Note

If any reaction occurs:
* Immediately blood transfusion is stopped and duty doctor is informed.
* Carry out the doctor's orders.
* The remains blood and blood sets send to the blood bank and documentation to be done.
* Recording and reporting of reactions if any, shall be done by the staff and consultant and then analyzed.
* The transfusion details will be recorded in the patient record.

INSERTION OF ENEMA AND SUPPOSITORIES

Definition

Enema is the procedure, which is used to refer to the process of instilling fluid through the anal sphincter into the rectum and lower intestine for a therapeutic purpose.

Purposes

- To stimulate peristalsis (involuntary contraction) and to evacuate stool from the rectum
- To administer medication
- To relive gaseous distention
- For diagnostic purposes
- To clean the bowl before some specific investigation or procedure
- To provoke anesthesia
- To reduce the temperature.

Equipments

A clean tray containing:
- Enema can with tubing's and clamp
- Suppositories or enema
- A pair of clean gloves
- Apron
- Mask
- Lubricant jelly
- Mackintosh
- Tissue paper
- Towels
- Bedpan.

Procedure

Procedure for enema and suppositories insertion is provided in Table 6.13.

Table 6.13: Procedure for enema and suppositories insertion

Sl No	Care action	Rationale
1.	Explain the procedure and its importance	To get acceptance from the patient
2.	Wash the hands and wear the gloves, apron and mask	To prevent the infection and unnecessary mess
3.	Before start the procedure ask the patient to void and collect the history from the patient about previous ano/rectal surgery or abnormalities	To prevent any add up to assault
4.	Arrange all the equipments in the procedure room	For the easy use and to minimize the contamination
5.	Adjust the intravenous (IV) stand height to hang the enema can at the required height	To ensure the free flow of water
6.	Connect all the tubing and clamp in the enema can and hung the can in the IV stand	To prevent any obstruction of fluid flow during the procedure
7.	Loose the pyjama and place the patient in the mackintosh	To prevent mess in the procedural area

Contd...

Contd...

Sl No	Care action	Rationale
8.	Position the patient on the bed on his or her left side with the top knee bent and pulled slightly upward toward the chin	To aid relaxation and minimize resistance, and discomfort on insertion
9.	Allow the small amount of fluid to run into the kidney tray by releasing the clamp	To check any leakage of the tube and let out the air from the tube
10.	Apply the lubricant jelly in the distal part of the enema tube (3–4 inch)	Easy to advance the tube into the rectal area
11.	Ask the patient take deep breath and advance the tube 3–4 inches in to the rectal area	To aid relaxation and minimize resistance and discomfort on insertion
12.	Release the clamp and allow the solution to go inside and the solution should be in room temperature	To minimize shock and prevent bowel spasms
13.	Ensure the prescribed amount of fluid has passed, once it does over clamp the tube	To prevent the air entry
14.	Gently remove the tube by using the adequate gauze pieces and hold the patient's buttocks together	To avoid the splashing the excretion of fluid
15.	Remove and discard the gauzes and other items, which are used for the procedure as per institutional policy	To minimize the risk of contamination
16.	Instruct the patient to hold the fluid 5–10 minutes until there is a strong urge to defecate	To facilitate the fecal matter soft and peristalsis movement
17.	If the patient wants to pass motion immediately, give bedpan or assess the patient to the toilet	To provide comfortable to the patients
18.	In case of suppositories administration: • Insert suppositories about 4 cm into the rectum, usually using the index finger • Clean the patient perianal area; ask the patient to retain the suppository • Ensure that assistance is available if patient is unable to walk to the toilet • A suppository will take about 20 minutes to dissolve	To prevent cross infection Some patient may prefer to insert the suppository themselves, if so the nurse should explain the procedure and be available to offer assistance, if necessary
19.	Document that the suppository has been given; monitor the patient and record the effects of the rectal enema	Easy to assess the patient condition

COLOSTOMY CARE

Definition

Colostomy care is the procedure, where the colostomy bag is emptying and cleaning regularly.

Indications

- To prevent tissue damage and skin excoriation
- To prevent infection and promote healing
- To check for the patency of the ostomy
- To assess the stoma and the surrounding regions
- Help to identify the complication in early stage
- To maintain personal hygiene
- To prevent odor and leakage from the ostomy bag.

Equipments

- Dressing tray
- Disposable gloves
- Mask
- Cleaning solution
- Ostomy pouch with clamp
- Tape or belt
- Skin barrier (powder or paste)
- Mackintosh
- Sponge cloth or tissue paper
- Towel
- Basin with warm water
- Kidney tray.

Procedure

Colostomy care is detailed in Table 6.14.

Table 6.14: Procedure for colostomy care

SI No	Care action	Rationale
1.	Explain the procedure to the patient	To get the cooperation from the patient
2.	Provide privacy	To make comfortable to the patient
3.	Gather all the equipment near the bedside	To prevent unnecessary contamination and easy to perform the procedure
4.	Place the mackintosh under the patient site of the stoma	To prevent soiling of the linen
5.	Place the patient in supine position and cover the patient appropriately	To make the patient feel comfortable and to prevent the contamination
6.	Wash the hands; wear gloves and mask	To reduce the risk of cross infection
7.	Release the clamp and empty the motion content from the bag to the bedpan	To prevent splashing of the fecal matter
8.	Remove the pouch and keep it aside	

Contd...

Contd...

SI No	Care action	Rationale
9.	Wash the skin around the stoma with water or normal saline and dry the area	Skin must be dry, pouch does not adhere to wet skin
10.	Observe the skin condition around the stoma side	Help to identify the complication in early stages
11.	Apply the skin barrier around the stoma site (paste or powder); allow 1–2 minutes for dry	It creates a flatter surface for pouch placement
12.	Measure the stoma size by measuring guide or stoma pattern according to that cut the Karaya sheet and prepares the pouch	To prevent the leakage from side of the stoma
13.	Peal the paper around the opening of the pouch; apply it to the non-covered shiny side of the Karaya sheet	Easy to stick over the area
14.	Remove the transparent layer from the Karaya sheet and apply it with the pouch as one unit, to the skin	Easy to attach around the stoma site
15.	Apply the belt as needed, to the edge of the faceplate over the Karaya sheet	Ensure the proper position for the bag
16.	Fold bottom edge of the pouch to fit clamp or devices	To prevent the leakage
17.	Dispose the waste material as per institutional policy	To prevent the contamination
18.	Remove the mackintosh and articles near the bedside	Make the environment clean and comfortable for the patient
19.	Remove the gloves and wash the hands	To reduce the risk of cross infection
20.	Make the patient comfortable	Ensure the patient comfortable
21.	Document the procedure in the nurse's record	Help to do the follow-up care for the patient

EXTRAVASATIONS

Definition

1. Extravasation is the inadvertent administration of drugs (vesicant solution or medication) into the surrounding tissues rather than into the intended vein, which can lead to tissue necrosis.
2. Extravasation is a complication of intravenous chemotherapy administration but in general condition that is often underdiagnosed, undertreated and under-reported.

Prevention of Extravasation

Focus

Safe intravenous technique and implementing appropriate strategies to minimize the risk. Forethought, planning and improved prevention measures can minimize the risk of extravasation:

1. Careful assessment of the most appropriate cannulation site should be undertaken before insertion. Siting the cannula over joints should be avoided, as tissue damage in these areas has serious consequences. If venous access proves difficult, the opinion of an experienced practitioner should be sought as placement of a central venous access device (CVAD) may be necessary.
2. Extravasations can occur in CVADs, often with delayed onset and can be recognized by the patient complaining of sudden pain, discomfort, inflammation or swelling around the extravasations site.
3. Some patient groups are at increased risk of extravasations. These include obese, elderly, pediatric patients, thrombocytopenic patients, diabetics with peripheral neuropathy and patients who have had previous chemotherapy/radiotherapy. Extra care should be taken with all these patient groups.
4. Vesicant drugs in a chemotherapy regimen must be given before the other cytotoxic agents.
5. When given peripherally, bolus doses (in syringes) of vesicants must be given via a fast running infusion of a compatible fluid. Continually assess the cannulation site throughout the administration for signs of swelling, pain or inflammation and monitor the fast running infusion for change in rate.
6. Only the following vesicant cytotoxics may be given by peripheral infusion (in bags), i.e. paclitaxel, vinca alkaloids, dacarbazine, streptozocin, treosulfan. However, the central venous route minimizes the extravasations risk and should be considered on an individual patient basis. Any other cytotoxic vesicant infusions (in bags) should be administered via CVAD.

Management of Extravasations of Cytotoxic Drugs

Administration of the vesicant drugs: It should be administered first since:
- The vascular integrity increases over time
- The vein is most stable and least irritated at the start of the treatment
- The initial assessment of vein patency is most accurate
- The vesicant drugs are irritant, increase the vein fragility and cause venous spasm masking the signs of extravasation, when administered last.

Signs and Symptoms

Extravasations should be suspected if one or more of the following symptoms have occurred:
1. The patient complains of burning, stinging or any discomfort/pain at the injection site.

2. This should be distinguished from a feeling of cold that may occur with some drugs.
3. Observation of swelling, redness or blistering at the injection site. This should be distinguished from the 'nettle rash' effect seen with anthracyclines.
4. No blood return is obtained. This is not a sign of extravasations, if found in isolation.
5. A resistance is felt on the plunger of the syringe of a bolus drug.
6. There is absence of free flow of the infusion.
7. If in any doubt, treat as extravasation.

Management of Extravasations

- Stop the chemotherapeutic drug infusion immediately
- Aspirate any residual drug and blood in IV tubing, needle and suspected infiltration site
- The peripheral access device can be left in situ or removed according to the physician order
- Apply hot or cold packs as indicated
- Administer antidote subcutaneously clockwise into the infiltrated area
- Elevate the limb to minimize the swelling
- Monitor the site frequently for pain, erythema, induration and necrosis
- Plastic surgeon consultation to remove the tissue containing the drug
- Surgical recommendation is required especially, when the lesion is greater than 2 cm
- There is significant residual pain 1–2 weeks after extravasations
- There is minimal healing 2–3 weeks after injury despite local therapeutic measures
- Document the extravasations management.

Documentation and Reporting

Purposes

- To provide an accurate account of what happened (in the event that there is litigation)
- To protect the healthcare professionals involved (showing they followed procedure)
- To gather information on extravasations, how and when they occurs—for audit purposes
- Highlight any possible deficits in practice, which require review.

Difference between extravasations from other conditions is given in Table 6.15.

Table 6.15: Distinguishing extravasations from other conditions

Characteristics	Flare reaction	Vessel irritation	Venous shock	Extravasations
Presenting symptoms	Itchy blotches or hives; pain and burning uncommon	Aching and tightness	Muscular wall of the blood vessel in spasm	Pain and burning are common at injection site; stinging may occur during infusion
Coloration	Raised red streak, blotches or 'hive-like' erythema along the vessel; diffuse or irregular pattern	Erythema or dark discoloration along vessel		Erythema around area of needle or around the venipuncture site
Timing	Usually appears suddenly and dissipates within 30–90 minutes	Usually appears within minutes after injection; coloration may only appear later in the process	Usually appears right after injection	Symptoms start to appear right after injection, symptoms endure
Swelling	Unlikely	Unlikely	None	Occurs often; does not dissolve for several days
Blood return	Usually, but not always intact	Usually, but not always intact	Often absent	Usually absent or sluggish

Poorly Managed Extravasation

Poorly managed extravasations leads to:
- Pain from the necrotic site
- Physical defect
- Increase in cost of hospitalization
- Delay in the treatment of disease
- Psychological distress.

Preparation and Administration

Equipment

- Clean tray or receiver in which to place drug and equipment
- Use 21 G needle(s) to ease reconstitution and drawing up, 23 G needle if from a glass ampule
- Ordered intravenous fluid
- Syringe(s) of appropriate size for amount of drug to be given
- Swabs saturated with 70% isopropyl alcohol
- Sterile topical swab, if drug is presented in ampule form
- Drug(s) to be administered
- Patient's prescription chart, to check dose, route, etc.
- Recording sheet or book as required by law or hospital policy

- Personal protective equipments (cap, mask, apron, industrial gloves, eye goggles)
- Drug labels.

Procedure

Extravasations procedure is given in Table 6.16.

Table 6.16: Procedure for extravasation

Sl No	Care action	Rationale
1.	Wash hands	To reduce risk of microbial contamination
2.	Put on a pair of disposable sterile gloves	To prevent the skin contact
3.	Wear cap, mask, apron with full sleeves and eye goggles	To prevent contact with skin/clothes in case of accidental spill
4.	Follow the six rights of drug administration	To prevent medication error
5.	Vials containing drugs requiring reconstitution should be vented	To reduce the internal pressure; this reduces the probability of spraying and spillage
6.	Use disposable syringe to draw the solvent from the solvent vial	To reduce risk of microbial contamination
7.	The external surface of the vial should be wiped with an alcohol swab	To reduce risk of microbial contamination
8.	The contents should be transferred aseptically into drug vial	To reduce risk of microbial contamination and to prepare the drug
9.	When opening the glass ampule, wrap and then snap at the break point using an alcohol swab; hold ampule away from your face	To reduce the possibility of injury and risk of contamination
10.	Reconstitution should be carried out within a laminar hood provided	To prevent skin contact
11.	Syringes and intravenous (IV) bottles containing cytotoxic drug should be labeled with patient identity, drug name, dose, date and time of starting; the prepared solutions should be stored separately from other medications	To prevent the administration error
12.	Explain the action, dose and expected adverse effect of the drug to the patient; administer the medicine	Patient has the rights to know the treatment
13.	Record the administration on appropriate charts	To maintain accurate records, provide point of reference in the event of any queries and prevent any duplication of treatment
14.	Contaminated needles, syringes, IV tubings, gloves, mask and cap should be disposed according to biomedical wastage policy; vials should be replaced in black cover and linen contaminated with drugs, patient excreta or body fluids should be handled separately; it must be sealed	To prevent aerosol generation and injury

CARE FOR NEUTROPENIC

Low Count Measures

- Proper handwashing before and after touching the patient and procedure
- Pulse/Temperature monitoring every 4th hourly; may need to be more frequent
- Mouth care: Hexidine/Listerine mouthwash after each feed/thrice a day
- Candid mouth painting twice daily
- Betadine scrub in axilla/groin and peripheral region and sitz bath daily
- Fucidin ointment in both nostrils twice a day (bd)
- Central venous catheter care if any (dressing to be changed in the alternative days)
- Sterile food (freshly cooked hot food and double boiled) from hospital preferably
- No fruits (unpeeled)/flowers
- No intramascular (IM) injections/enema/per rectal (PR) examination
- Weight recording once daily
- Neosporin powder in axilla and groin bd
- Limited visitors
- Complete blood count (CBC), renal parameter as applicable daily and liver function test (LFT) thrice a week
- Wash the hands before examining the patient, blood products to be given through the leukocyte filters only
- Use N95 mask for the patient (to prevent further infection)
- Use alcohol swab before using any port
- Use clave connecter for all lines
- Use sterile gloves, mask, cap and apron for each procedure.

MODIFIED EARLY WARNING SIGNS

Terms and Definition

Scoring systems were developed in response to studies that showed patients, who suffered in-hospital cardiac arrest, often had abnormal physiologic values charted in the preceding hours. Modified early warning signs (MEWS) provided in Table 6.17.

Table 6.17: Modified early warning signs

Score	3	2	1	0	1	2	3	Total
Glasgow coma scale				15	14	9–13	Less than or equal to 8	

Contd...

Contd...

Score	3	2	1	0	1	2	3	Total
Respiratory rate (breath per minute)		Less than 8		9–14	15–20	21–29	Greater than 30	
Heart rate (beats per minute)		Less than 40	40–50	51–100	101–110	111–130	Greater than 130	
Systolic blood pressure (mm Hg)	Less than 70	71–80	81–100	101–180	181–200	201–220	Greater than 220	
Temperature (°F)	Less than 93.2	93.2–95		95.18–99.5	99.68–101.3	101.48–104	Greater than 104	
Oxygen saturation with appropriate oxygen therapy (%)	Less than 90	91–93		94–100				
Urine output (mL/h)	Less than 10	Less than 20						
Total score								

Any single score of 3 in any category or a total score of 4 indicate the need to initiate 'rapid response call (MET)'.

Rapid response call alert is the call given by the unit/ward nurses to the medical emergency team (MET) for early decision and management (Fig. 6.1).

Purpose

To decrease unexpected mortality by early recognition of a patient's condition and intervene before the patient either goes to arrests or requires transfer to intensive care unit (ICU).

Aim

To empower nurses to call rapid response for whatever level of help is required.

Most Common Abnormalities in Ward to ICU

- Tachypnea and an altered level of consciousness
- Also derangement of heart rate, arterial blood pressure, arterial oxygen saturation and urinary output.

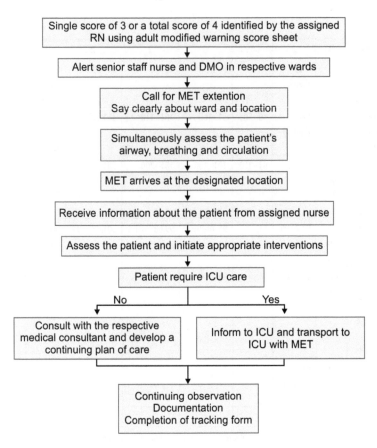

FIGURE 6.1: Modified early warning signs and rapid response (DMO, duty medical officer; ICU, intensive care unit; MET, medical emergency team; RN, registered nurse).

Criteria to Call the MET

- Respiratory rate of more than 25 or less than10 breaths per minute
- Arterial systolic blood pressure of less than 90 mm Hg
- Heart rate of more than110 or less than 55 beats per minute
- Not fully alert and oriented
- Oxygen saturation of less than 90%
- Urine output over the last 4 hours of less than100 mL
- Respiratory rate more than 35 breaths or a heart rate more than140 beats per minute.

Rapid Response Call Team Members

1. Specialist on call for service: Assesses, collaborates and initiates appropriate interventions.
2. Intensive care unit nurse: Guides and assists the primary nurse in the assessment and nursing management for the patient.

3. Respiratory therapist: Assesses, collaborates and initiates appropriate respiratory interventions.

Interpretation

- The greater the physiologic deviation from the normal parameters, the higher the point scores
- Clinical deterioration is subsequently detected and medical intervention can be implemented at an early stage in the patient's illness.

BASIC LIFE SUPPORT

Definition

Cardiopulmonary resuscitation (CPR) is a basic emergency procedure of manual external cardiac message and artificial respiration.

Basic life support (BLS) acts to slow down the deterioration of the brain and the heart until defibrillation or advanced cardiac life support (ACLS) can be provided.

Chain of Survival

The chain of survival refers to a series of actions that, when put into action, reduce the mortality associated with cardiac arrest. The four interdependent links in the chain of survival are explained in Figure 6.2.

Working of CPR

The air we breathe in travels to our lung, where oxygen is picked up by our blood and then pumped by the heart to tissue and organs. When a person experiences cardiac arrest whether due to heart failure in adults and the elderly or an injury such as near drowning, electrocution or severe trauma in a child, the heart goes from a normal best to an arrhythmic pattern and eventually ceases to beat altogether.

This prevents oxygen from circulating throughout the body, rapidly killing cells and tissue in essence, cardio (heart) pulmonary (lung) resuscitation (revive, revitalize) serves as an artificial heart beat and artificial respiration.

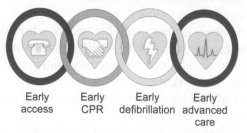

FIGURE 6.2: Chain of survival for cardiac arrest (CPR, cardiopulmonary resuscitation).

The CPR may not save the victim even when performed properly, but if started within 4 minutes of cardiac arrest and defibrillation is provided within 10 minutes it is possible to save one's life.

The CPR consist of four main components:
1. Circulation.
2. Airway.
3. Breathing.
4. Defibrillation.

Before you start any rescue efforts you must remember to check the responsivenss by taping the victims shoulder and shout 'are you okay'.

For infants: Tap the infant's foot and shout, if the victim has no response activates emergency response system.

Circulation

After checking response, locate the carotid pulse.

Steps to locate the carotid artery pulse
The steps to locate the carotid artery pulse in adults are the following:
• Maintain a head tilt with one hand on the victim's forehead
• Locate the trachea using two or three fingers into the other hand
• Slide these two or three fingers into the groove between the trachea and the muscle at the side of the neck, where you can feel the carotid pulse
• Palpate the artery for at least 5 seconds and not more than 10 seconds.

Steps to locate the brachial artery pulse
The steps to locate the brachial artery pulse in infants as follows:
• Place two or three fingers on the inside of the upper arm, between the infants elbow and shoulder
• Press the index and middle fingers gently on the upper arm for at least 5 second and not more than 10 second when attempting to feel the pulse.

Chest compression technique
If no pulse, start cycle of:
• In 1 and 2: Rescuer adult and child CPR
• Ratio: Comperession of 30:2
• Rate: 100/min
• Depth: At least 2 inches.

Steps to perform chest compression on an adult
1. Position yourself at the victim's side.
2. Make sure the victim is lying on his/her back on a firm, flat surface. If the victim is lying face down, carefully roll him into his/her back.
3. Move or remove all clothing covering the victim's chest. You need to be able to see the victim's skin.
4. Put the heel of first-hand. Straighten your arms and position your shoulder directly over your hands.
5. Push hard and fast, press down at least 2 inches with each compression make sure you push straight down on the victim's breastbone.

6. At the end of each compression, make sure you allow the chest recoil or re-expand completely. Full chest recoil will reduce the blood flow created by chest compression.
7. Deliver compression in a smooth fashion at a rate of 100 compression per minute.

Steps to perform chest compression on an infant
- In 1: Rescuer infant CPR
- Ratio: Comperession 30:2
- Rate:100/min
- Depth: At least 1.5 inches
- Draw an imaginary line between the nipples place two fingers on the breastbone just below this line. This will allow you to compress on the lower half of the breastbone. Do not press on the xiphoid process.

Rescue infants CPR (2 thumb-encircling hands technique)

Steps includes the following:

1. Draw an imaginary line between the nipples. Place both thumbs side by side in the center of the infant's chest on the breastbone, just below this line. This will allow you to compress on the lower half of the breastbone. Do not press on the xiphoid. The thumps may overlap in very small infants.
2. Encircle the infant's chest and support the infants back with the fingers of both hands.
3. With your hands encircling the chest, use both thumbs to depress the breast approximately at least 1.5 inches the depth of the infant's chest. As you push down with your thumbs, squeeze the infant's chest with your fingers.
4. After each compression completely release the pressure on the breastbone and chest and allow the chest to fully recoil.
5. Deliver compression in a smooth fashion at a rate of 100 compression per minute.
6. After every 15 compression, pause briefly for the second rescuer to open the airway with head tilt-chin lift and give two breaths. Coordinate compression and ventilation to avoid simultaneous deliver and to ensure adequate ventilation and chest expansion, especially when the airway is unprotected.

Airway

1. After giving the chest compression you need to make sure that his airway is clear of any obstruction. The breath may be faint and shallow.
2. Look, listen and feel for any signs of breathing. If you determine that the victim is not breathing then something may be blocking the air passage. The tongue is the most common airway obstruction in an unconscious person.
3. Open the victims airway with a head tilt-chin lift maneuver and look for the chest rise and fall, place your ear near the victim's mouth and nose

and listen for air escaping during exhalation, feel for flow of air against your cheek.

4. If the victim is not breath adequately, use a barrier device to give two breath or by mouth–to-mouth resuscitation.

Steps to give mouth-to-mouth breath to adults
- Hold the victim's airway open with a head tilt-chin lift
- Pinch the nose closed with our thumb and index finger
- Take a regular breath and seal your lips around the victim's mouth, creating an airtight seal
- Give one breath (blow for 1 second) watch for the chest to rise as you give the breath
- Give the second breath like the same as above.

Steps to give mouth-to-mask breath to adults
- Position yourself at the victim's side
- Place the mask on the victim's face using the bridge of the nose as a guide for correct position
- Seal the mask against the face
- Using your hand that is closer to the top of the victim's head that closer to the top of the victim's head, place the index finger and thumb along the border of the mask
- Place the thumb of your other hand along the lower margin of the mask
- Place the remaining fingers of your hand closer to the victim's neck along the bony margin of the jaw and lift to open the airway
- While you lift the jaw, press firmly and completely around the outside margin of the mask to seal the mask against the face.

Techniques for giving mouth-to-mouth breath to infants
- Hold the victim's airway open with a head tilt-chin lift
- Place your mouth over the infants mouth and nose create an airtight seal
- Give one breath (blow for 1 second) watch for the chest to rise as you give the breath
- Give the second breath like the same as above.

Steps to give mouth-to-mask breath to infants
- Same maneuver for adult.

Procedure

Procedure of CPR (basic life support) is given in Table 6.18.

Table 6.18: Procedure for cardiopulmonary resuscitation

Sl No	Care action	Rationale
1.	Note time of arrest	Lack of cerebral perfusion for approximately 3–4 minutes can lead to irreversible brain damage

Contd...

Contd...

SI No	Care action	Rationale
2.	Call for help; if second nurse is available can call for cardiac arrest team	Cardiopulmonary resuscitation (CPR) is more effective if two rescuer is present One is responsible for inflating the lung and the other is giving chest compression
3.	Place cardiac table under the patient	Effective cardiac massage can be performed only on a hard surface
4.	If the patient is in bed, remove head end rail and ensure adequate space between back of bed and wall	To allow easy access of patients head in order to facilitate ventilation
5.	Check for the carotid pulse with two or three fingers	To know circulation is present or not
6.	If the circulation is not present place the heel of one hand in the center of the sternum and place the other on top, ensuring that the hand is on the center of the sternum and only the heel of the dominant hand is touching the sternum	To ensure the cardiac compression and reduce the delay in commencing cardiac compression
7.	The sternum should be depressed sharply 4–5 cm; cardiac compression should be forceful and sustained at a rate of 100 per min	This produced a cardiac output by applying direct downward force of compression
8.	Maintain cardiac compression and ventilation ratio 30:2, this must be continue until the cardiac output returns or handed over the patient to advanced cardiac life support (ACLS) team	To maintain circulation and ventilation Thus reducing the risk of damage to vital organs
9.	Ensure a clear airway this is best achieved by head tilt-chin lift maneuver	To establish and maintain airway, thus facilitate ventilation
10.	If breath is not present give artificial respiration	For adequate oxygenation and ventilation
11.	When the cardiac arrest team arrives, it will assume responsibility for the arrest in coordination with ward staff	To ensure an effective team coordinates the resuscitation
12.	Attach patient to electrocardiogram (ECG) monitor using three electrodes defibrillator patches	To obtain adequate ECG signal Accurate recording of cardiac rhythm will determine the appropriate treatment
Intubation		
13.	Continue to ventilate and oxygenate the patient before intubation	The risk of cardiac arrhythmias due to hypoxia is decreased
14.	Equipment for intubation should be checked before handing to appropriate medical or nursing staff	To provide continuity of care

Contd...

Contd...

Sl No	Care action	Rationale
15.	Recommence ventilation and oxygenation once intubation is completed	Intubation should be interrupt resuscitation only for a maximum of 16 seconds to prevent the occurrence of cerebral anoxia
16.	Once the patient intubated, chest compression at the rate of 100/min, should continue and ventilation should continue at 10–12 breath per minute	Uninterrupted compression result in a substantially higher mean coronary perfusion pressure A pause in chest compression allows the coronary pressure to fall
Intravenous access		
17.	Venous access must be established through the large vein as soon as possible	To administer cardiac drug and fluid replacement
18.	Asepsis should be maintained throughout the procedure	To prevent local and systemic infection
19.	The correct rate of infusion is required	To ensure maximum drug and solution effectiveness
20.	Document in detail the proceedings in the CPR track sheet and in the nurse's record and document the condition of the patient with time, medications used, response and interventions done	To monitor differences and detect trends; any irregularities should be brought to the attention of the appropriate senior nursing and medical teams

ADVANCED CARDIAC LIFE SUPPORT

In ACLS, the specific treatment of a given dysrhythmias or condition depends on the patient's hemodynamic status.

Patient Assessment

In general, patients can be divided into four categories to determine treatment priorities:
1. Asymptomatic.
2. Stable symptomatic.
3. Unstable symptomatic.
4. Pulseless.

Asymptomatic patients do not receive treatment, but should be monitored for changes in condition. Any patient with symptoms (even apparently mild symptoms such as palpitations) should be assessed to determine if they are stable or unstable. Determination of a patient's level of hemodynamic compromise can include several factors.

General Appearance

The first indication of hemodynamic status comes from a patient's general appearance, including skin signs, level of activity and work of breathing. If a patient shows signs of compensation (e.g. pale cool or diaphoretic skin) or acute distress, they are unstable.

Level of Consciousness

Interaction with the patient allows the provider to evaluate the patient's level of consciousness based on the patient's activity, awareness of their surroundings and ability to provide information. If a patient shows any level of mental deficit, family or friends should be consulted to determine if this state differs from the patient's baseline. If the mental deficit is acute, the patient should be considered unstable.

Vital Signs

Vital signs provide a diagnostic evaluation of the patient. Blood pressure is the primary indicator. A systolic blood pressure above 90 mm Hg usually indicates that the patient is stable (although the provider should be alert for changes in blood pressure that might indicate an unstable patient even if blood pressure is normal).

Other vital signs may be useful, but should not be relied upon exclusively. Pulse oximetry can be useful, especially if it rises or falls, but providers should remember that various conditions (such as CO_2 poisoning) can make changes in blood oxygen levels and that high O_2 saturation may be present in unstable patients (such as those in shock). Additionally, heart rate is of no use in determining if a patient is stable or unstable; a patient with a heart rate of 80 can be severely unstable, while a patient with a heart rate of 210 can be stable if they are still perfusing well.

Assessment Findings

If a patient's general appearance, level of consciousness and vital signs are all normal, the patient is stable. If possible, treatment should be rendered starting with the least invasive that is appropriate for that patient's hemodynamic status. In ACLS, the preferential treatment is symptomatic, but a stable patients is generally medications, while the preferential treatment for unstable patients is generally electrical therapy.

Once treatment is rendered, the provider must reassess the patient. If the patient remains symptomatic, the appropriate treatment (medications or electricity) should be given again depending on the patient's heart rhythm and current hemodynamic status (thus, if a patient was stable before, but becomes unstable after administration of a drug, the patient should receive electrical therapy to continue treating the dysrhythmia rather than additional doses of a medication).

If a patient's general appearance indicates that they may be unconscious, then should check for responsiveness. If the patient is unresponsive, get help [send someone to call 911 and bring back an external defibrillator (AED), call a code, etc.]. The BLS algorithm should then be followed— open the airway, check for breathing, and assess circulation. If the patient is apneic, rescue breathing should be started; if the patient is pulseless, rescuers should begin CPR.

Once you determine that a patient is pulseless, an automated AED or ECG monitor should be attached as soon as possible. CPR should be continued with minimal interruptions. After each rhythm check, the patient should be defibrillated if appropriate [for ventricular fibrillation (V-Fib or VF) and pulseless ventricular tachycardia (V-Tach or VT)]. Regardless of the heart rhythm, medications should be given as soon as possible after CPR is resumed (the specific medication determined by the patient's exact status and heart rhythm).

Algorithm Review of ACLS

Always start with the CABD survey. CABD stands for circulation, airway, breathing, defibrillation.

Acute Coronary Syndromes

Algorithm: Consider MONA for patients with suspected acute coronary syndrome (ACS) [angina or acute myocardial infarction (AMI)]:
- Morphine
- Oxygen
- Nitroglycerine
- Aspirin.

Bradycardia

Algorithm: Steps given below:
1. Atropine 0.5 mg intravenous pyelogram (IVP) for sinus bradycardia and 1°, 2° type I arteriovenous (AV) Block.
2. Transcutaneous pacing (preferred for 2° type II and 3° heart block); do not delay pacing in symptomatic patients (even those in sinus bradycardia or low-degree heart blocks).
3. Dopamine 5–10 µg/kg/min (if patient unresponsive to atropine/pacing).
4. Epinephrine drip 2–10 µg/min (if patient unresponsive to atropine/pacing).

Note: Atropine is not indicated for 2° type II and 3° heart blocks, proceed directly to pacing if the patient is symptomatic, although atropine can be considered if pacing is delayed.

Tachycardia

Algorithm: Tachycardia with pulses. If the patient is unstable, go directly to synchronized cardioversion. Otherwise:
1. For regular narrow complex tachycardia [probable supraventricular tachycardia (SVT)]:
   - Obtain 12-lead ECG; consider expert consultation
   - Attempt vagal maneuvers
   - Adenosine 6 mg rapid IV push. If no conversion, give up to two more doses at 12 mg each.

2. For irregular narrow complex tachycardia [probable artrial fibrillation (A-Fib)]:
   - Obtain 12-lead ECG; consider expert consultation
   - Control rate with diltiazem or beta blockers.
3. For regular wide complex tachycardia (probable V-Tach):
   - Obtain 12-lead ECG; consider expert consultation
   - Convert rhythm using amiodarone—150 mg over 10 minutes
   - Elective cardioversion.
4. For irregular wide complex tachycardia:
   - Obtain 12-lead ECG; consider expert consultation
   - Consider antiarrhythmics
   - If torsades de pointes, give magnesium sulfate 1–2 g over 5–60 minutes.

Ventricular Fibrillation/Pulseless Ventricular Tachycardia

Algorithm: Pulseless arrest (shockable).

Stage I
1. CPR: Start immediately. Push hard and push fast.
2. Shock: Analyze rhythm and shock if in VF/pulseless VT.
3. CPR: Resume CPR immediately after shock delivery. Continue for 5 cycles/2 minutes.
4. Vasopressor: Epinephrine 1 mg q 3–5 min (can replace 1st or 2nd dose of epinephrine with 40 units vasopressin). Give as soon as possible after resuming CPR, circulate with chest compressions.

Stage II
1. Shock: Analyze rhythm, and shock if in VF/pulseless VT.
2. CPR: Resume CPR immediately after shock delivery. Continue for 5 cycles/2 minutes.
3. Antiarrhythmic: Amiodarone 300 mg IV/IO or lidocaine 1–1.5 mg/kg up to 3 mg/kg. Give as soon as possible after resuming CPR, circulate with chest compressions.

Stage III
1. Shock: Analyze rhythm and shock if in VF/pulseless VT.
2. CPR: Resume CPR immediately after shock delivery. Continue for 5 cycles/2 minutes.

Note: Minimize interruptions to chest compressions; do not check a pulse or evaluate the heart rhythm after a shock. After each shock, resume CPR immediately and continue for 5 cycles prior to rhythm analysis and possible pulse check. After a second dose of epinephrine, a second antiarrhythmic dose (amiodarone 150 mg or lidocaine 0.5–0.75 mg/kg) may be given after the next rhythm check.

Pulseless Electrical Activity

Algorithm: Pulseless arrest (not shockable) [pulseless electrical activity (PEA)]:
1. Possible causes (consider the 6 H's and 5 T's).
2. Epinephrine 1 mg q 3–5 min (can replace 1st or 2nd dose of epinephrine with 40 units vasopressin). Give as soon as possible after resuming CPR, circulate with chest compressions.

3. Atropine 1 mg intravenous/introsseous (IV/IO) q 3–5 min to maximum 3 mg (only if electrical rate is < 60). Give as soon as possible after resuming CPR, circulate with chest compressions.

Note: In PEA, the electrical system of the heart is functioning, but there is a problem with the pump, pipes or volume—a mechanical part of the system is not working. You can use the 6 H's and 5 T's to remember the most common reversible causes of PEA.

H's

- Hypovolemia
- Hypo- or hyper-kalemia
- Hydrogen ion (acidosis)
- Hypothermia
- Hypoxia
- Hypoglycemia.

T's

- Tension pneumothorax
- Tamponade (cardiac)
- Trauma
- Toxins
- Thrombosis (coronary or pulmonary).

Asystole

Algorithm: Pulseless arrest (not shockable) (Dead?):

1. Determine whether to initiate resuscitation.
2. Epinephrine 1 mg q 3–5 min (can replace 1st or 2nd dose of epinephrine with 40 units vasopressin). Give as soon as possible after resuming CPR, circulate with chest compressions.
3. Atropine, 1 mg IV/IO q 3–5 min to maximum 3 mg. Give as soon as possible after resuming CPR, circulate with chest compressions.
4. Differential diagnosis or discontinue resuscitation: Are they still dead? Consider the 6 H's and 5 T's (refer above); check blood glucose; check core temperature; consider Naloxone, etc.

Electrocardiogram and Electrical Therapy Review

The ECG tracing represents electrical activity through the heart. The P-wave represents depolarization of the atria; the QRS complex represents depolarization of the ventricles and the T-wave represents the later stage of repolarization of the ventricles. The interval from the first deflection of the P-wave to the beginning of the QRS complex is the PR interval (PRI) and should be between 0.12 and 0.20 seconds. A normal QRS complex has duration of 0.12 seconds or less, a longer duration (wide QRS) indicates delayed conduction through the ventricles, often as the result of a ventricular pacemaker focus.

The horizontal axis of the ECG strips measures time. Each large box represents 0.20 seconds; each small box represents 0.04 seconds.

To obtain a 3-lead ECG tracing, place the white [right arm (RA)] electrode on the right chest just below the clavicle, the black electrode [left arm (LA)] on the left chest just below the clavicle and the red electrode [left leg (LL)] laterally on the lower left abdomen. Pacer pads go in the anterior/posterior positions. Defibrillation pads go on the upper right chest and lower left abdomen, although on children and other small patients the pads may need to be placed in the middle of the anterior and posterior chests.

Rhythm disturbances treat the patient, not the dysrhythmia. Always assess your patient for pulses, perfusion and level of consciousness—is the patient stable, unstable or pulseless? Next, assess the rhythm—is it fast or slow? Is it life-threatening? As you treat the patient, try to discover the cause of the dysrhythmia, for many patients, their only chance of survival is if you can identify and treat a reversible cause. There are many possible causes of rhythm disturbances or PEA. Common causes include sympathetic stimulation, stress, hypoxia, ischemia, drugs/toxins and electrolyte disturbances. Although laboratory draws can be useful, a history of the patient and the current event obtained from a family member or caregiver is often more useful.

Defibrillation (Unsynchronized Shock)

Fibrillation is a disorganized rhythm that, if present in the ventricles, is life-threatening. Immediate CPR combined with early defibrillation is critical to survival from sudden cardiac arrest. Defibrillation terminates all electrical activity in the pulseless heart, hopes that it will resume beating in a coordinated fashion. A shock should be delivered about once every 2 minutes if the patient remains in ventricular fibrillation. With a monophasic monitor, the recommendation is to deliver a single shock at 360 joules. If a biphasic monitor is used, the recommended dosage is machine dependent and should appear on the front of the monitor. If optimal shock dosage is not known, the consensus is to defibrillate at 200 J.

Synchronized Cardioversion

Synchronized cardioversion is the preferred treatment for unstable patients with a tachycardia such as atrial fibrillation, V-Tach with a pulse or supraventricular tachycardia (SVT). The shock is timed by the monitor to be delivered in coordination with the QRS complex of the heart. If the patient is conscious, consider sedation prior to cardioversion; however, synchronized cardioversion should not be delayed while waiting for sedation in severely symptomatic patients.

With a monophasic monitor, the initial shock is delivered at 100 J; if the rhythm does not terminate, deliver additional shocks in stepwise fashion (200 J, 300 J and 360 J for subsequent shocks). With a biphasic monitor, dosage and steps are device dependent; if optimal doses are unknown, begin at 100 J and step up from there.

Transcutaneous Pacing

External cardiac pacing is the recommended treatment for symptomatic bradycardia. If the patient is conscious, consider sedation; however, pacing should not be delayed while waiting for sedation. Begin pacing at zero milliampere, slowly increasing until capture is achieved. Then, set the rate at 20 beats per minute (bpm) above the monitored heart rate, with a minimum rate of 50 bpm.

Medications Review of ACLS

This information on medications meets the standard set by the 2005 American Heart Association (AHA) for advanced cardiac life support. It does not supersede local protocols or medical control; consult with your medical director for the most up-to-date guidelines on medication administration where you work.

Intravenous/intraosseous medications should be administered in a peripheral line during CPR, as soon as possible after a rhythm check. It is recommended that you flush with 20 mL of fluid after each drug administration and elevate the extremity. Always use large bore catheters if possible.

A note on endotracheal administration of medications: This route of medication administration is being de-emphasized by the AHA; the IV or 10 routes are preferred. However, the endotracheal (ET) route can still be used if providers are unable to gain access by IV/IO. Use the mnemonic 'NAVEL' to remember, which drugs can be administered via this route:

- Narcan
- Atropine
- Vasopressin
- Epinephrine
- Lidocaine.

If using the ET route, the drug dosage must be increased, typically 2–2.5 times the IV/IO bolus dosage (although there is no consensus on epinephrine or vasopressin dosing via this route), followed by a 10 mL normal saline flush.

Adenosine

Class: Endogenous nucleoside.

Indicated for: Paroxysmal supraventricular tachycardia (PSVT)/Regular narrow complex tachycardia.

Intravenous bolus dosage: Includes the following:
- Rapid IV push 6 mg—1st dose
- Rapid IV push 12 mg—2nd dose
- Rapid IV push 12 mg—3rd dose.

Notes: Doses are followed by a saline flush. Two subsequent doses of 12 mg each may be administered at 1–2 minutes intervals. Use the port closest to cannulation. The AHA recommends that the dose be cut by half if administering through a central line or in the presence of dipyridamole or carbamazepine. Larger doses may be required in the presence of caffeine or theophylline.

Amiodarone

Class: Antiarrhythmic.

Indicated for: V-Fib/pulseless V-Tach.

Intravenous/Intraosseous bolus dosage: Are as follows:
- 300 mg—1st dose
- 150 mg—2nd dose.

Arrhythmias: Dosage are the following:
- 360 mg over 6 hours (slow)
- 150 mg over 10 minutes (rapid) infusion dose
- 540 mg IV/IO over 18 hours (0.5 mg/min).

Notes: Cumulative doses more than 2.2 g/24 hours are associated with significant hypotension. Do not administer with other drugs that prolong QT interval (i.e. procainimide). Terminal elimination is extremely long half-life lasts up to 40 days. During arrest, IV bolus should be delivered slowly, over 1–3 minutes.

Aspirin

Class: Non-steroidal anti-inflammatory drug (NSAID).

Indicated for: Chest pain/acute coronary syndrome (ACS).

Per os (PO) dosage (no IV/IO): 160–325 mg.

Suppository dose: 300 mg.

Notes: In suspected ACS, Aspirin can block platelet aggregation and arterial constriction. Also helps with pain control. May cause or exacerbate gastrointestinal (GI) bleeding.

Atropine

Class: Parasympathetic blocker.

Indicated for: Bradycardia, asystole and slow PEA.

Intravenous/Intraosseous bolus dosage: Includes the following:
- 0.5 mg every 3–5 minutes as needed
- 1 mg every 3–5 minutes (up to 3 mg).

Notes: Used only in symptomatic bradycardia or in PEA with heart rate less than 60 (not indicated in 2° type II or 3° heart block). Doses less than 0.5 mg may result in paradoxical slowing of the heart. ET route discouraged, but can be used if IV/IO access not available.

Dextrose/Glucose

Class: Carbohydrate.

Indicated for: Hypoglycemia.

Intravenous/Intraosseous bolus dosage: 25 g (50 mL) of dextrose 50% in water (D50W).

Notes: Used to reverse documented hypoglycemia in patients with symptomatic bradycardia or during cardiac arrest. Should not be used routinely during cardiac arrest.

Dopamine

Class: Catecholamine.

Indicated for: Symptomatic bradycardia hypotension.

Intravenous infusion: These are the following:
- 2–10 µg/kg/min, cardiac dose
- 10–20 µg/kg/min, vasopressor dose.

Notes: Titrate to patient response. Correct hypovolemia with volume replacement before initiating dopamine. It may cause tachyarrhythmias. Do not mix with sodium bicarbonate.

Epinephrine

Class: Catecholamine.

Indicated for: Pulseless arrest.

Intravenous/Intraosseous bolus dosage: 1 mg (1:10,000) every 3–5 minutes.

Symptomatic bradycardia infusion: 1 mg in 500 mL of D5 W or NaCl at 1 µg/min titrated to effect.

Notes: First line drug in all pulseless rhythms. Increases myocardial oxygen demand and may cause myocardial ischemia or angina. ET route is discouraged, but if used give 2–2.5 mg of a 1:1,000 solution diluted in 10 mL normal saline.

Fluid Administration

Example: Normal saline/NaCl.

Class: Fluid volume.

Indicated for: Hypovolemia.

Intravenous/Intraosseous bolus dosage: 250–500 cc bolus (repeat as needed).

Notes: Use to treat specific reversible causes such as hypovolemia. Routine administration of fluids during a resuscitation is not indicated, as it can reduce coronary perfusion pressure.

Heparin (Unfractionated)

Class: Anticoagulant.

Indicated for: ST-segment elevation acute myocardial infarction (STEMI) (AMI).

Intravenous/Intraosseous bolus dosage: These are as follows:

Initial dose: 60 IU/kg (maximum 4,000 IU).

Infusion: 12 IU/kg/h (maximum 1,000 IU/h).

Notes: Do not use in patients with active bleeding or bleeding disorders, severe hypertension or recent surgery. Monitor activated partial thromboplastin time (aPTT) and platelet count, while administering.

Lidocaine

Class: Antiarrhythmic.

Indicated for: V-Fib/pulseless V-Tach, stable V-Tach.

Intravenous/Intraosseous bolus dosage: 1–1.5 mg/kg (1st dose).

Infusion: 1–4 mg/min (30–50 μg/kg/min).

Notes: May repeat at 0.5–0.75 mg/kg every 5–10 minutes to a maximum dose of 3 mg/kg. Use with caution in presence of impaired liver; discontinue if signs of toxicity develop. Prophylactic use in AMI is contraindicated. ET route discouraged, but can be used if IV/IO access not available.

Magnesium Sulfate

Class: Electrolyte.

Indicated for: Torsades de pointes or hypomagnesemia.

Intravenous/Intraosseous bolus dosage: 1–2 g in 10 mL D5W over 5–20 minutes.

Notes: A fall in blood pressure may be noted with rapid administration. Dose is given over 5–20 minutes during cardiac arrest, 5–60 minutes in living patients. Use with caution in renal failure.

Morphine Sulfate

Class: Opiate/Analgesic.

Indicated for: Chest pain and pulmonary edema.

Intravenous/Intraosseous bolus dosage: 2–4 mg every 5–30 minutes.

Notes: Administer slowly and titrate to effect; may cause hypotension. May cause respiratory depression; be prepared to support ventilations. Naloxone is the reversal agent.

Nitroglycerin

Class: Vasodilator.

Indicated for: Chest pain/ACS.

Intravenous bolus dosage: 12.5–25 µg in D5W or NaCl.

Sublingual dose: 0.3–0.4 mg.

Notes: Most commonly given sublingually as tablet or spray, repeat up to 3 doses at 5 minute intervals. Hypotension may occur. Do not use with Viagra or other phosphodiasterase inhibitors; with severe bradycardia or tachycardia; or in presence of right ventricular (RV) infarction or inferior MI. Do not mix with other drugs.

Sodium Bicarbonate

Class: Buffer.

Indicated for: Acidosis, hyperkalemia.

Intravenous bolus dosage: 1 mEq/kg.

Notes: Not recommended for routine use in cardiac arrest patients. If available, use arterial blood gas analysis to guide bicarbonate therapy.

Vasopressin

Class: Hormone.

Indicated for: Pulseless arrest.

Intravenous/Intraosseous bolus dosage: 40 U IV/IO.

Notes: Only given one time to replace the first or second dose of epinephrine; epinephrine dosing can continue 3–5 minutes after vasopressin is administered. Vasopressin should not replace antiarrhythmics (such as amiodarone). May cause cardiac ischemia and angina. Not recommended for responsive patients with coronary artery disease. ET route discouraged, but can be used if IV/IO access not available.

Verapamil

Class: Calcium channel blocker.

Indicated for: A-Fib/A-flutter, paroxysmal supraventricular tachycardia (PSVT).

Intravenous bolus dosage: 2.5–5 mg over 2–5 minutes.

Notes: Alternative drug after adenosine to terminate PSVT with adequate blood pressure and preserved left ventricular (LV) function can cause peripheral vasodilatation and hypotension. Use with extreme caution in patients receiving oral beta blockers.

GLASGOW COMA SCALE

Definition

Glasgow coma scale (GCS) is a standardized neurological scale that aims to give a reliable, objective way of recording the conscious state of a patient following a traumatic brain injury for initial as well as subsequent assessment.

Purposes

1. Gives an overview of the patient's level of consciousness (LOC).
2. The GCS allows health practitioner to quickly and easily communicate the severity of a patient's head injury in the 1st hours or days after the trauma.
3. The GCS is a good prognostic indicator to identify the patient condition.
4. To assess the level of consciousness in any patient, who has altered sensorium.
5. To track the prognosis of patients, who have been admitted with altered sensorium.

Equipments

- Glasgow coma scale scoring sheet (Table 6.19)
- Pen torch.

Table 6.19: Glasgow coma scale sheet

Activity	Response	Score
Eye opening		
None	Even to supraorbital pressure	1
To pain	Pain from sternum/limb/supraorbital pressure	2
To speech	Non-specific response, not necessarily to command	3
Spontaneous	Eyes open, not necessarily aware	4
Motor response		
None	To any pain; limbs remain flaccid	1
Extension	Shoulder adducted and shoulder and forearm internally rotated	2
Flexor response	Withdrawal response or assumption of hemiplegic posture	3
Withdrawal	Arm withdraws to pain, shoulder abducts	4
Localizes pain	Arm attempts to remove supraorbital/chest pressure	5
Obeys commands	Follows simple commands	6
Verbal response		
None	No verbalization of any type	1
Incomprehensible sound	Moans/groans, no speech	2
Inappropriate	Intelligible, no sustained sentences	3
Confused	Converses but confused, disoriented	4
Oriented	Converses and oriented	5

Contd...

Contd...

Activity	Response	Score
Total score		3–15
Mild head injury 13–15 Moderate head injury 9–12 Severe head injury (coma) 8 or less		

Procedure

Glasgow coma scale procedure is given in Table 6.20.

Table 6.20: Procedure for Glasgow coma scale

Sl No	Action	Rationale
1.	Keep the patient in a comfortable position	To evaluate responses accurately
2.	Score response in the Glasgow coma scale sheet	Grades the level of conscious of the patient

Assisting Procedures

ABDOMINAL PARACENTESIS

Definition

Paracentesis is a procedure to take out fluid that has collected in the abdomen (peritoneal fluid). The fluid is taken out using a long, thin needle put through the abdomen. Paracentesis also may be done to take the fluid out to relieve belly pressure or pain in people with cancer or cirrhosis.

Purposes

1. Find the cause of fluid buildup in the abdomen.
2. Diagnose an infection in the peritoneal fluid.
3. Check for certain types of cancer such as liver cancer.
4. Remove a large amount of fluid that is causing pain or difficulty in breathing or that is affecting how the kidneys or the intestines (bowel) are working.
5. Check for damage after an abdominal injury.

Equipments

- Sterile abdominal paracentesis set
- Sterile dressing pack
- Sterile specimen container
- Tincture benzoin
- Xylocaine injection (2%)
- Disposable needle and syringe
- Sterile gloves
- Tape measure
- Weighing machine
- Disposable plastic apron
- Mask
- Mackintosh
- Appropriate antiseptic solution (Betadine)
- Underpad/Disposable clean pad
- Adhesive plaster
- Clean intravenous (IV) bottle.

Procedure

Procedure of abdominal paracentesis is given in Table 7.1.

Table 7.1: Procedure of abdominal paracentesis

Sl No	Care action	Rationale
1.	Explain the procedure to the patient/patient's relative	Ensure that the patient and the relative understand the procedure, and to get the valid consent
2.	Before starting the procedure, check whether the patient is on anticoagulant therapy	To prevent the complication of bleeding after the procedure
3.	Arrange all the needed articles near the bedside	To prevent unnecessary contamination and easy to perform the procedure
4.	Tell the patient to empty his/her bladder before the procedure	To prevent the puncture of the bladder, while doing the trocar insertion
5.	Place the mackintosh under patient's back and hip	To prevent soiling of the linen
6.	Check abdominal girth and weigh patient before and after the procedure and record the readings	This provides an indication of fluid shift and how much fluid has reaccumulated
7.	Place patient in supine position with head elevated 20°–30°; select and mark a position on the abdominal wall for puncture	Helps for the removal of fluid from the abdomen by gravity
8.	Drape the patient appropriately and expose the abdomen puncture site	To make the patient feel privacy and comfortable
9.	Wear sterile gown, gloves and mask	To prevent the contamination
10.	Use skin preparation solution to cleanse skin over the proposed puncture site and drape to define a sterile field	To prepare sterile environment for the procedure
The following procedure will be done by the doctor; the nurse will assist		
11.	Anesthetize the skin over the proposed puncture site with the Xylocaine drawn up in the 5 cc syringe with the attached 25 gauge needle Anesthetize down to the peritoneum Aspirate periodically; if ascitic fluid returns, withdraw the needle slightly to re-enter tissue before further anesthetic is infiltrated	To prevent the local/systemic infection
12.	Insert the 18 gauge needle/trocar perpendicularly through the anesthetized abdominal wall, and advance until hub of needle is 5 mm to1cm from the skin surface	To prevent injury to the abdominal wall
13.	Ascitic fluid is collected (20–200 mL as per the requirement of therapeutic/diagnostic purpose/both)	If necessary to diagnose the cause of ascitis

Contd...

Contd...

Sl No	Care action	Rationale
14.	Once the fluid is withdrawn, collect it in the appropriate specimen container Once a biopsy is taken, transfer the biopsy specimen into a container with 10%–12% formalin	To preserve tissue status
	Collect sample in the labeled container	To ensure correct identity of the specimen
15.	If for therapeutic purpose, a large volume of fluid has to be drained in the drainage bottle	To promote comfort by reducing the fluid pressure
Nurse's responsibilities		
16.	Check the vital status of the patient (BP*, pulse, respiration, temperature, SpO_2†)	To assess any signs of complication
17.	To change vacuum bottles, as they become full, close the clamp on the tubing gently and remove full bottle, and reinsert into empty bottle; reopen clamp to start fluid flow again	To prevent misplacement of the needle in the abdomen
18.	Once the paracentesis is done, simply remove needle from abdominal wall; place a small pressure dressing on puncture site and instruct the patient to remain supine for 2–4 hours	To arrest leak of abdominal fluid
19.	Comfort patient and replace all equipments used	To make them ready for the next usage
20.	Wash the hands	To prevent the risk of cross infection
21.	Document the procedure in the nurse's record in detail	To maintain accurate records, provide a point of reference in the event of any queries

*BP, blood pressure; †SpO_2, peripheral oxygen saturation.

THORACENTESIS

Definition

Thoracentesis is a procedure to take out fluid that has collected in the pleural cavity of the lungs (plural fluid). The fluid is taken out using a long, thin needle put through the thoracic cavity.

Purposes

1. It is used diagnostically to establish the cause of a pleural effusion.
2. To relieve pneumothorax, hemothorax and pyothorax.
3. Diagnose an infection in the pleural fluid.
4. Remove a large amount of fluid that is causing pain or difficulty in breathing.

Equipments

- Sterile thoracentesis set (trocar and cannula)
- Sterile dressing pack
- A 3–way adopter
- Sterile specimen container
- Drainage bottle
- Tincture benzoin
- Xylocaine injection (2%)
- Disposable needle and syringe
- Sterile gloves
- Disposable plastic apron
- Mask
- Mackintosh
- Appropriate antiseptic solution (Betadine)
- Underpad/Disposable clean pad
- Adhesive plaster.

Procedure

The procedure of thoracentesis is detailed in Table 7.2.

Table 7.2: Procedure for thoracentesis

Sl No	Care action	Rationale
1.	Explain the procedure to the patient	Ensure that the patient understand the procedure and to get the valid consent
2.	Tell the patient to empty his/her bladder before the procedure	To avoid interruption during the procedure
3.	Arrange all the needed articles near the bedside	To prevent unnecessary contamination; and to easily perform the procedure
4.	Place the mackintosh under the patient's back and hip	To prevent the soiling of the linen
5.	Assess the respiratory rate and depth; symmetry of chest on inspiration and expiration; cough and sputum	To obtain the baseline data
6.	Place patient in sitting position with head leaning forward on the cardiac table (Fig. 7.1), lateral decubitus or supine with head elevated 45°; select and mark a position on the chest wall for puncture	Helps for the removal of fluid from the lungs by gravity and increase the intercostal space
7.	Drape the patient appropriately and expose the chest puncture site	To make the patient feel privacy and comfortable
8.	Wear sterile gown, gloves and mask	To prevent the contamination

Contd...

Contd...

SI No	Care action	Rationale
9.	Use skin preparation solution to cleanse skin over the proposed puncture site and drape to define a sterile field	To prepare sterile environment for the procedure
The following procedure will be done by the doctor; the nurse will assist		
10.	Anesthetize the skin over the proposed puncture site with the Xylocaine drawn up in the 5 cc syringe with the attached 25 gauge needle	To prevent local/systemic infection
11.	Insert the 18 gauge needle/trocar through the anesthetized chest wall	To remove the excess fluid in the thoracic cavity
12.	Connect the 3-way adapter with the trocar and collect the required quantity of pleural fluid in the specimen container	To send it to the laboratory
13.	If for therapeutic purpose, a large volume of fluid has to be drained in the drainage bottle	To promote comfort by normal lung function
Nurse's responsibilities		
14.	Check the vital status of the patient (BP*, pulse, respiration, temperature)	To assess any signs of complication
15.	Observe for sudden shortness of breath, tracheal deviation and decreased oxygen saturation	It indicates the complication
16.	Once the thoracentesis is done, simply remove needle from chest wall; place a small pressure dressing on puncture site; instruct the patient to remain supine for 2–4 hours	To arrest leak of abdominal fluid
17.	Remove the mackintosh from the patient side	To make the patient comfortable
18.	Wash and replace the equipments; send the specimen to the laboratory with all patient details	To make them ready for the next usage
19.	Document the procedure and patient parameters (during and after the procedure) in the nurse's record	To maintain accurate records, provide a point of reference in the event of any queries

*BP, blood pressure.

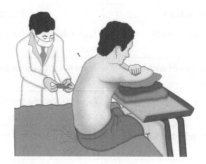

FIGURE 7.1: Position for thoracentesis

ASSISTING WITH LUMBAR PUNCTURE

Definition

A lumbar puncture is a diagnostic and at times therapeutic procedure that is performed in order to collect a sample of cerebrospinal fluid (CSF) for biochemical, microbiological and cytological analysis or very rarely as a treatment (therapeutic lumbar puncture) to relieve increased intracranial pressure (ICP).

Purposes

- To detect possible infection in the CSF
- To measure the pressure in the CSF
- To measure the level of chemicals in the CSF
- To collect CSF for diagnostic purposes
- To detect the spinal subarachnoid block.

Equipments

- A sterile tray [lumbar puncture (LP) set]
- Antiseptic skin cleaning agents (e.g. Betadine or chlorhexidine)
- Local anesthetic (Xylocaine injection)
- Sterile gloves
- Appropriate size of lumbar puncture needles
- Sterile specimen bottles (these bottles should be labeled as bottle 1, 2, 3 with patient's profile)
- Tincture benzoin
- Mackintosh
- Adhesive plaster.

Procedure

The procedure of lumbar puncture assisting is described in Table 7.3.

Table 7.3: Procedure of lumbar puncture

SI No	Care action	Rationale
1.	Explain the procedure to the patient	To get valid consent from the patient/patient's relatives
2.	Ensure that the patient passed urine before starting the procedure	To ensure comfort of the patient
3.	Arrange needed articles near the bedside	Easy to perform the procedure and to prevent unnecessary contamination
4.	Place the mackintosh and draw sheet under the lumbar region	To prevent the soiling of the linen

Contd...

Contd...

Sl No	Care action	Rationale
5.	Position the patient in lateral knee-chest position at the edge of the cot (universal flexion)	To ensure maximum expand of the intervertebral spaces and thus easier access to the subarachnoid space; easy to perform the procedure
6.	Place the pillow under the head and between the knees	To maintain the position and comfort of the patient and avoid sudden movement by the patient
7.	Drape the patient properly	To provide privacy to the patient
8.	Wash the hands	To minimize the infection
9.	Provide sterile gloves to the consultant	To prevent infection, as it is an invasive procedure
10.	Assist the doctor during the procedure	
11.	Communicate the patient in between the procedure and observe the hemodynamic level during the procedure	To give psychological support to the patient and identify the early signs of abnormalities
12.	The following step will be done by the doctors: • Prepare and drape the area after identifying landmarks; use anesthetic agent to anesthetize the skin and the deeper tissues under the insertion site • Insert Quincke needle bevel up through the skin and advance through the deeper tissues between the second and third lumbar vertebrae, and into the subarachnoid space • When CSF* flows, attach the 3-way stopcock and manometer; measure ICP[†] • Collect the suitable specimens of CSF for analysis and filling collection tubes 1–3 with 1–2 mL of CSF each • If intrathecal medication is to be instilled, drug and dose must be checked and administered safely	Anesthetic agent prevents pain sensation
13.	As soon as the needle is removed, assist the doctor in applying tincture benzoin seal or Healex spray and put the dressing on the punctured area	To prevent the leakage of the CSF fluid
14.	Make the patient in supine position without pillow at least for 4–6 hours	To avoid complication such as headache and reduction in CSF pressure
15.	Monitor the vital signs of the patient	To identify the abnormalities immediately
16.	Remove the mackintosh form the patient side	To make the patient comfortable
17.	Wash and replace the equipments	To make them arranged for next usage
18.	Send the specimen to the laboratory with all patient details	To do the analysis
19.	Document the procedure and patient parameters (during and after the procedure) in the nurse's record	For follow-up care of the patient

*CSF, cerebrospinal fluid; [†]ICP, intracranial pressure.

┌─ *Points to Note* ─────────────────────────────────────┐

• Monitor the vital signs of the patient every 15 minutes for the first 1 hour, followed by every ½ hour for 6 hours.
• Encourage fluid intake as per physician order.
• Observe for the complications such as headache, nausea, vomiting and loss of sensation or movement in lower limbs.
• Check puncture site frequently for CSF leakage.

└──┘

LIVER BIOPSY

Definition

Liver biopsy is the removal of small sample of tissue from the liver.

Methods

• Percutaneous needle biopsy
• Laparoscopic or open surgical biopsy.

Purposes

• Investigation of suspected diffuse liver disease
• Investigation of focal liver disease, e.g. hepatoblastoma, sarcoma
• Management of liver transplant.

Contraindications

• A patient who is too unstable or critically ill to undergo this procedure
• Significant coagulopathy
• Significant thrombocytopenia
• Ascites.

Equipments

• A sterile tray (liver biopsy set)
• Antiseptic skin cleaning agents (e.g. Betadine or chlorhexidine)
• Local anesthetic (Xylocaine injection)
• A 5 mL syringe and needle
• Sterile gloves
• Appropriate size of liver biopsy needles
• Sterile specimen bottles (these bottles should be labeled as bottle 1, 2, 3 with patient's profile)
• Tincture benzoin
• Adhesive plaster
• Mackintosh.

Procedure

The procedure of liver biopsy is given in Table 7.4.

Table 7.4: Procedure of liver biopsy

Sl No	Care action	Rationale
1.	Explain the procedure to the patient; obtain informed consent from the patient	To get valid consent from the patient/patient relatives
2.	Make sure whether the patient has completed 6 hours fasting	To prevent gastrointestinal complications during procedure
3.	Obtain and check the coagulation studies and blood glucose levels	To prevent the complication of bleeding and hypoglycemia after the procedure
4.	Arrange all the needed articles near the bedside	Easy to perform the procedure and to prevent unnecessary contamination
5.	Tell the patient to empty his/her bladder before the procedure	To ensure comfort of the patient
6.	Obtain a premedication order and give sedation	To avoid interruption during the procedure
7.	Place the patient in a supine position	To ensure comfort during the procedure
8.	Use skin preparation solution to cleanse skin over the liver biopsy site and drape to define a sterile field	To prevent infection and to make the patient feel privacy and comfortable
9.	Wear sterile gown, gloves and mask	To prevent infection, as it is an invasive procedure
The procedure will be done by the doctor; the nurse will assist		
10.	Anesthetize the skin over the proposed biopsy site with the Xylocaine drawn up in the 5 cc syringe with the attached 25 gauge needle	To prevent the local/systemic infection
11.	Ask the patient to hold the breath and insert the liver biopsy needle through the anesthetized abdominal wall	To prevent injury to the liver tissue
12.	Biopsy is taken as per the requirement	To send it to the lab for histopathological examination
13.	Once the biopsy is taken, place it in the appropriate medium; normally it is a very small amount of sterile normal saline in a sterile specimen container	To prevent the growth of microorganisms
Nurse's responsibilities		
14.	Check the vital status of the patient (blood pressure, pulse, respiration, temperature)	To identify the abnormalities immediately
15.	Once the biopsy is done, simply remove needle from abdominal wall; place several layers of pressure dressing on puncture site Instruct the patient to roll on to the right side and advise him to remain in the same position for 1–2 hours	To prevent bleeding and bile leakage complications

Contd...

Contd...

SI No	Care action	Rationale
16.	Remove the mackintosh from the patient side	To make the patient comfortable
17.	Wash and replace the equipments	To make them arranged for next usage
18.	Send the specimen to the laboratory with all patient details	To do the analysis
19.	Document the procedure and patient parameters (during and after the procedure) in the nurse's record	To maintain accurate records; provide a point of reference in the event of any queries

BONE MARROW ASPIRATION AND BIOPSY

Definition

A bone marrow aspiration involves the removal of a small amount of marrow, the liquid material from the bone. Bone marrow biopsy takes a small sample of bone and bone marrow using a needle.

Purposes

To diagnose the conditions and diseases that can affect our bone marrow, which include:
1. Anemia or a low red blood cell count.
2. Bone marrow diseases such as myelofibrosis or myelodysplastic syndrome.
3. Blood cell conditions such as leukopenia or polycythemia.
4. Cancers of the bone marrow or blood such as leukemias or lymphomas.
5. Hemochromatosis, a genetic disorder in which iron builds in the blood.

Equipments

- A sterile tray (bone marrow aspiration set)
- Antiseptic skin cleaning agents (e.g. Betadine or chlorhexidine)
- Local anesthetic (Xylocaine injection)
- Sterile gloves
- Appropriate size of bone marrow biopsy needle
- Sterile specimen bottles and slides (these bottles should be labeled as bottle 1, 2, 3 with patient's profile)
- Tincture benzoin
- Adhesive plaster
- Mackintosh.

Procedure

Procedure of the bone marrow aspiration and biopsy is detailed in Table 7.5.

Table 7.5: Procedure of the bone marrow aspiration and biopsy

Sl No	Care action	Rationale
1.	Explain the procedure to the patient; explain to client that pain may occur when the bone marrow is aspirated	To get valid consent from the patient/patient's relatives
2.	Arrange all the needed articles near the bedside	Easy to perform the procedure and to prevent unnecessary contamination
3.	Tell the patient to empty his/her bladder before the procedure	To ensure comfort of the patient
4.	Obtain a premedication order and give sedation	To avoid interruption during the procedure
5.	Assist client in maintaining correct position (Fig. 7.2)	To ensure comfort during the procedure
6.	Drape the patient appropriately and expose the bone marrow aspiration site	To make the patient feel privacy and comfortable
7.	Wear sterile gown, gloves and mask	To prevent infection, as it is an invasive procedure
8.	Use skin preparation solution to cleanse skin over the proposed bone marrow aspiration site and drape to define a sterile field	To prevent infection and to make the patient feel privacy and comfortable
The procedure will be done by the doctor; the nurse will assist		
9.	Anesthetize the skin over the proposed puncture site with the Xylocaine drawn up in the 5 cc syringe with the attached 25 gauge needle	To prevent the local/systemic infection
10.	Insert the bone marrow aspiration needle through the anesthetized pelvic wall	To prevent sensation of pain
11.	Bone marrow fluid is aspirated as per the requirement	To send it to the laboratory for investigation
12.	Once the fluid is withdrawn, collect in an appropriate labeled specimen container	To send it to the laboratory
Nurse's responsibilities		
13.	Check the vital status of the patient (BP*, pulse, respiration, temperature, SpO$_2$†)	To identify the abnormalities immediately
14.	Once the bone marrow aspiration is done, simply remove needle from pelvic wall and place a small pressure dressing on puncture site; instruct the patient to remain supine for 2–4 hours	To prevent bleeding
15.	Remove the mackintosh from the patient side	To make the patient comfortable
16.	Wash and replace the equipments	To make them arranged for next usage
17.	Send the specimen to the laboratory with all patient details	To do the analysis
18.	Document the procedure and patient parameters (during and after the procedure) in the nurse's record	To maintain accurate records, provide a point of reference in the event of any queries

*BP, blood pressure; †SpO$_2$, peripheral oxygen saturation.

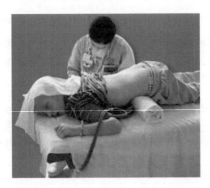

FIGURE 7.2: Position of the patient for bone marrow aspiration and biopsy

KIDNEY BIOPSY

Definition

A biopsy is a procedure performed to remove tissue or cells from the body for examination under a microscope. During a kidney biopsy, tissue samples are removed with a special needle to determine if cancer or other abnormal cells are present, or to determine how well the kidney is working.

Types of Kidney Biopsy

There are two types of kidney biopsies:
1. Needle biopsy: After a local anesthetic is given, the doctor inserts the special biopsy needle into the kidney to obtain a sample. Ultrasound (high-frequency sound waves) or computerized tomography (CT) scan may be used to guide the biopsy needle insertion. Most kidney biopsies are performed using this technique.
2. Open biopsy: After a general anesthetic is given, the doctor makes an incision in the skin and surgically removes a piece of the kidney.

Purposes

- Determine the reason for poor kidney function
- Determine if a tumor in the kidney is malignant (cancerous) or benign
- Evaluate how well the transplanted kidney is working.

Equipments

- A sterile tray (kidney biopsy set)
- Antiseptic skin cleaning agents (e.g. Betadine or chlorhexidine)
- Local anesthetic (Xylocaine injection)
- Sterile gloves
- Appropriate size of renal biopsy needle
- Sterile specimen bottles (these bottles should be labeled as bottle 1, 2, 3 with patient's profile)

- Tincture benzoin
- Adhesive plaster
- Mackintosh.

Procedure

Procedure of kidney biopsy is described in Table 7.6.

Table 7.6: Procedure of kidney biopsy

Sl No	Care action	Rationale
1.	Explain the procedure to the patient; obtain informed consent from the patient	To get valid consent from the patient/patient relatives
2.	Make sure whether the patient has completed 6 hours fasting	To prevent gastrointestinal complications during procedure
3.	Obtain and check the coagulation studies	To prevent the complication of bleeding after the procedure
4.	Arrange all the needed articles near the bedside	Easy to perform the procedure and to prevent unnecessary contamination
5.	Tell the patient to empty his/her bladder before the procedure	To ensure comfort of the patient
6.	Obtain a premedication order and give sedation	To avoid interruption during the procedure
7.	Place the patient in a prone position	To reach the kidney easily
8.	Use skin preparation solution to cleanse skin over the liver biopsy site and drape to define a sterile field	To prevent infection and to make the patient feel privacy and comfortable
9.	Wear sterile gown, gloves and mask	To prevent infection, as it is an invasive procedure
The procedure will be done by the doctor; the nurse will assist		
10.	Anesthetize the skin over the proposed biopsy site with the Xylocaine drawn up in the 5 cc syringe with the attached 25 gauge needle	To prevent the local/systemic infection
11.	Ask the patient to hold the breath and insert the kidney biopsy needle through the anesthetized abdominal wall	To prevent the movement of the diaphragm during the procedure
12.	Biopsy is taken as per the requirement	To send it to the laboratory for histopathological examination
13.	Once the biopsy is taken, place it in the appropriate medium; normally it is a very small amount of sterile normal saline in a sterile specimen container	To prevent the growth of microorganism
Nurse's responsibilities		
14.	Check the vital status of the patient (blood pressure, pulse, respiration, temperature)	To identify the abnormalities immediately

Contd...

Contd...

Sl No	Care action	Rationale
15.	Once the biopsy is done, simply remove needle from abdominal wall; place a several layers of pressure dressing on puncture site and instruct the patient to lie down in a supine position and advise to remain in the same position for 1–2 hours	To prevent bleeding
16.	Remove the mackintosh from the patient side	To make the patient comfortable
17.	Wash and replace the equipments	To make them arranged for next usage
18.	Send the specimen to the laboratory with all patient details	To do the analysis
19.	Observe the urine	To check for bleeding
20.	Document the procedure and patient parameters (during and after the procedure) in the nurse's record	To maintain accurate records, provide a point of reference in the event of any queries

ASSISTING FOR CENTRAL VENOUS CATHETERIZATION

Definition

A central venous catheter (central line, CVC, central venous line or central venous access catheter) is a catheter placed into a large vein in the neck (internal jugular vein), chest (subclavian vein or axillary vein) or groin (femoral vein). It is used to administer medication or fluids, obtain blood sample for the tests (specifically the mixed venous oxygen saturation), and directly obtain cardiovascular measurements such as the central venous pressure (CVP).

Purposes

- Venous access is needed for IV fluids or antibiotics
- For CVP measurement
- For the administration of certain chemotherapeutic drugs or total parenteral nutrition (TPN)
- For hemodialysis or plasmapheresis.

Equipments

- A sterile tray (CVP set)
- Antiseptic skin cleaning agents (e.g. Betadine or chlorhexidine)
- Local anesthetic (Xylocaine injection)
- Sterile gloves
- Appropriate size of central line catheters
- Labeled specimen container
- Tincture benzoin
- Adhesive plaster
- Mackintosh.

Procedure

The procedure of central venous catheterization is given in Table 7.7.

Table 7.7: Procedure of central venous catheterization

Sl No	Care action	Rationale
1.	Explain the procedure to the patient	To get valid consent from the patient/patient's relatives
2.	Ensure that the patient passed urine before starting the procedure	To ensure comfort of the patient
3.	Arrange needed articles near the bedside	Easy to perform the procedure and to prevent unnecessary contamination
4.	Place the mackintosh and draw sheet under the head and neck	To prevent the soiling of the linen
5	Remove the pillow; place the patient in prolonged Trendelenburg position (15°–30° head down) and turn the head in the opposite direction of the insertion site	To ensure easy to identify the visible veins and easy to perform the procedure To reduce the chance of an air embolism
6.	Place a rolled towel or sheet between the shoulder blades and place the arms to the sides of the patient	To make the clavicles more prominent
7.	Wash the hands	To minimize the infection
8.	Provide sterile gloves to the consultant	To prevent infection, as it is an invasive procedure
9.	Assist the doctor during the procedure	
10.	Observe the hemodynamic level during the procedure	To identify the early signs of abnormalities
11.	The following step will be done by the doctors: • Prep and drape the area after identifying landmarks; use anesthetic agent to anesthetize the skin and the deeper tissues under the insertion site • Use 22 gauge needle (seeker needle) on a 3 cc syringe to locate the vein, aspirating as the needle is advanced until a flush of blood returns • Use 18 gauge needle on a 5 cc syringe to follow the path of the seeker needle, aspirating as the needle is advanced; entry into the vein is marked by a flush of blood • Stabilizing the needle with the thumb and forefinger, remove the syringe and immediately occlude the hub of the needle • Thread the J wire into the 18 gauge needle leaving about half of the wire extruding from the needle • Secure the J wire with a fingertip and remove the 18 gauge needle over the exposed, remaining portion of the J wire • Make a small cut in the skin adjacent to the entry site of the J wire using a scalpel, thread the silastic dilator over the wire • Advance the dilator fully into the chest and remove the dilator, while still leaving the J wire in place • Remove the hub from the long central catheter; thread the long central catheter over the wire into the vein	To prevent local and systemic infection and pain

Contd...

Contd...

SI No	Care action	Rationale
	• Leave 5–10 cm of the catheter outside the skin and carefully remove the J wire • Attach intravenous (IV) tubing to the catheter; lower the IV bag below the level of the patient to observe for blood return	
12.	As soon as possible, position the catheter; assist the doctor for suturing the line	To prevent the misplacement of the catheter
13.	Discontinue the Trendelenburg position and make the patient to lying down	To ensure the comfort of the patient
14.	Collect the needed blood sample in the labeled container	For analysis
15.	Monitor the vital signs of the patient	To identify the abnormalities immediately
16.	Remove the mackintosh form the patient side	To make the patient comfortable
17.	Wash and replace the equipments	To make them arranged for next use
18.	Send the specimen to the laboratory with all patient details	To do the analysis
19.	Document the procedure and patient parameters (during and after the procedure) in the nurse's record	To follow-up care for the patient

Points to Note

✦ The rolled towel, which is used for the clavicles position, should not over accentuate this position, since it might move the clavicle closer to the first rib, making cannulation of the subclavian vein more difficult.

ASSISTING WITH ENDOTRACHEAL INTUBATION

Definition

Endotracheal intubation is a medical procedure in which a tube is placed into the windpipe (trachea) through the mouth or the nose. In most emergency situations, it is placed through the mouth.

Purposes

- Protection from gastric aspiration and secretions
- Access and maintenance in difficult airway and difficult surgical positions/ procedures
- Provide positive pressure ventilation can be done for shorter periods with a mask or Oxylog
- Oxygenation to provide a controlled concentration of oxygen up to 100%, also provides for complete scavenging
- Secretions facilitates removal of secretions via suctioning.

Equipments

- Cardiac monitor
- Pulse oximeter
- Laryngoscope (check light)
- Adult blades No. 3 and No. 4
- Magill forceps
- Lubricant
- Connector: Body/Elbow (may be required)
- Flexible introducer
- Syringe 10 mL
- Clamp
- Appropriate size of airway
- Tape for ties
- Licorice stick
- Appropriate endotracheal tubes:
  - Size of tube is dependent on size of patient
  - The 'universally accepted' size is 7.5 mm for an unknown victim
  - Men are comparatively taller, therefore 8.0 mm tube may be appropriate
  - Females are usually smaller, therefore 7.0 mm tube may be appropriate.
- Means of inflating lungs: Air Viva, anesthetic machine
- Suction apparatus with Yankauer nozzle and endotracheal suction catheter
- Container for used laryngoscope, face mask
- Sterile gloves
- Mask
- Mackintosh and drawsheet.

Procedure

The procedure of endotracheal intubation is given in Table 7.8.

Table 7.8: Procedure of endotracheal intubation

Sl No	Care action	Rationale
1.	Explain the procedure to the patient's relatives	To get valid consent from the patient's relatives
2.	Determine whether the patient requires endotracheal (ET) intubation	For baseline assessment
3.	Assemble required equipment near the bedside	To prevent unnecessary contamination
4.	Place the mackintosh and draw sheet under the head and neck	To prevent the soiling of the linen
5.	If patient is in bed, remove head end rail; make sure there is adequate space between the back of bed and wall	To allow easy access to patient's head in order to facilitate intubation

Contd...

Contd...

SI No	Care action	Rationale
6.	Position of the patient: • Supine • Pillow under head • Flexion of the neck	To complete direct visualization of the vocal cords
7.	Open the mouth by separating the lips and pulling on the upper jaw with the index finger	To get direct visualization of the vocal cords
8.	Check for any loose teeth or dentures; if found, remove with Magill forceps	To prevent the obstruction during the procedure
9.	Suction the patient (no longer than 12 second)	To maintain a patent airway
10.	Oxygenate patient for 1 minute with 100% oxygen using the Ambu bag	To prevent hypoxia
11.	Provide the laryngoscope to the doctor (switched on)	To visualize the larynx and the epiglottis
12.	Hold the laryngoscope in the left hand and insert the laryngoscope into the mouth with blade directed to the right tonsils; once the right tonsil is reached, sweep the blade to the midline, keeping the tongue on the left	To insert the ET tube easily and visualize the larynx and the epiglottis clearly
13.	Advance the laryngoscope blade till it reaches the angle between the base of the tongue and the epiglottis Insert the ET tube through the cords only till the cuff is just below the cords First inflate the ET tube cuff and check for any air leak; if no leak is present, deflate the ET tube cuff Inflate the cuff of the ET tube with 10 mL of air	To prevent leakage of the tube and misplacement of the tube
14.	Auscultate, listen/feel for airflow through the tube and observe for bilateral chest movements	To identify any displacement of the tube
15.	Connect the Ambu bag with oxygen to the ET tube and continue bagging	To prevent hypoxia
16.	Fix the ET tube in position by adhesive strips, securing the ET tube over the bridge of the nose/cheek	To prevent dislodgement of the tube
17.	Connect to ventilator	To prevent hypoxia
18.	Document the procedure in the nurse's record in detail	To maintain accurate records, provide a point of reference in the event of any queries

APPLICATION OF SKIN TRACTION

Definition

Skin traction is the traction on a body part maintained by an apparatus affixed by dressings to the body surface. Skin traction requires pressure on the skin to maintain the pulling force across the bone.

Purposes

- Helps to reduce the fracture
- Helps to reduce the muscle spasm
- To keep the suitable alignment of an injured part
- Helps to prevent the deformities
- Helps to stretch the muscles and obtain more working space within the joint prior to the total hip replacement surgery.

Equipments

- Cotton roll
- Roller bandages
- Spreader
- Rope
- Pulley
- Required weight
- Bed blocks
- Appropriate size of adhesive plaster
- Tincture benzoin
- Disposable gloves
- Kidney tray
- Mackintosh and draw sheet.

Procedure

The skin traction procedure is detailed in Table 7.9.

Table 7.9: Procedure of skin traction

Sl No	Care action	Rationale
1.	Explain the procedure to the patient	To ensure that the patient should understand the procedure and give valid consent
2.	Arrange all the needed articles near the patient bedside	Easy to perform the procedure and minimize unnecessary contamination
3.	Wash the hands	To reduce the cross infection
4.	Place the mackintosh and draw sheet under the limb area	To prevent the soiling of the linen
5.	Wear gloves and clean the area with soap and water, and dry it	To reduce the infection and contamination
6.	Collect the history from the patient whether he/she have any adhesive tape allergy before applying; measure the appropriate length of adhesive strapping and place it on a level surface with the adhesive side up	Helps to support the part entirely

Contd...

Contd...

SI No	Care action	Rationale
7.	Place a square wooden spreader of about 7.5 cm (with a central hole) in the middle of the adhesive strapping	Helps to maintain the traction position correctly
8.	Gently elevate the limb off the bed, while applying longitudinal traction; apply the strapping to the medial and lateral sides of the limb, allowing the spreader to project 15 cm below the sole of the foot	Helps to place the traction downward
9.	Pad bony areas with felt or cotton wool; wrap the crepe or ordinary gauze bandage firmly over the strapping	Helps to support the strapping
10.	Elevate the end of the bed and attach a traction cord through the spreader with the required weight; the weight should not exceed 5 kg	To prevent the compartment syndrome
11.	Make the patient comfortable	To ensure the comfort of the patient
12.	Clean and replace the equipments properly	To make them ready for next use
13.	Remove the gloves, discard as per institutional policy and wash the hands	To minimize the contamination
14.	Document the procedure in the nurse's record	To do the follow-up care for the patient

> **Points to Note**
>
> Check the whole system of traction for its work order:
> - The rope and pulley are in straight alignment.
> - The weight is freely hanging without touching the bed or floor.
> - The force of pull is felt by the patient.
> - The toes are freely movable.

APPLICATION OF PELVIC TRACTION

Definition

Pelvic traction is applied to the lower spine with a belt around the waist.

Purposes

- The conservative management for prolapsed lumbar intervertebral disk
- To stretch muscle and ligaments
- To separate vertebral bodies in the spine.

Equipments

- Pelvic unit and belt
- Spreader
- Rope
- Required weight
- Bed locks.

Procedure

The application procedure of pelvic traction is detailed in Table 7.10.

Table 7.10: Procedure of pelvic traction

Sl No	Care action	Rationale
1.	Explain the procedure to the patient	To ensure that the patient should understand the importance of the procedure and give valid consent
2.	Arrange all the needed articles near the patient bedside	Easy to perform the procedure and minimize unnecessary contamination
3.	Wash the hands	To reduce the cross infection
4.	Wear gloves	To reduce the cross infection
5.	Place the patient in supine position and remove the pillow from the head end	To make the patient comfortable and easy to perform the procedure
6.	Spread the pelvic belt underneath the lumbar region; take the belt to the front on the abdomen and secure it tightly	To maintain the position and to apply the traction easily
7.	Elevate the foot end of the bed, as needed	Helps to hang the weight appropriately
8.	Connect the belt to spreader and pass the rope through the pulley	Helps to maintain the position by placing the weight
9.	Apply the weight as per doctor's order and provide a small pillow under the knee	Helps to support the knee joint
10.	Make the patient comfortable	To ensure the comfort of the patient
11.	Wash and replace the articles	To make them ready for next usage
12.	Remove the gloves, discard as per institutional policy and wash the hands	To minimize the contamination
13.	Document the procedure in the nurse's record	To do the follow-up care for the patient

Points to Note

◆ Clear instruction should be given to the patient that, not to fold the lower limbs or turn while on traction for too long period.

ASSISTING FOR SKULL TRACTION

Definition

Use skull traction for traumatic and infectious conditions in the cervical spine. Apply it to the skin using head halter traction, or to the skull bones using Gardner-Wells tongs or a halo device.

Purposes

- To regain normal length and alignment of involved bone
- To reduce the fracture and immobilize a fractured bone.

Equipments

- Spreader
- Rope
- Pulley
- Required weight
- Dressing pack
- Appropriate size of adhesive plaster
- Tincture benzoin
- Disposable gloves
- Kidney tray
- Mackintosh
- Appropriate skull traction set
- Razor
- Antiseptic solution
- Disposable apron.

Procedure

The assisting procedure of skull traction application is given in Table 7.11.

Table 7.11: Procedure of skull traction

SI No	Care action	Rationale
1.	Explain the procedure to the patient/patient's relatives	To ensure that the patient should understand the procedure and give valid consent
2.	Arrange all the needed articles near the patient bedside	Easy to perform the procedure and minimize unnecessary contamination
3.	Wash the hands	To reduce the cross infection
4.	Place the mackintosh and draw sheet under the head	To prevent the soiling of the linen
5.	**Gardner-Wells tongs technique** Place the pins below the brim of the skull in line with the external auditory meatus, 2–3 cm above the top of the pinna	Helps to place the traction in accurate place
6.	Prepare the patient's scalp by shaving the hair and washing the skin with an antiseptic solution	To minimize the infection
7.	Position the tongs correctly and mark the pin entrance points	To perform hole accurately
8.	Infiltrate the pin sites with 1% lidocaine and make stab wounds through the skin and down to the bone; insert the pins by alternately tightening one side and then the other, until 3.6 kg of torque is applied and determine the tightness with a special torque screwdriver or by tightening the pins using two fingers only—to grip the screwdriver	To prevent mobility and misplacement traction

Contd...

Contd...

Sl No	Care action	Rationale
9.	Dress the wounds with sterile gauze and apply the appropriate traction weight; tighten the pins once again on the following day, then leave those alone unless they are loose	To minimize the unnecessary contamination
10.	**Halo traction technique** Determine the ring size by measuring the head circumference or by trial; the clearance should be 1–2 cm at all points	Helps to fit the traction accurately
11.	Cautiously place the patient's head off the end of the bed and hold it with a special head holder or with an assistant; the halo should be just above the eyebrows and ears	Easy to place the traction correctly
12.	Use two pins posterolaterally and two in the lateral third of the forehead; these may be placed as far back as the hairline for cosmetic reasons, but should be anterior to the temporal muscle	Helps to prevent the mobility
13.	Advance the pins to finger tightness while keeping the halo placement symmetrical; ask the patient to keep his/her eyes closed during the procedure	To avoid pulling the skin upward and preventing eye closure, once the pins are tight
14.	Next, tighten the pins sequentially across the diagonals; if a torque screwdriver is available, tighten the screws to 34–45 cm/kg; if not, twist the screws tight by holding the screwdriver with two fingers	To place the traction accurately
15.	Tighten the screws once after 1–2 days and thereafter, only if loose; traction can now be applied or the patient can be placed in a halo jacket	To prevent the mobility
16.	Make the patient comfortable	To ensure the comfort of the patient
17.	Clean and replace the equipments properly	To make them ready for next use
18.	Remove the gloves, discard as per institutional policy and wash the hands	To minimize the contamination
19.	Document the procedure in the nurse's record	To do the follow-up care for the patient

ASSISTING FOR SKELETAL TRACTION

Definition

Apply skeletal traction by placing a metal pin through the metaphyseal portion of the bone and apply weight to the pin.

Purposes

- Helps to reduce overlying space of fractured bones
- Helps to maintain the reduction of the fracture
- Helps to reduce muscle spasms, friction between bony surfaces and pain
- Helps to separate bone surface.

Equipments

- Dressing pack
- Rope
- Pulley
- Required weight
- Bed blocks
- Appropriate size of sterile skeletal traction set
- Disposable gloves
- Kidney tray
- Mackintosh
- Xylocaine injection (2%)
- Disposable syringe.

Procedure

The assisting procedure for skeletal traction given in Table 7.12.

Table 7.12: Assisting procedure for skeletal traction

Sl No	Care action	Rationale
1.	Explain the procedure to the patient	To ensure that the patient should understand the procedure and give valid consent
2.	Arrange all the needed articles near the patient bedside	Easy to perform the procedure and minimize unnecessary contamination
3.	Place the mackintosh and draw sheet under the limb area	To prevent the soiling of the linen
4.	Wash the hands	To reduce the cross infection
5.	Cover the surrounding area with sterile drapes; infiltrate the skin and soft tissues down to the bone with 2% Xylocaine both the entrance and exit sides	To prepare the sterile environment and to minimize the contamination
6.	Make a small stab incision in the skin and introduce the pin through the incision horizontally and at right angles to the long axis of the limb; proceed until the point of the pin strikes the underlying bone	Helps to make the pathway for the hand drill
7.	Insert the pins with a T-handle or hand drill; advance the pin until it stretches the skin of the opposite side and make a small release incision over its point	Helps to apply the traction equally in the area

Contd...

Contd...

Sl No	Care action	Rationale
8.	Dressing the skin wounds separately with sterile gauze attach a stirrup to the pin, cover the pin ends with guards and apply traction	To minimize the contamination
9.	Apply countertraction by elevating the appropriate end of the bed or by placing a splint against the root of the limb	To prevent the mobility
10.	Make the patient comfortable	To ensure the comfort of the patient
11.	Clean and replace the equipments properly	To make them ready for next use
12.	Remove the gloves, discard as per institutional policy and wash the hands	To minimize the contamination
13.	Document the procedure in the nurse's record	To do the follow-up care for the patient

ASSISTING FOR PAPANICOLAOU TEST

Definition

Papanicolaou test or the Pap smear is a gynecological examination procedure, where the cells or tissues collected from the cervix are examined under a microscope.

Purposes

- To detect the presence of certain abnormality such as cancer of the cervix
- Helps to confirm or rule out the abnormal changes in the cells and tissues that occur in case of cancer.

Equipments

- Dressing tray
- Vaginal speculum
- Wooden spatula or cotton swab
- Slide: One slide with office clips
- Preservatives (alcohol 50 mL)
- Permanent marker
- Spotlight
- Mackintosh and draw sheet
- Antiseptic solution
- Kidney tray.

Procedure

Pap smear test procedure is given in Table 7.13.

Table 7.13: Procedure of Pap smear

SI No	Care action	Rationale
1.	Explain the procedure to the patient	To get valid consent from the patient/patient's relatives
2.	Ensure that the patient passed urine before starting the procedure	To ensure comfort of the patient
3.	Arrange needed articles near the bedside	Easy to perform the procedure and to prevent unnecessary contamination
4.	Place the mackintosh and draw sheet under the buttocks	To prevent the soiling of the linen
5.	Wash the hands	To reduce the cross-contamination
6.	Place the patient in lithotomy position	Easy to visualize the part and perform the procedure
7.	Drape the patient appropriately	To ensure the privacy for the patient
8.	Assist the doctor during the procedure	
9.	Communicate with patient in between the procedure	To give psychological support to the patient
10.	Collect the specimen in labeled container	For analysis
11.	Make the patient comfortable	To ensure the comfort of the patient
12.	Check the vitals of the patient	Helps to identify any subnormal parameter early
13.	Send the specimen to the laboratory	To do the analysis
14.	Wash and replace the equipments	To make them arrange for the next use
15.	Document the procedure and patient parameters (during and after the procedure) in the nurse's record	To follow-up care for the patient

ASSISTING FOR DILATATION AND CURETTAGE

Definition

Dilatation and curettage is a surgical procedure usually performed under local anesthesia in which the cervix is dilated and the endometrial lining of the uterus is scraped with a curette; it is performed to obtain tissue samples, to stop prolonged bleeding, to remove small tumors, to remove fragments of placenta after childbirth or as a method of abortion.

Purposes

1. To identify the causes of dysfunctional uterine bleeding.
2. To obtain the specimen for biopsy with incomplete abortion, hydatidiform mole, inevitable abortion, dysfunctional uterine bleeding, polyps, misplaced intrauterine contraceptive devices, medical termination of pregnancy.

Equipments

- Big dressing tray or dressing bin
- Small towel
- Posterior vaginal wall Sims' speculum
- Vulsellum
- Uterine sound
- Graduated cervical canal dilators (Hegar's dilator)
- Ovum forceps
- Anterior vaginal wall retractor
- Uterine curette
- Thumb forceps
- Sedative as per doctor's order
- Disposable syringe
- A sterile gown
- Sterile hand towels
- Sterile leggings
- Sterile big towel
- Antiseptic solution, spirit swab.

Procedure

Procedure of dilatation and curettage is described in Table 7.14.

Table 7.14: Procedure of dilatation and curettage

Sl No	Care action	Rationale
1.	Explain the procedure to the patient and patient's relatives	To get valid consent from the patient/patient's relatives
2.	Wash the hands	To reduce the infection
The following steps will be performed by the doctor		
3.	After adequate anesthesia has been administered, the patient's legs are parted and flexed, and comfortably put up on a stirrup in a position that is called 'lithotomy' position	This ensures a good view of the genital area for the surgeon or gynecologist to operate
4.	The vagina and cervix are scrubbed with an antibacterial solution; that maybe iodine or chlorhexidine	To reduce the infection
5.	The cervix is visualized using speculum Lights are adjusted to visualize the cervix, so that its upper lip can be grasped with 'vulsellum'	Helps to stabilize and bringing the cervix down toward the vaginal opening to ease with rest of the procedure
6.	Dilatation is next done using sequential metal, round, tapered dilators and the opening to the uterus is gradually widened to about the size of a large pencil	Easy to visualize and perform the procedure
7.	The spoon-like curette is inserted into the uterine cavity and is used to gently scrape the lining of the uterus	Helps to remove the tissue or part from the uterus

Contd...

Contd...

Sl No	Care action	Rationale
8.	When the surgeon feels the gritty layer of cells just above the muscle of the uterus, then he/she knows that the scraping has gone deep enough to sample the tissue adequately	If any part remained inside, it may cause the infection
9.	This scraping is done throughout the uterus and the tissue that is removed, sent to a pathologist for microscopic examination	To do the analysis and identify any abnormalities
10.	Depending on the indication for the procedure, the surgeon terminates the procedure once he/she feels that enough tissue has been obtained or that the entire cavity has been sampled or scrapped	For therapeutic purposes
11.	Collect the specimen in an appropriate labeled sample container if needed	To do the analysis
12.	Monitor the patient's hemodynamic level or any signs of bleeding	To identify the complications or abnormalities in an early stage
13.	Transfer the patient to the bed and make comfortable	To ensure the comfort of the patient
14.	Send the specimen to the laboratory	To do the analysis
15.	Wash and replace the articles	To make them ready for next usage
16.	Document the procedure and patient's parameters (during and after the procedure) in the nurse's record	To follow-up care for the patient

ASSISTING FOR SUPRAPUBIC CATHETERIZATION

Definition

A urinary bladder catheter inserted through the skin about 1 inch above the symphysis pubis. It is inserted under a general or local anesthetic. It is used for closed drainage and may be left in place for a time, sutured to the abdominal skin.

Purposes

1. To lower the incidence of urinary tract infection.
2. To turn away the flow of urine from the urethra in case of traumatic and pathological condition of the bladder and urethra is observed.
3. After gynecological surgery, wherein bladder dysfunction is likely to occur.

Equipments

A tray containing:
- Antiseptic solution
- Sterile catheterization set
- Gloves
- Disposable syringe and needle

- Water for injection or sterile water
- Sterile suturing set
- Xylocaine injection (2%)
- Appropriate size of Foley catheter and urosac set
- Sterile specimen container (if needed)
- Mackintosh and draw sheet
- Kidney tray
- Measuring jar
- Adhesive tape and scissors.

Procedure

Procedure of suprapubic catheterization is detailed in Table 7.15.

Table 7.15: Procedure of suprapubic catheterization

SI No	Care action	Rationale
1.	Explain the procedure to the patient	To get valid consent from the patient/ patient's relatives
2.	Arrange needed articles near the bedside	Easy to perform the procedure and to prevent unnecessary contamination
3.	Shave the suprapubic area if the patient is hairy	To avoid the entry of the hair, while doing the insertion
4.	Place the mackintosh and draw sheet under the back and buttocks	To prevent the soiling of the linen
5.	Place the patient in lying down position	Easy to perform the procedure
6.	Drape the patient appropriately	To provide privacy to the patient
7.	Wash the hands	To minimize the infection
8.	Provide sterile gloves to the consultant	To prevent infection, as it is an invasive procedure
9.	Assist the doctor during the procedure	
10.	Communicate the patient in between the procedure and observe the hemodynamic level during the procedure	To give psychological support to the patient and identify the early signs of abnormalities
11.	The following step will be done by the doctors: • Provide adequate parenteral analgesia with or without sedation • Clean the lower abdominal wall by applying an antiseptic solution from the pubis to the umbilicus; repeat the application of the antiseptic solution more than two times and allow the area to dry • Apply sterile drapes and verify the insertion site by palpating the anatomic landmark • Fill the 10 mL syringe with a local anesthetic agent and use the 25 gauge needle to raise a skin at the insertion site	To prevent local and systemic infection and pain

Contd...

Contd...

SI No	Care action	Rationale
	• Advance the needle through the skin, subcutaneous tissue, rectus sheath and retropubic space, while alternating injection and aspiration, until urine enters the syringe; note the direction and depth required to enter the bladder • By using No. 11 blade, make a 4-mm stab incision at the insertion site with the blade facing inferiorly • Insert the needle obturator into the Malecot catheter and lock it into the port by twisting it, so that the needle tip projects 2.5 mm from the distal end of the catheter • Connect the 60 mL syringe to the port of the needle obturator • Place the tip of the catheter-obturator unit into the skin incision and direct it caudally and at a 20°–30° angle from true vertical toward the patient's legs • The practitioner's non-dominant hand should be placed on the lower abdominal wall, and the unit should be stabilized between the thumb and index fingers • The dominant hand should be used to advance the unit, while aspirating, until urine enters the syringe • Once urine enters the syringe, advance the unit 3–4 additional centimeters into the bladder • While securing the unit with the non-dominant hand, unscrew the obturator from the catheter • Advance the catheter approximately 5 additional centimeters over the obturator and then completely withdraw the obturator needle • Connect the extension tubing to the catheter and connect the tubing to a urinometer or a leg bag • Gently withdraw the catheter to lodge the wings against the bladder wall • Apply drain dressings around the catheter at the insertion site • Tape the catheter to the skin (leaving a mesentery between the skin and catheter) or stitch the catheter to the skin	
12.	Collect the specimen in a labeled container if needed	For analysis
13.	Make the patient in comfortable position	To ensure the patient's comfort
14.	Monitor the vital signs of the patient	To identify the abnormalities immediately
15.	Remove the mackintosh form the patient side	To make the patient comfortable
16.	Wash and replace the equipments	To make them ready for the next use
17.	Send the specimen to the laboratory with all patient details	To do the analysis
18.	Document the procedure and patient parameters (during and after the procedure) in the nurse's record	To follow-up care for the patient

---

Points to Note

* To observe for hematuria, bladder or abdominal distension.
* Check for kinks and patency of the tubings.
* Instruct the patient to avoid tension on the catheter site.

Infection Control Procedures

HAND HYGIENE

Definition

The art of cleansing the hands with water or other liquid, with or without the inclusion of soap or other detergent, for the purpose of removing soil, dirt or microorganism.

Standard Handwashing Procedure

According to Occupational Safety Health Administration (OSHA) standards regarding bloodborne pathogens, handwashing should be performed, at a minimum:
- Before and after every patient contact
- After removing gloves and other protective wear
- After handling blood or other body fluids
- When visibly contaminated with blood or tissues
- Before leaving the patient area
- Before and after eating, applying makeup, using the bathroom
- Handling contact lenses, handling equipment.

Purposes
- To remove visible soiling from hands
- To prevent transfer of bacteria from the home to the hospital
- To prevent transfer of bacteria from the hospital to the home
- Preventing the risk of cross infection
- Protecting the patients, visitors, healthcare workers from healthcare-associated infection (HAI)
- Importance of handwashing to reduce nosocomial infections
- Reduces spread of disease from patient-to-patient
- Reduces spread of disease from patient to healthcare professional
- Reduces spread of disease from healthcare professional to patient
- Reduces spread of disease from healthcare professional to other healthcare professionals
- Reduce spread of disease to visitors in the healthcare facility.

Procedure

Step 1: Palm-to-palm (Fig. 8.1A).

Step 2: Right palm over left dorsum and left palm over right dorsum (Fig. 8.1B).

Step 3: Palm-to-palm fingers interlocked (Fig. 8.1C).

Step 4: Back of fingers to opposing palms with fingers interlocked (Fig. 8.1D).
Step 5: Rotational rubbing of right thumb clasped in left palm and vice versa (Fig. 8.1E).

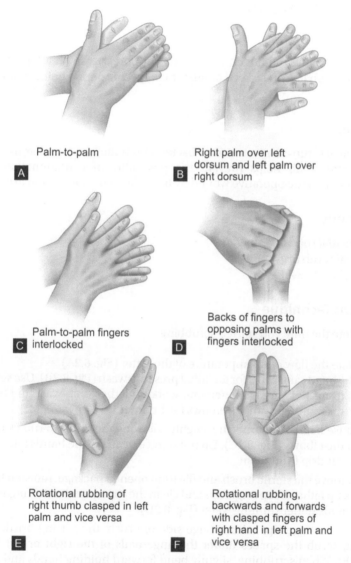

FIGURES 8.1A to F: Procedure of handwashing

Step 6: Rotational rubbing back and forwards with clasped fingers of right hand in left palm and vice versa (Fig. 8.1F).

Points to Note

- Keep short nails and pay attention to them when washing hands.
- Avoid wearing rings.
- Do not wear artificial nails, nail polish.
- Remove wrist watches, bracelets, bangles, roll up long sleeves.

SURGICAL SCRUBBING

Definition

The act of washing the fingernails, hands and forearms with a bactericidal soap or solution in a prescribed manner for a specific period before a surgical procedure.

Purposes

1. Surgical scrub is the removal of bacteria from the hands and arms.
2. Surgical scrub helps prevent the possibility of contamination and infection of the operative wound by bacteria on the hands and arms.

Equipments

- Germicidal soap or detergent
- Surgical scrub brush
- Sterile hand towel.

Scrub Up Technique

Step 1: Note the time you started scrubbing.
Step 2:
- Regulate the flow and temperature of the water (Fig. 8.2A)
- Wet the hands and arms for an initial prescrub wash (Fig. 8.2B). Use several drops (5 mL) of surgical detergent, work up lather then wash the hands and arms thoroughly to the elbows for 1 minute.

Step 3: Rinse hands and arms thoroughly, allowing the water to run from the hands to the elbows (Fig. 8.2C). Do not retrace or shake the hands and arms, let the water drip from them.

Step 4: Remove the sterile brush and file from opened package, moisten brush and work up lather. Soap fingertips and clean the spaces under the fingernails of both hands under running water (Fig. 8.2D).

Step 5: Lather fingertips with sponge side of brush, then using bristle side of brush, scrub the spaces under the fingernails of the right or left hand (Fig. 8.2E). When scrubbing, slightly bend forward holding hands and arms above the elbow, and keep arms away from the body.

Step 6: Lather fingers (Fig. 8.2F); wash on all four sides of each finger. Only nails should be brushed as brushing of other areas has been shown to be damaging to the skin surface causing abrasions.

Step 7: Begin with the thumb or little finger on the right or left hand. Wash one hand and arm completely before moving on to the other hand and arm:
1. Lather palm, back of hand, heel of hand and space between thumb, and index finger washing each surface. Move up the forearm, lather then wash to the elbow (subsequent washes should encompass two thirds of the forearm only).
2. Repeat for the other arm. Discard brush and rinse hands and arms without retracing. Allow the water to drip from elbows before approaching gown pack.

Step 8: Slightly bend forward, pick up a hand towel from the top of the gown pack and step back from the table:
1. Grasp the towel and open it; do not allow the towel to touch any unsterile object or unsterile parts of the body.
2. Hold hands and arms higher than the elbows, and keep arms away from the body (Fig. 8.2G).

Step 9: Holding one end of the towel with one hand, dry the other hand and arm with a blotting, rotating motion (Fig. 8.2H).

Step 10: Work from fingertips to the elbow (Fig. 8.2I); do not retrace any area. Dry all sides of the fingers, the forearm and the arms thoroughly (Fig. 8.2J).

Step 11: Grasp the other end of the towel, dry the other hand and arm in the same manner as above.

Step 12: Discard the towel into an appropriate receptacle.

Points to Note
- Rinse as often as possible using one direction only. Start from the hand going to the arm, taking care not to touch the faucet and the sink.
- A person with cut or burn should not scrub because of the high bacterial count.
- The hands and arms can never be rendered sterile no matter how long or how strong the antiseptics.
- Surgical scrub is most effective when firm motion is applied. Short horizontal or circular stroke could be used.
- Use an sufficient supply of antiseptics.
- Since the hands are to be cleaner than any other area, after the initial hand wash, they are held higher than the elbows, during the rest of the procedure to prevent water from running back the scrubbed hands.

Preparation before doing surgical scrub
- Attend to your personal needs.
- Adjusts your cap and mask properly. The hair should be confined inside the cap. The mask should cover the nose, mouth, cheek and chin.
- Roll up sleeves of the uniform 3 inches above the elbow if sleeves are long.
- Check on the liquid soap and brush dispenser.
- Remove your jewelry.
- Check on your fingernails. They must be kept clean and short to reduce the bacteria count and to prevent the puncturing or tearing of gloves.

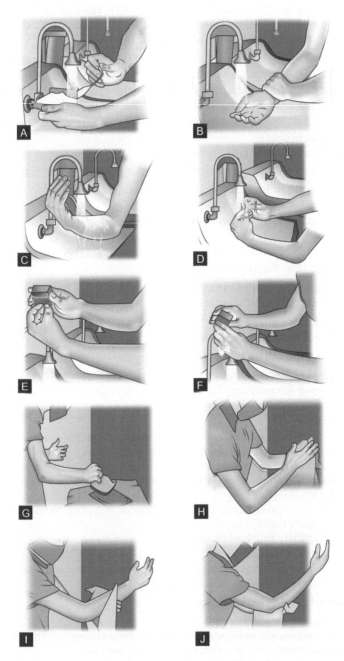

FIGURES 8.2A to J: Scrub up technique. **A.** Regulate the flow and temperature of water; **B.** Prescrub wash; **C.** Allow the water to run from hands to elbow; **D.** Cleaning the finger nails; **E.** Later fingertips with brush; **F.** Cleaning the nails with brush; **G.** Grasping the towel from the gown pack; **H.** Drying the hand with the towel; **I.** Dry the hands from finger tips to elbow; **J.** Dry all sides of the hands and arm.

GOWNING

Definition

Wearing of sterile gown over theater clothing, before assisting surgical patient.

Purpose

The sterile gown is worn in order to permit the wearer to come within the sterile field and carry out sterile technique during an operative procedure.

Equipments

- Gown
- Surgical towel.

Technique

Step 1: With one hand, pick up the entire folded gown from the wrapper by grasping the gown through all layers, being careful to touch only the inside top layer, which is exposed. Step back from the trolley/shelf (Fig. 8.3A).

Step 2: Hold the gown in the manner shown in Figure 8.3B near the gown's neck and allow it to unfold being careful that it does not touch either the body or other unsterile objects. Grasp the inside shoulder seams and open the gown with the armholes facing.

Step 3: Slide arms part way into the sleeves of the gown keeping hands at shoulder level away from the body (Fig. 8.3C).

Step 4: Slide arms further into the gown sleeves and when the fingertips are level with the proximal edge of the cuff, grasp the inside seam at the juncture of gown sleeve and cuff using thumb and index finger (Fig. 8.3D). Be careful that no part of the hand protrudes from the sleeve cuff.

Step 5: The circulating person should assist at this point to position, the gown over the shoulders by grasping the inside surface of the gown at the shoulder joint. They can then adjust the gown over the scrub person's shoulders. The circulating person's hands are only in contact with the inside surface of the gown (Fig. 8.3E).

Step 6: The circulating person then prepares to secure the gown, the neck and back may be secured with a Velcro tab or ties. The circulating person then ties the gown at waist level at the back. This technique prevents the contaminated surfaces at the back of the gown from coming into contact with the front of the gown (Fig. 8.3F).

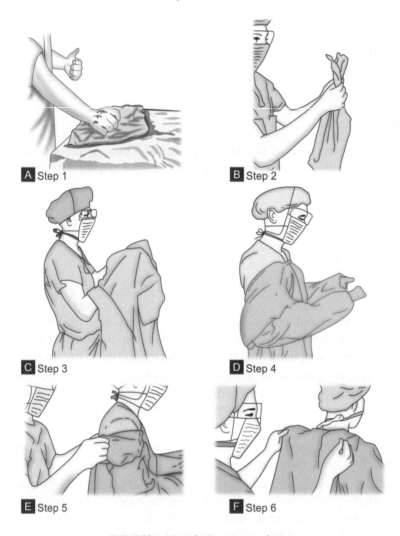

A Step 1 B Step 2 C Step 3 D Step 4 E Step 5 F Step 6

FIGURES 8.3A to F: Gowning technique

Points to Note

- This is done after the surgical scrub.
- Use an oscillating motion pat dry in drying the hands and arms. Start from the hand going to the arms.
- Do not dry hand then arms and return to the same hand.
- In drying the hand and arms, a towel could be used. If a towel is used, dry one hand and arm on one end of the towel and use the opposite end to dry the other hand and arm.
- In serving the gown, do not turn your back on the sterile field to prevent contamination.
- In picking the gown from a sterile linen pack, be careful not to touch any other articles in the pack with.

MASKING

Definition

Wearing a disposable mask over nose and mouth.

Purpose

- To prevent dispersal of droplet from wearer to environment and patient.

Equipment

Disposable or clean mask.

Procedure

To Wear the Mask

- Wash hands
- Hold mask by top two strings or loop, keeping top edge above bridge of nose (Fig. 8.4A)
- Tie both string at the top of back of head firmly above ears (Fig. 8.4B)
- Tie two lower strings snugly at the back of neck (Fig. 8.4C)
- Gently press nose clip of the disposable mask for a snug fit (Fig. 8.4D)
- Change surgical mask when contaminated (Fig. 8.4E)
- Dispose the mask after use (Fig. 8.4F).

To Remove the Mask

- Wash hand
- Untie lower strings first, then top once and pull mask away from face
- Hold mask by string and discard into appropriate receptacle.

GLOVING TECHNIQUE

Gloving is done after the gowning technique.

Purpose

Gloves are worn to complete the sterile dress in order that the one, who wears them may handle sterile equipment.

Technique

Step 1: Open the inner package containing the gloves and pick up one glove by the folded cuff edge with the sleeve-covered hand (Fig. 8.5A).

Step 2: Place the glove on the opposite gown sleeve palm down, with the glove fingers pointing toward the shoulder. The palm of the hand inside the gown sleeve must be facing upward toward the palm of the glove (Figs 8.5B and C).

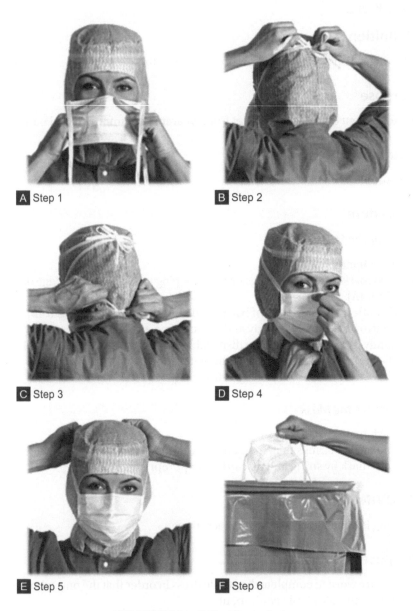

A Step 1

B Step 2

C Step 3

D Step 4

E Step 5

F Step 6

FIGURES 8.4A to F: Masking technique

Step 3: Place the glove's rolled cuff edge at the seam that connects the sleeve to the gown cuff. Grasp the bottom rolled cuff edge of the glove with the thumb and index finger (Fig. 8.5D).

Step 4: While holding the glove's cuff edge with one hand, grasp the uppermost edge of the glove's cuff with the opposite hand (Fig. 8.5E). Take care not to expose the bare fingers, while doing this.

Step 5:
- Continuing to grasp the glove, stretch the cuff of the glove over the hand (Fig. 8.5F)
- Using the opposite sleeve covered hand, grasp both the glove cuff and sleeve cuff seam and pull the glove onto the hand. Pull any excessive amount of gown sleeve from underneath the cuff of the glove.

Step 6: Using the hand that is now gloved put on the second glove in the same manner. When gloving is completed no part of the skin has touched the outside surface of the gloves. Check to make sure that each gown cuff is secured and covered completely by the cuff of the glove. Adjust the fingers of the glove as necessary, so that they fit snugly.

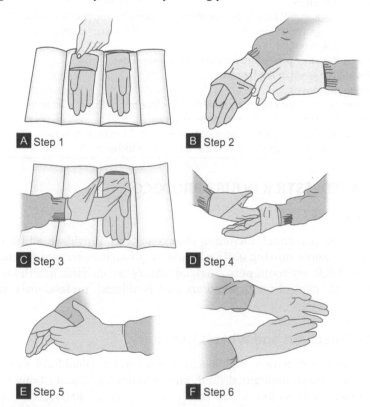

FIGURES 8.5A to F: Gloving technique. **A.** Pick up one glove with thumb and forefinger; **B.** Pull glove on hand; **C.** Slip partially gloved hand under cuff of second glove; **D.** Pull second glove over other hand and pull glove up to gowned wrist; **E.** Slip fingers of completely gloved hand under cuff of first hand, pull glove to gowned wrist; **F.** Gloving procedure completed.

Points to Note

- Not to contaminate the outside surface of the glove.
- In serving the gloves, the nurse must have a wide base of support by putting her foot apart.
- Always serve the right hand glove first.
- In serving, get the right glove with the left and the left hand glove with the right hand.
- Always keep gloved hands at waist level or above.
- Keep gloved hands away from your mask.

Removing the gown and the gloves
- Regardless of whether the scrub nurse assists in a case or contaminated case remove gown first and then the gloves. Wash the gloved hands, if they are grossly contaminated before removing the gown.

Removing the gown
- With the gloves still in, ask the circulating nurse to loosen the ties and the belt.
- Grasp the right shoulder of the gown and slip off the arm allowing use sleeves to turn inside out.
- Repeat the same procedure for the opposite shoulder.
- Discard the gown in the hamper.

Removing the gloves
- With the gloved right hand, remove the left glove by holding it at its outer surface and pull off (this is the glove to glove technique).
- To remove the right glove, insert your thumb or three fingers between the skin and the glove and pull off (this is the skin to skin technique).

POST NEEDLESTICK INJURY PROTOCOL

Who is at Risk?

All healthcare personnel, including emergency care providers, all hospital employees, interns, nursing staff and students, physicians, surgeons, dentists, labour and delivery room personnel, laboratory technicians, health facility sanitary staff, clinical waste handlers and healthcare professionals at all levels.

What is Infectious and What is Not?

Exposure to blood, semen, vaginal secretions, cerebrospinal fluid, synovial, pleural, peritoneal, pericardial fluid, amniotic fluid and other body fluids contaminated with visible blood can lead to infection. Exposure to tears, sweat, saliva, urine and feces is non-infectious unless these secretions contain visible blood.

The risk of acquiring human immunodeficiency virus (HIV) infection following percutaneous needle stick injury and after mucous membrane exposure has been estimated to be 0.3%–0.09%. This is because of the low concentration of virus in the blood of HIV patients.

The risk of acquiring hepatitis B virus (HBV) infection is related to the hepatitis B e-antigen (HBeAg) status of the source person. The risk associated with a single parental exposure to blood from a source patient ranges from 6% in HBeAg negative patients to as high as 40% in HBeAg positive patients.

The average risk of seroconversion following needle stick injury from an hepatitis C virus (HCV) infected patient is about 2%.

Immediate Care

First Aid in Management of Exposure

For skin

If the skin is broken after a needle stick or sharp instrument:

- Immediately wash the wound and surrounding skin with water, soap and rinse
- Do not scrub
- Do not use antiseptics or skin washes (bleach, chlorine, alcohol, Betadine).
  After a splash of blood or body fluids on unbroken skin:
- Wash the area immediately
- Do not use antiseptics.

For the eye

- Irrigate exposed eye immediately with water or normal saline. Sit in a chair, tilt head back and ask a colleague to gently pour water or normal saline over the eye.

For mouth

- Spit fluid out immediately
- Rinse the mouth thoroughly, using water or saline and spit again. Repeat this process several times.

Reporting

All sharps injury (break of skin with any sharp instrument such as hypodermic needle previously used on a patient) and mucosal exposure (blood or body fluids coming into contact with eye, mouth, etc.) should be reported to the hospital infection control nurse, nursing supervisors, floor managers and to the medical superintendent.

Protocol

After needle stick injury or blood/body fluid exposure, follow the below protocols.

Incident

Needle sticks injury or blood/body fluid exposure (exposure means contact with mucous membranes, intact or breached skin).

Procedure

Procedures to be followed after needle stick injury:

- Do not panic
- Do not put pricked finger in mouth
- Do not squeeze wound to bleed
- Wash the hands with soap and water
- Do not use bleach, chlorine, alcohol, Betadine, iodine, any antiseptic or detergent.

Process Flow

- Inform the floor manager/supervisor of the respective department
- File a report within half an hour form needle stick injury (NSI) available at intensive care unit (ICU), accident and emergency department and operation theater (OT)
- Go to the emergency department
- Get assessed by duty medical officer (DMO)/physician within 2–6 hours
- Proceed with the treatment suggested
- Review for the follow-up care as advised.

Instructions for the Staff

Standard Precautions

1. Wash hands after patient contact and after removing gloves.
2. Wash hands immediately, if hands are contaminated with body fluids.
3. Wear gloves when contamination of hands with body substances is anticipated.
4. Protective eyewear and masks should be worn when splashing with body substances is anticipated.
5. All healthcare workers should take precautions to prevent injuries during procedures and when cleaning or during disposal of needles or other sharp instruments.
6. Needles should not be recapped.
7. Needles should not be purposely bent or broken by hand and not removed from disposable syringes nor manipulated by hand.
8. After using disposable syringes and needles, scalpel blades and other sharp instruments should be placed in a puncher resistant container.
9. Healthcare worker who have lesions or dermatitis should refrain form direct patient care and from handling equipment.
10. All needle stick injuries should be reported to the emergency room (ER), who in turn will inform infection control nurse.
11. Handle and dispose of sharps safely.
12. Clean and disinfect blood/body substances spills with appropriate agents.
13. Adhere to disinfection and sterilization standards.
14. Vaccinate all clinical and laboratory workers against hepatitis B.
15. Other measures are double gloving, changing surgical techniques to avoid 'exposure prone' procedures, use of needleless systems and other safe devices.

BIOMEDICAL WASTE MANAGEMENT

Definition

The waste generated during the diagnosis, treatment or immunization of human beings or animals or in research activities pertaining to or in the production of testing biologicals.

Purposes

- Ensure occupational health safety
- Avoid illegal reuse
- Favors recycling
- Reduce the cost of treatment and disposal.

Color Code of Biomedical Waste Management

Details about color code and usage is given in Table 8.1:
- Yellow
- Red
- Black
- Green
- Blue
- Puncture proof container.

Table 8.1: Color code of biomedical waste management

Color	Waste category	Location	Treatment
Yellow	Human anatomical and body parts	Operation theater (OT) and labor room	Incineration/Burial
Red	Infectious gauze, cotton, plastic tubing, syringes, other infected plastics, etc.	All wards/nursing stations	Autoclave
Blue	Vials and bottles	All wards/nursing stations	Autoclave
Puncture proof container	Sharp	All wards/nursing stations	Sharp pit
Green	General wastes	Separately kept from biomedical waste bins	Composing/Handed over to municipal corporation
Black	Cytotoxic drugs, expiry medicines	All wards/nursing stations	Return to original supplier, incineration at high temperatures

Yellow Bag (Infectious)

- Postoperative human body parts
- Placenta
- Pathological waste.

Red Bag (Infectious Plastics)

- All types of intravenous (IV) sets and tubes/bags
- Gloves, blood bags, urine bags
- Disposable syringes (without needle)
- Catheters
- All kinds of drains and aprons (like cotton, swabs and bandages)
- Dialysis kits.

Green Bag (General Waste)

- Paper and plastic packing
- Disposable cups and plates, etc.
- Cans and tins
- Food items.

Black Bag

- Chemotherapy waste
- Acids and alkalis
- Phenol
- Expiry medicines.

Puncture Proof Container (Infectious)

- All kinds of broken glasses, tools and ampules
- All kinds of sharps like scalpels, needles, blades, IV catheters, etc.
- Clinical and pathological slides
- Guide wires
- Venflon needles, etc.

Tips for Safe-sharp Disposal

- Avoid recap
- Empty the sharp container once the fill is three fourth
- The container should be filled with 1% hypochloride solution always
- Avoid the use of burner or needle cutter
- Avoid the store rage of needle in the kidney tray after use. It should be discarded immediately after use.

Treatment Options of Biomedical Waste

Treatment options of biomedical waste is given in Table 8.2.

Table 8.2: Treatment method of biomedical waste

Sl No	Waste type	Treatment method
1.	Body parts	Incineration/Deep burial
2.	Bandages/Cotton/Linen	Incineration/Autoclaving/Microwaving
3.	Gloves/Surgical gowns/ Needles/Sharps	Chemicals/Disinfection/Autoclaving/Microwaving
4.	Intravenous (IV) bottles/Plastic tubing/Blood bags/Urine bags/Items used in hemodialysis units	Autoclaving/Microwaving
5.	IV sets/Catheters	Chemicals/Disinfection/Autoclaving
6.	Syringes/Vacutainer tubes	Autoclaving/Chemicals/Disinfection
7.	Unused drugs	Return to manufacturer
8.	Waste chemicals	Incineration
9.	Culture fluids/Lavage fluids/Blood/Urine samples/Other body fluids	Chemicals/Disinfection/Autoclaving
10.	Culture plates/vials	Autoclaving/Microwaving

Index

Page numbers followed by *t* refer to table and *f* refer to figure

Fundamentals of
NURSING
Clinical Procedure Manual

Fundamentals of
NURSING
Clinical Procedure Manual

JC Helen Shaji

MA (Psychology) MSc (Nursing) PhD (Nursing)

Professor
Department of Nursing
College of Applied Medical Sciences, Majmaah University
Kingdom of Saudi Arabia

Ex-Principal and Professor
St. Isabel's College of Nursing
Mylapore, Chennai, Tamil Nadu, India

Foreword
Nalini Jeyavanth Santha

(JAYPEE) *The Health Sciences Publisher*

New Delhi | London | Philadelphia | Panama

Jaypee Brothers Medical Publishers (P) Ltd

Headquarters

Jaypee Brothers Medical Publishers (P) Ltd
4838/24, Ansari Road, Daryaganj
New Delhi 110 002, India
Phone: +91-11-43574357
Fax: +91-11-43574314
Email: jaypee@jaypeebrothers.com

Overseas Offices

J.P. Medical Ltd
83 Victoria Street, London
SW1H 0HW (UK)
Phone: +44 20 3170 8910
Fax: +44 (0)20 3008 6180
Email: info@jpmedpub.com

Jaypee-Highlights Medical Publishers Inc
City of Knowledge, Bld. 237, Clayton
Panama City, Panama
Phone: +1 507-301-0496
Fax: +1 507-301-0499
Email: cservice@jphmedical.com

Jaypee Medical Inc
The Bourse
111 South Independence Mall East
Suite 835, Philadelphia, PA 19106, USA
Phone: +1 267-519-9789
Email: jpmed.us@gmail.com

Jaypee Brothers Medical Publishers (P) Ltd
17/1-B Babar Road, Block-B, Shaymali
Mohammadpur, Dhaka-1207
Bangladesh
Mobile: +08801912003485
Email: jaypeedhaka@gmail.com

Jaypee Brothers Medical Publishers (P) Ltd
Bhotahity, Kathmandu, Nepal
Phone +977-9741283608
Email: kathmandu@jaypeebrothers.com

Website: www.jaypeebrothers.com
Website: www.jaypeedigital.com

© 2015, Jaypee Brothers Medical Publishers

The views and opinions expressed in this book are solely those of the original contributor(s)/author(s) and do not necessarily represent those of editor(s) of the book.

All rights reserved. No part of this publication may be reproduced, stored or transmitted in any form or by any means, electronic, mechanical, photocopying, recording or otherwise, without the prior permission in writing of the publishers.

All brand names and product names used in this book are trade names, service marks, trademarks or registered trademarks of their respective owners. The publisher is not associated with any product or vendor mentioned in this book.

Medical knowledge and practice change constantly. This book is designed to provide accurate, authoritative information about the subject matter in question. However, readers are advised to check the most current information available on procedures included and check information from the manufacturer of each product to be administered, to verify the recommended dose, formula, method and duration of administration, adverse effects and contraindications. It is the responsibility of the practitioner to take all appropriate safety precautions. Neither the publisher nor the author(s)/editor(s) assume any liability for any injury and/or damage to persons or property arising from or related to use of material in this book.

This book is sold on the understanding that the publisher is not engaged in providing professional medical services. If such advice or services are required, the services of a competent medical professional should be sought.

Every effort has been made where necessary to contact holders of copyright to obtain permission to reproduce copyright material. If any have been inadvertently overlooked, the publisher will be pleased to make the necessary arrangements at the first opportunity.

Inquiries for bulk sales may be solicited at: jaypee@jaypeebrothers.com

Fundamentals of Nursing: Clinical Procedure Manual

First Edition: **2015**

ISBN 978-93-5152-637-7
Printed at Repro India Limited

Dedicated to

*The nursing students and registered nurses
who have always been the source of inspiration
and make a difference in patients'
life every day and every moment*

Foreword

It gives me immense pleasure, and it is a great privilege and honor to write the foreword for this book *Fundamentals of Nursing: Clinical Procedure Manual* written by Dr JC Helen Shaji.

The initiative and effort taken toward bringing up this manual is commendable. The contents of the book cover the curriculum prescribed by Indian Nursing Council, which sustains uniform standard of nursing education in the country. The author states that the primary purpose of this work is to provide a textbook for young nursing students who are studying to become qualified professional nurses. This book also serves as a ready reference source for the practicing nurses.

This book has detailed information to understand fundamental and advanced medical and surgical nursing procedures, which would benefit students and graduates to maintain high standard of nursing practice for humanitarian service, and the dignity and status of the profession. In order to enhance the quality of nursing, it is essential to maintain standard of care in nursing education and nursing practice. This manual will help the nursing students to maintain standard and high quality patient care in the healthcare setting. Through this manual, wide knowledge and fine nursing skills can be transferred to the nursing students very effectively.

Nalini Jeyavanth Santha PhD (N)
Principal
Sacred Heart Nursing College, Ultra Trust
Madurai, Tamil Nadu, India

Preface

I am extremely happy to present this book *Fundamentals of Nursing: Clinical Procedure Manual* to the nursing students and registered nurses in India as well as overseas. The primary objective of this book is to prepare competent nurses to meet the challenging situations of nursing, since it is prepared according to the curriculum of Indian Nursing Council as well as the syllabus adopted by various universities overseas. The nursing students will find it as a 'textbook' for learning nursing procedures.

The nurse educators will find it easy to teach their students and prepare them well for the examination. Moreover, the present-day practicing nurses also find this book as a ready reference source for better understanding of basic and advanced medical and surgical nursing procedures. This book will also bring a uniform standard of the nursing education in India.

It will be much appreciated, if readers send their criticism, suggestions and corrections if any for further improvement of this book.

JC Helen Shaji

Acknowledgments

I am highly indebted to Dr Nalini Jeyavanth Santha, for writing the foreword. I am grateful to my husband G David Rajesh, my children Daleesh, Prajol and Sharon, for their invaluable assistance and dedication during the preparation of this book. I am also grateful to some of my colleagues in profession who has encouraged me throughout, for writing this book.

I am thankful to Shri Jitendar P Vij (Group Chairman), Mr Ankit Vij (Group President), Mr Tarun Duneja (Director–Publishing) and all the staff of Bengaluru Branch of M/s Jaypee Brothers Medical Publishers (P) Ltd, New Delhi, India, for bringing out this book in a professional manner.

Contents

Section
1

Basic Nursing Care Procedures

- ❏ Bed Making
- ❏ Checking Vital Signs
- ❏ Performing Hygienic Procedures and Other Basic Procedures
- ❏ Specimen Collection
- ❏ Administration of Medications

Bed Making

MAKING AN UNOCCUPIED BED

Definition

A bed prepared to receive a new patient is an unoccupied bed.

Purposes

1. To provide clean and comfortable bed for the patient.
2. To reduce the risk of infection by maintaining a clean environment.
3. To prevent bed sores by ensuring that there are no wrinkles to cause pressure points.

Equipments Required

- Mattress: 1
- Bed sheets: 2
  - Bottom sheet: 1
  - Top sheet: 1.
- Pillow: 1
- Pillow cover: 1
- Mackintosh: 1
- Draw sheet: 1
- Blanket: 1
- Savlon water or Dettol water in basin
- Sponge cloth: 4
  - To wipe with solution: 1
  - To dry: 1
  - When bed making is done by two nurses, sponge cloth is needed two each.
- Kidney tray or paper bag: 1
- Laundry bag or hamper bag: 1
- Trolley: 1.

Procedure

Bed making procedure is detailed in Table 1.1.

Table 1.1: Bed making procedure

Sl No	Care action	Rationale
1.	Explain the purpose and procedure to the client	Providing information fosters cooperation
2.	Perform hand hygiene	To prevent the spread of infection
3.	Prepare all required equipments and bring the articles to the bedside	Organization facilitates accurate skill performance
4.	Move the chair and bedside locker	It makes space for bed making and helps effective action
5.	Clean the bedside locker: • Wipe with wet and dry	To maintain the cleanliness
6.	Clean the mattress: • Stand in right side • Start wet wiping from top to center and from center to bottom in right side of mattress • Gather the dust and debris to the bottom • Collect them into kidney tray • Give dry wiping as same as procedure 2 • Move to left side • Wipe with wet and dry the left side • Move to right side	To prevent the spread of infection
7.	Bottom sheet: • Place and slide the bottom sheet upward over the top of the bed leaving the bottom edge of the sheet • Open it lengthwise with the center fold along the bed center • Fold back the upper layer of the sheet toward the opposite side of the bed • Tuck the bottom sheet securely under the head of the mattress (approximately 20–30 cm) • Make a mitered corner: – Pick up the selvage edge with your hand nearest to the hand of the bed – Lay a triangle over the side of the bed – Tuck the hanging part of the sheet under the mattress – Drop the triangle over the side of the bed – Tuck the sheet under the entire side of bed • Repeat the same procedure at the end of the corner of the bed • Tuck the remainder in along the side	Unfolding the sheet in this manner allows you to make the bed on one side A mitered corner has a neat appearance and keeps the sheet securely under the mattress Tucking the bottom sheet will be done by turning the corner of top first and the corner of the bottom later To secure the bottom sheet on one side of the bed
8.	Mackintosh and draw sheet: • Place a mackintosh at the middle of the bed (if used), folded half, with the fold in the center of the bed • Lift the right half and spread it forward to the near side • Tuck the mackintosh under the mattress • Place the draw sheet on the mackintosh • Spread and tuck as same as procedure 1–3 • Move to the left side of the bed	Mackintosh and draw sheet are additional protection for the bed, and serves as a lifting or turning sheet for an immobile client

Contd...

Contd...

Sl No	Care action	Rationale
9.	Bottom sheet, mackintosh and draw sheet: • Fold and tuck the bottom sheet as in the above procedure 7 • Fold and tuck both the mackintosh and the draw sheet under the mattress, as given in the above procedure 8 • Return to the right side	Secure the bottom sheet, mackintosh; and draw the bottom sheet, mackintosh and draw sheet
10.	Top sheet and blanket: • Place the top sheet evenly on the bed, centering it in the below 20–30 cm from the top of the mattress • Spread it downward • Cover the top sheet with blanket in the below 1 foot from the top of the mattress and spread downward • Fold the cuff (approximately 1 foot) in the neck • Tuck all these together under the bottom of mattress; miter the corner • Tuck the remainder in along the side	A blanket provides warmth Making the cuff at the neck part prevents irritation from blanket edge Tucking all these pieces together saves time and provides a neat appearance To save time in this manner
11.	Repeat the same as in procedure 10 for the left side Return to the right side	
12.	Pillow and pillow cover: • Put a clean pillow cover on the pillow • Place a pillow at the top of the bed in the center with the open end away from the door	A pillow is a comfortable measure Pillow cover keeps cleanliness of the pillow and neat The open end may collect dust or organisms The open end away from the door is also maintained neat
13.	Return the bed, chair and bedside table to their proper place	Bedside necessities will be within easy reach for the client
14.	Replace all equipments in proper place	It makes well-setting for the next procedure
15.	Discard lines appropriately	Proper linen disposal prevents the spread of infection
16.	Perform hand hygiene	To prevent the spread of infection

Nursing Alert

1. Do not let your uniform touch the bed and the floor not to contaminate yourself.
2. Never throw soiled linens on the floor not to contaminate the floor.
3. Staying one side of the bed until one step is completed, save steps and time to do effectively.

CHANGING AN OCCUPIED BED

Definition

The procedure of changing used linens of a hospitalized patient is an occupied bed.

Purposes

1. To provide clean and comfortable bed for the patient.
2. To reduce the risk of infection by maintaining a clean environment.
3. To prevent bed sores by ensuring that there are no wrinkles to cause pressure points.

Equipments Required

- Bed sheets: 2
  - Bottom sheet (or bed cover): 1
  - Top sheet: 1.
- Draw sheet: 1
- Mackintosh: 1 (if contaminated or needed to change)
- Blanket: 1 (if contaminated or needed to change)
- Pillow cover: 1
- Savlon water or Dettol water in bucket
- Sponge cloth: 2
  - To wipe with solution: 1
  - To dry: 1
  - When the procedure is done by two nurses, sponge cloth is needed two each.
- Kidney tray or paper bag: 1
- Laundry bag or bucket:1
- Trolley: 1.

Procedure

Procedure for changing an occupied bed is detailed in Table 1.2.

Table 1.2: Procedure for changing an occupied bed

Sl No	Care action	Rationale
1.	Check the client's identification and condition	To assess necessity and sufficient condition
2.	Explain the purpose and procedure to the client	Providing information fosters cooperation
3.	Perform hand hygiene	To prevent the spread of infection
4.	Prepare all required equipments and bring the articles to the bedside	Organization facilitates accurate skill performance
5.	Close the curtain or door of the room; put screen	To maintain the client's privacy
6.	Remove the client's personal belongings from bedside and put them into the bedside locker or in safe place	To prevent personal belongings from damage and loss
7.	Lift the client's head and move pillow from center to the left side	Pillow is a comfortable measure for the client
8.	Assist the client to turn toward left side of the bed; adjust the pillow and leave top sheet in place	Moving the client as close to the other side of the bed as possible, which give more room to make the bed

Contd...

Contd...

Sl No	Care action	Rationale
		Top sheet keeps the client warm and protect his/her privacy
9.	Stand in right side; loose bottom bed linen and fanfold (or roll) soiled linens from the side of the bed and wedge them close to the client	Placing folded (or rolled) soiled linen close to the client allows more space to place the clean bottom sheets
10.	Wipe the surface of mattress by sponge cloth with wet and dry	To prevent the spread of infection
11.	Bottom sheet, mackintosh and draw sheet: • Place the clean bottom sheet evenly on the bed, folded lengthwise with the center fold as close to the client's back as possible • Adjust and tuck the sheet tightly under the head of the mattress, making mitered the upper corner • Tighten the sheet under the end of the mattress making mitered the lower corner • Tuck in alongside • Place the mackintosh and the draw sheet on the bottom sheet and tuck in them together	Soiled linens can easily be removed and clean linens are positioned to make the other side of the bed
12.	Assist the client to roll over the folded (rolled) linen to right side of the bed; readjust the pillow and top sheet	Moving the client to the bed's other side allows to make the bed on that side
13.	Move to left side; discard the soiled linens appropriately; hold them away from the uniform and place them in the laundry bag (or bucket)	Soiled linens can contaminate the uniform, which may come into contact with other clients
14.	Wipe the surface of the mattress by sponge cloth with wet and dry	To prevent the spread of infection
15.	Bottom sheet, mackintosh and draw sheet: • Grasp clean linens and gently pull them out from under the client • Spread them over the bed's unmade side; pull the linens taut • Tuck the bottom sheet tightly under the head of the mattress and miter the corner • Tighten the sheet under the end of the mattress and make mitered the lower corner • Tuck in alongside • Tuck the mackintosh and the draw sheet under the mattress	Wrinkled linens can cause skin irritation
16.	Assist the client back to the center of the bed; adjust the pillow	Pillow is a comfort measure for the client
17.	Return to right side: • Clean the top sheet, blanket • Place the clean top sheet at the top side of the soiled top sheet	Tucking these pieces together saves time and provides neat, tight corners

Contd...

Contd...

SI No	Care action	Rationale
	• Ask the client to hold the upper edge of the clean top sheet • Hold both the top of the soiled sheet and the end of the clean sheet with right hand and withdraw to downward; remove the soiled top sheet and put it into a laundry bag (or a bucket) • Place the blanket over the top sheet; fold top sheet back over the blanket over the client • Tuck the lower ends securely under the mattress; miter corners • After finishing the right side, repeat for the left side	
18.	Remove the pillow, replace the pillow cover with clean one and reposition the pillow to the bed under the client's head	Pillow is a comfortable measure for the client
19.	Replace personal belongings back; return the bedside locker and the bed as usual	To prevent personal belongings from loss and provide safe surroundings
20.	Return all equipments to proper place	To prepare for the next procedure
21.	Discard linens appropriately; perform hand hygiene	To prevent the spread of infection

MAKING A POSTOPERATIVE BED

Definition

Postoperative bed is a special bed prepared to receive and take care of a patient returning from surgery.

Purposes

1. To receive the postoperative client from surgery and transfer him/her from a stretcher to a bed.
2. To arrange client's convenience and safety.

Equipments Required

- Bed sheets:
  - Bottom sheet: 1
  - Top sheet: 1.
- Draw sheet: 1–2
- Mackintosh or rubber sheet: 1–2 (according to the type of operation, the number required of mackintosh and draw sheet is different)
- Blanket: 1
- Hot water bag with hot water (104°F–140°F): 1 (if needed)
- Tray: 1
- Thermometer, stethoscope, sphygmomanometer: 1 each

- Spirit swab
- Artery forceps: 1
- Gauze pieces
- Adhesive tape: 1
- Kidney tray: 1
- Trolley: 1
- Intravenous (IV) stand
- Client's chart
- According to doctor's orders:
    - Oxygen cylinder with flow meter
    - Oxygen cannula or simple mask
    - Suction machine with suction tube
    - Airway, tongue depressor
    - Electrocardiogram (ECG), SpO_2 (peripheral O_2 saturation) monitor.

Procedure

Procedure for making a postoperative bed is detailed in Table 1.3.

Table 1.3: Procedure for making postoperative bed

Sl No	Care action	Rationale
1.	Perform hand hygiene	To prevent the spread of infection
2.	Assemble equipments and bring to bedside	Organization facilitates accurate skill performance
3.	Strip bed; make foundation bed as usual with a large mackintosh and cotton draw sheet	Mackintosh prevents bottom sheet from wetting or soiled by sweat, drain or excrement Place mackintosh according to operative technique Cotton draw sheet makes the client feel dry or comfortable without touching the mackintosh directly
4.	Place top bedding as for closed bed, but do not tuck at foot	Tuck at foot may hamper the client to enter the bed from a stretcher
5.	Fold back top bedding at the foot of bed	To make the client's transfer smooth
6.	Tuck the top bedding on one side only	Tucking the top bedding on one side stops the bed linens from slipping out of place
7.	On the other side, do not tuck the top sheet: • Bring head and foot corners of it at the center of bed and form right angles • Fold back suspending portion in one third and repeat folding top bedding twice to opposite side of bed	The open side of bed is more convenient for receiving client than the (other) closed side
8.	Remove the pillow	To maintain the airway
9.	Place a kidney tray on bedside	To receive secretion
10.	Place intravenous (IV) stand near the bed	To prepare it to hang IV soon

Contd...

Contd...

Sl No	Care action	Rationale
11.	Check locked wheel of the bed	To prevent moving the bed accidentally, when the client is shifted from a stretcher to the bed
12.	Place hot water bags (or hot bottles) in the middle of the bed and cover with fan-folded top, if needed	Hot water bags (or hot bottles) prevent the client from taking hypothermia
13.	When the patient comes, remove hot water bags if put before	To prepare enough space for receiving the client
14.	Transfer the client: • Help lifting the client on to the bed • Cover the client by the top sheet and blanket immediately • Tuck top bedding and miter a corner in the end of the bed	To prevent the client from chilling and/or having hypothermia

Checking Vital Signs

CHECKING ORAL AND AXILLARY TEMPERATURE

Definition

The temperature is defined as the expression of heat or coldness in terms of a specific scale; a measure of the average kinetic energy due to thermal disturbance of the particles in a system.

Purposes

1. To assess the progress and recovery of the patient from illness.
2. To diagnose significant conditions.
3. To ensure fitness of patient prior to procedures/surgeries.
4. To assess the patient response to medication and treatment.

Equipments

- A tray containing a bottle of disinfectant and a bottle of water (if glass thermometer)
- Thermometer (mercury in glass thermometer, electronic thermometer, tympanic thermometer)
- Clean cotton balls
- Towel/tissue paper.

Procedure

The procedure for checking axillary temperature and oral temperature are detailed in Tables 2.1 and 2.2.

Table 2.1: Procedure for checking axillary temperature

Sl No	Care action	Rationale
1.	Explain the procedure to the patient	To ensure that the patient understands the procedure and give consent
2.	Carry out handwashing	To prevent cross infection
3.	Place the patient in a comfortable position	To reduce uneasiness

Contd...

Contd...

SI No	Care action	Rationale
4.	Read mercury level, while gently rotating thermometer at eye level; grasp thermometer with thumb and forefinger, and shake gently by snapping the wrist in a downward motion to move mercury to a level until reading lowers mercury level to 35.6°C (96°F)	To get the accurate value, as the brisk shaking lowers mercury level in the glass tube
5.	Clean and dry axilla with towel	To get the exact value; moisture may also alter the temperature
6.	Place the thermometer in axilla, the bulb of thermometer is well in contact with the skin, while the patient's hand is held across chest	Ensures correct contact with the blood vessels in the axilla
7.	Wait for 5 minutes	To trace the temperature correctly
8.	Remove the thermometer, clean from stem to bulb and read at eye level	Reduces transmission of microorganisms to the bulb
9.	Shake gently the thermometer so that the mercury level falls below 35°C (95°F)	Keeps it set for use again
10.	Place the thermometer in disinfectant solution	To reduce cross infection
11.	Discard used tissue paper/cotton balls	Reduce transmission of microorganisms
12.	Record temperature on the graph sheet of temperature, pulse, respiration (TPR) record	Provides proper data for clinical data analysis

Points to Note

- Collect the history from the patient/relatives about the bathing time; the bath just before taking axillary temperature can alter the reading.

Table 2.2: Procedure for checking oral temperature

SI No	Care action	Rationale
1.	Explain the procedure to the patient	To ensure that the patient understand the procedure and to reduce the anxiety
2.	Wash the hands	To prevent cross infection
3.	Place the patient in a comfortable position (sitting or lying down)	To relieve anxiety
4.	Read mercury level, while gently rotating thermometer at eye level; shake it until reading lowers mercury level to 35.6°C (96°F)	To get the accurate readings
5.	Ask the patient to open the mouth and gently place thermometer under tongue in posterior sublingual pocket lateral to center of lower jaw	Ensures proper contact with the blood vessels in the mouth
6.	Wait for 3 minutes	To record the temperature accurately
7.	Remove the thermometer, clean from stem to bulb and read at eye level	Reduces transmission of microorganisms to the bulb

Contd...

Sl No	Care action	Rationale
8.	Shake gently so that mercury level falls below 35°C (95°F)	Keeps it set for use again
9.	Place the thermometer in disinfectant solution	To reduce cross infection
10.	Discard used tissue paper/cotton balls	Reduce transmission of microbes
11.	Record temperature on the graph sheet of temperature, pulse, respiration (TPR) record	Provides proper data for clinical data analysis

Points to Note

- Collect the details from the patient or relative about if he/she has taken any cold or hot food or fluids, or has smoked. If yes, the nurse is supposed to wait for 30 minutes to prevent the false reading.

OBSERVATION OF PULSE

Definition

Pulse is the rhythmic expansion and contraction of an artery caused by the impact of blood pumped by the heart. The pulse can be felt with the fingers at different pulse pressure points throughout the body.

Purposes

1. To ensure an accurate and effective assessment of the rate, rhythm and amplitude (strength) of the pulse.
2. To identify any trends/discrepancies and/or to detect early signs of alteration of cardiovascular function.

Equipments

- A watch
- A stethoscope.

Procedure

The procedure for observation of pulse is detailed in Table 2.3.

Table 2.3: Procedure for observation of pulse

Sl No	Care action	Rationale
1.	Explain the procedure to the patient	To get the consent and cooperation
2.	Wash and dry hands thoroughly	To prevent cross infection
3.	Encourage the patient to relaxed	To provide consistent readings
4.	Explain and discuss the procedure with the patient	To ensure that the patient understands the procedure and gives his/her valid consent

Contd...

Contd...

SI No	Care action	Rationale
5.	If supine, place patient's forearm straight or across lower chest or abdomen with wrist extended straight If sitting, bend patient's elbow 90° and support lower arm on chair; slightly flex the wrist with palm down	Relaxed position of lower arm and flexion of wrist permits full exposure of radial artery for palpation
6.	Place second and/or third finger tips over radial artery and press gently until the pulse is felt	Fingertip is the most sensitive part of hand to palpate pulse
7.	Determine pulse amplitude and rhythm	Strength reflects volume of blood ejected against arterial wall with each heart contraction
8.	When pulse has been detected, look at watch's and count pulse rate for 60 seconds	Adequate time is essential to detect irregularities or any other defect
9.	Document any abnormalities in amplitude and rhythm	To maintain accurate records, and allow for monitoring and detection of trends
10.	Use disinfectant hand rub, once the procedure is over	To minimize cross infection risks between patients
11.	Document any relevant evaluation or changes in patient's record	To provide ongoing evaluation
12.	For the assessment of apical pulse, give details to the patient that expose sternum and left side of chest and position the diaphragm of the stethoscope over the point of maximal impulse (PMI) at the left fifth intercostal space, medial to the midclavicular line; if the heart beat is regular, count for 30 seconds and multiply by 2; if irregular, auscultate for one full minute	It provides a more accurate assessment

Points to Note

* Collect the details from the patient/relative, if he/she has been mobilized or done any such motion within the previous 15 minutes. Activity and anxiety can elevate heart rate. These activities may alter pulse rate.
* Thumb and forefinger are not equal, as they have their own pulse.
* Pulse is more accurately assessed with moderate pressure. Too much pressure can occlude pulse and impairs blood flow.

Pulse Sites

Sites of pulse is detailed in Table 2.4.

Table 2.4: Sites of pulse

Site	Location	Assessment criteria
Temporal	Above temporal bone of head, above and lateral to the eye	Easily accessible site to assess pulse in children
Carotid	Along medial edge of sternocleidomastoid muscle in neck	Easily accessible, used during physiological shock or cardiac arrest when other sites are not palpable
Brachial	Groove between biceps and triceps muscles at antecubital fossa	Site used to assess pulse rate; site used to auscultate blood pressure
Radial (commonly used)	Radial or thumb side of forearm at wrist	Common site used to assess character of pulse peripherally and assess status of circulation to hand
Femoral	Below inguinal ligament; midway between symphysis pubis and anterior superior iliac spine	Site used to assess character of pulse during physiological shock or cardiac arrest when other pulses are not palpable
Popliteal	Behind knee in popliteal fossa	Site used to auscultate lower extremity blood pressure
Posterior tibial	Inner side of ankle, below medial malleolus	Site used to assess circulation to foot
Dorsalis pedis	Along top of foot, between extension tendons of great and first toe	Site used to assess circulation to foot

OBSERVATION OF RESPIRATION

Definition

Monitoring the exchange of oxygen and carbon dioxide between the atmosphere and the body cells, including ventilation (inhalation and exhalation).

Purposes

1. To reveal the deviation from the normal body function.
2. To identify any changes in the condition of the patient.
3. To obtain specific information, which will help in the diagnosis of disease, the result of treatment, medications and nursing care.

Equipment

- A watch that has a second's hand.

Procedure

The procedure for observation of respiration is detailed in Table 2.5.

Table 2.5: Procedure for observation of respiration

SI No	Care action	Rationale
1.	Explain the procedure to the patient	To gain consent and cooperation
2.	Patient shall be in sitting or supine position in a quiet environment	Optimum position for recording respiration
3.	Allow the patient to rest for at least 5 minutes before the reading is taken	To gain an accurate reading; respiratory rate settles on rest
4.	Instruct the patient to stop talking during the procedure	Activity, including talking will cause an inaccurate respiratory rate
5.	Promote the patient to place his/her hand over the abdomen or chest, or place nurse's hand directly over patient's upper abdomen	Sufficient time is required to detect irregularities or other defects
6.	Watch complete respiratory cycle (inspiration and one expiration)	Rate is correctly determined only after the nurse had viewed respiratory cycle
7.	Count the respirations for 60 seconds	To observe the abnormality of rate, quality or rhythm
8.	Observe abnormal breathing patterns	To observe any deterioration in patient's respiratory pattern
9.	Observe for regularity of chest movement	To observe for abnormalities in chest movement
10.	Record the respirations on the observation chart as soon as possible	Do not rely on memory; each reading is a vital recording for each patient to maintain accurate records, and allow for monitoring and detection of trends

MEASUREMENT OF BLOOD PRESSURE

Definition

Arterial blood pressure is the force exerted by the blood on the wall of a blood vessel as the heart pumps (contracts) and relaxes. Systolic blood pressure is the degree of force when the heart is pumping (contracting). The diastolic blood pressure is the degree of force when the heart is relaxed.

Indications

1. To determine the patient's blood pressure at initial assessment as a base for subsequent evaluation.
2. To monitor fluctuations in blood pressure.
3. To assess the cardiac status.
4. To identify and monitor changes resulting from a disease process and medical/surgical therapy.
5. To determine patient's hemodynamic status.

Equipments

- Sphygmomanometer
- Stethoscope

- A bowl with spirit cotton swab
- Kidney tray.

Procedure

The procedure for measurement of blood pressure is detailed in Table 2.6.

Table 2.6: Procedure for measurement of blood pressure

Sl No	Care action	Rationale
1.	Wash and dry the hands	To prevent cross infection
2.	Explain the procedure to the patients	Gain consent and cooperation, and ensure the patient is comfortable
3.	Make the patient preferably in supine position or sitting position, if not contraindicated	Tense muscles can raise diastolic pressure hence the need to support the limbs
4.	Position the sphygmomanometer at the level of the heart with palm facing upwards	To ensure an accurate reading is obtained
5.	The meniscus of mercury should be read at the eye level and more than 3 feet away	To prevent errors in recording values
6.	Remove tight clothing from the limb to be used and support the limb	To obtain correct reading
7.	Apply the correct-sized sphygmomanometer cuff 2.5 cm above the antecubital fossa directly over the patient's skin and in level with the heart	The incorrect position of the cuff can lead to inaccuracy of 0.8 mm Hg/cm above or below heart level (Hill and Grim, 1991); the cuff should be sufficient enough to nearly/completely encircle arm and too smaller cuff raises blood pressure artificially
8.	Ensure the level of mercury in the manometer; it should be within zero	To get correct value
9.	Close the valve of the pump; palpate the radial artery gently with the non-dominant hand and inflate the cuff, and note the point where the pulsations disappear (palpation method)	This recognizes a predictable value of systolic pressure, which helps to reduce errors caused by auscultatory gap (a gap occurring when Korotkoff sounds disappear after K5 and reappear after a gap of 5–40 mm Hg)
10.	Palpate the brachial artery with the fingers and place the stethoscope in the ear, and keep the diaphragm of stethoscope over the brachial artery gently; do not allow the stethoscope to touch the clothing or the cuff	Hearing of the pulsation sound should be clear; the pressure of the inflated cuff will prevent blood flow through the artery and light pressure on the stethoscope maintains full skin contact, but when excessive, it distorts/lengthens Korotkoff sounds
11.	Inflate the cuff until the mercury rises up to 2–3 mm Hg/s; the deflation should not be too fast or too slow	If the deflation is too fast, it gives false low reading; if it is too slow, it causes venous congestion and arm pain can result in false high reading and discomfort to the patient
12.	Note the point at which the sound become clear and louder; read the pressure to the closest even number and continue deflating the cuff, and observe the point	To get the exact value of the patient's blood pressure and the markings on the sphygmomanometer at 2 mm Hg intervals; so, rounding up/down to 5 mm Hg factors leads to errors, which could give rise to inappropriate or inconsistent treatment

Contd...

Contd...

SI No	Care action	Rationale
13.	Do not show evidence of panic on the face when a considerably low or high reading is obtained	To prevent the anxiety of the patient
14.	To double check the reading, deflate the cuff fully and repeat the steps 9–14 after 30–60 seconds	To avoid patient discomfort To avoid the misconception of the values
15.	Allow the remaining air to escape quickly; remove the cuff and fold and keep it in place	To ensure the patient is comfortable To keep it ready for use again
16.	Record the systolic and diastolic pressures in the nurses' chart and on the vitals record	Documentation is necessary to identify the variances in future recordings

Points to Note

- Collect the history from the patient or relatives whether he/she ingested caffeine or has smoked within 30 minutes prior to measurement. These activities may alter the blood pressure. Factors such as a recent meal, full bladder and cigarette smoking can affect blood pressure. Ideally they should have rested 5–15 minutes preprocedure.
- The nurse should instruct the patient to keep their feet flat. Crossing of feet may increase the blood pressure.

Contraindications

- The arm has intravenous line
- The arm has got affected with any injury, e.g. fracture, burns, open wound, etc.
- The arm has a shunt or fistula for renal dialysis
- The side on which a breast or axillary surgery is done.

Performing Hygienic Procedures and Other Basic Procedures

MOUTH CARE

Definition

Mouth care is defined as the scientific care of the teeth and mouth by using antiseptic solutions.

Purposes

1. To keep the mucosa clean, soft, moist and intact.
2. To keep the lips clean, soft, moist and intact.
3. To prevent oral infections.
4. To remove the food debris as well as dental plaque without damaging the gum.
5. To alleviate pain, discomfort and enhance oral intake with appetite.
6. To prevent halitosis or relieve it and freshen the mouth.

Equipments

A clean tray containing:
- Sterile dressing tray
- Mackintosh and towel
- Toothbrush and paste/tooth powder (if needed)
- Mouthwash solution
- Cup of water (needed amount)
- Face towel
- Sponge cloth
- A tongue depressor/spatula
- A pair of gloves
- Gauze pieces
- Emollient
- Kidney tray
- A bowl with clean water (for dentures as applicable).

Procedure

The procedure for mouth care is detailed in Table 3.1.

Table 3.1: Procedure for mouth care

SI No	Care action	Rationale
1.	Explain the procedure to patient	To reduce the unease and get the cooperation from the patient
2.	Wash hands	To reduce transmission of microorganisms
3.	Gather all equipment near the patient side	To promote efficiency
4.	Discuss procedure with patient	To discover hygiene preferences
5.	Wear clean gloves	To prevent contact with microorganisms or body fluids
6.	Assess oral mucosa, teeth and throat	To determine status of oral cavity and patient's need for care and teaching
7.	Take the patient to the edge of bed and if possible in semi-Fowler, if it is not contraindicated	For no difficulty of doing the procedure and to prevent the aspiration
8.	Put a small mackintosh with a face towel on the patient's chest and tuck it under the chin	To prevent the soil and make the patient comfortable
9.	Place kidney tray against the cheek and directly under the mouth	To dispose the used gauze
10.	Raise the head end of the bed to 45°	To avoid the aspiration
11.	If the patient is unconscious, with help of tongue depressor, gently open the jaw	To prevent injury and bleeding
12.	Examine the patient's oral cavity completely with the help of torch, tongue depressor or spatula and gauze	To identify any changes in moisture, cleanliness, infection or bleeding, ulcers in the oral cavity
13.	Pour antiseptic solution into a cup and soak gauze in solution, and squeeze nicely with help of artery forceps	To prevent the infection and easy to do the procedure
14.	Clean teeth from incisors to molars using up and down movements, from gums to crown	To promote the circulation and proper cleanliness
15.	Use one clamp to pick up gauze and the other to clean (avoid interchanging of clamps)	To avoid cross-contamination
16.	Clean oral cavity from proximal to distal, using one gauze for each stroke with wet gauze	To avoid cross-contamination
17.	For supportive and oriented patients, toothbrush might be used to clean the teeth	This facilitates the patient to involve in self-care
18.	Discard used gauze into K-basin	To help for proper disposal and make the patient comfortable
19.	Provide a tumbler of water and instruct the patient to gargle mouth	Rinsing takes away loosened debris and make the mouth taste and fresher
20.	Position K-basin properly	To prevent the spillage to other area
21.	Clean tongue from inner to outer aspect, folding rag piece in such a way that the tip of clamp is completely protected	To prevent injury and remove the bad taste in the mouth
22.	Provide water to rinse mouth	Rinsing removes loosened debris and make the mouth taste fresher

Contd...

Contd...

Sl No	Care action	Rationale
23.	Lubricate lips using swab stick	To prevent dry lips and lip cracks
24.	Wipe face with towel	To make the patient comfortable and promote the positive body image
25.	Rinse used articles and replace equipment	To promote the safe and comfortable environment to the patient

> **Points to Note**
>
> * Common antiseptic solutions (dentifrices) used:
>   * Thymol glycerin.
>   * Sodium bicarbonate (1%).
>   * Borax glycerin.
>   * Vaseline.
> * Pay more attention to lips, buccal mucosa, lateral and ventral surfaces of the tongue, floor of the mouth and soft palate.
> * Ask the patient about taste changes, changes in saliva production and composition, oral discomfort or any problem in swallowing.

HAIR COMBING

Purposes

- To keep the hair clean and healthy
- To appear neat and make the patient comfortable
- Help to observe the scalp
- To promote growth of the hair and reduce hair fall
- To prevent itching and infection of the scalp
- To prevent the accumulation of dirt and dandruff
- To provide the sense of well-being
- To wipe out the pediculi.

Equipments

A clean tray containing:
- Towel
- Clean comb with coarse and fine teeth
- Kidney tray
- Oil in container (if necessary).

Procedure

The procedure for hair combing is described in Table 3.2.

Table 3.2: Procedure for hair combing

Sl No	Care action	Rationale
1.	Explain the procedure to the patient	To get the cooperation
2.	Wash your hands	To prevent cross-contamination
3.	If possible, make the patient to sit on a bed/chair/stool	To make the patient comfortable for the procedure
4.	Place a towel across the pillow if the patient is in bed; for the sitting patient, place a towel around shoulders	To prevent hair accumulation on the bed/surrounding area
5.	Ensure each half of the hair is treated separately	To make the patient comfortable and to make the procedure painless
6.	Separate the hair in small strands	To enable too easy comb
7.	Hold the strands above the part to be combed (anchoring)	To enhance the comfort
8.	Comb the tangles out from the ends first and then go up gradually	Easy to remove the tangles and ensure the comfort of the patient
9.	Brush from the scalp toward hair end	To promote the circulation and feel the patient comfortable
10.	If tangles are more, use the fingers to take apart small lock of hair, comb loose end of the hair	Easy to remove the tangles and ensure the comfort of the patient
11.	Comb one side of patient's head and repeat the same for other side	To make the patient neat and comfortable
12.	Discard loose hair into kidney tray	To make the area clean
13.	Secure the plait, it should not be too tight	To avoid the discomfort for the patient
14.	Remove the towel and kidney tray	To promote the patient comfort

Points to Note

♦ For patients who can be assisted with hair care, the nurse should advocate timely combing of hair and make sure that they are presentable.

HAIR WASH

Definition

Giving hair wash, while patient is bedridden.

Purposes

- To improve the scalp condition
- To keep the hair clean and healthy
- To reduce the hair loss
- To prevent dandruff and infection
- To increase the patient cleanliness and neat appearance.

Equipments

A tray containing:
- Shampoo
- Comb
- Small bowl
- Mackintosh
- Bath towel
- Sponge towel
- Rag pieces
- Bucket to collect waste water
- Jugs of hot and tepid water
- Basin
- Mug
- Non-absorbent cotton
- Kidney tray.

Procedure

The procedure for hair wash is detailed in Table 3.3.

Table 3.3: Procedure for hair wash

Sl No	Care action	Rationale
1.	Explain the procedure to the patient	To relieve the anxiety and to get the cooperation
2.	Place the mackintosh and towel under the neck, head and shoulder	To prevent the soiling of linen
3.	Consign the patient diagonally across the bed over the mackintosh, so that the head and shoulder are at the edge of the bed; other end of the mackintosh should be placed in the bucket	To make the patient comfortable for the procedure and to prevent the water spill over the floor
4.	Check the temperature of the water before starting the procedure	To prevent the burs and to promote comfort of the patient
5.	Place the small towel over the eyes and plug ears with the cotton balls	To prevent the entry of water into the ears
6.	Wear the personal protective equipment (PPE), i.e. apron, gloves, etc.	To protect the uniforms
7.	Loosen the hair and remove tangles, and wet the hair with warm water; apply the shampoo equally on the scalp	To enable proper washing
8.	Work up foam with both hands and start at hair line and work in the direction of back of neck by massage of all the scalp area	To promote circulation and to ensure that all the areas are cleaned
9.	Immerse the hair into the bucket, shower the water slowly and wash the hair, raise the head to some extent with one hand and rinse the back side of the head and squeeze the water thoroughly	To take away the shampoo comprehensively and prevent the water spill over the floor

Contd...

.

.

.

.

Contd...

Sl No	Care action	Rationale
10.	Apply the shampoo again, if the hair is found dirty	To ensure the cleanliness of the hair
11.	Drape the hair with towel and remove the water away	To make the patient comfortable and to ensure cleanliness of the area
12.	Fold the mackintosh into the bucket	To prevent the spill of water on the floor
13.	Remove the ear plugs and towel, which has covered the eyes; dry the neck and hair thoroughly	To make the hair waterless of hair and ease
14.	Spread the hair on the pillow for some time	To dry completely
15.	Wipe face with towel thoroughly after the bath; dry the hair	To keep the patient comfortable
16.	Replace the articles; discard dirty water and wash the hands	To maintain a safe environment

Points to Note

+ For patients who can be assisted with hair care, the nurse should advocate timely washing of hair and make sure that they are presentable.

EYE CARE

Definition

Eye care is the procedure of assessing, cleaning or irrigating the eye and/or instillation of prescribed ocular preparations.

Purposes

- To relieve pain and discomfort
- To prevent or treat infection
- To prevent or treat injury to the eye
- To detect disease at an early stage
- To detect drug-induced toxicity at an early stage
- To prevent damage to the cornea in sedated or unconscious patients.

Equipments

Sterile tray containing:
- Cotton balls
- Thumb forceps
- Bowl
- Kidney tray
- Towel
- Sterile 0.9% sodium chloride.

Procedure

The procedure for eye care is detailed in Table 3.4.

Table 3.4: Procedure for eye care

Sl No	Care action	Rationale
1.	Explain the procedure to the patient	To get consent from the patient
2.	Place the patient head well supported with tilted back	To make the patient comfortable and easy to do the procedure
3.	Wash hands thoroughly using bactericidal soap	To reduce the risk of cross infection
4.	Make sure enough light source is available	For the better observation
5.	For all time, treat uninfected or uninflamed eye first	To reduce the risk of cross infection
6.	Take two cotton balls, dip in sterile 0.9% normal saline and squeeze them nicely; start to clean the eye from inner canthus to outer canthus in a straight single stroke	If the swab is not squeezed properly, the solution will run downward to the patient's cheek; this may induce the risk of cross infection and cause the patient discomfort
7.	Ensure to use new swab each time; repeat the procedure until all the discharge has been removed	To reduce the risk of cross infection
8.	Once both eyelids have been cleaned and dried out, make the patient comfortable	To ensure patient's comfort
9.	Discard the waste according to the hospital policy	To minimize the cross-contamination
10.	Replace the equipment	To arrange and keep for next use
11.	Wash hands	To reduce the cross infection
12.	Record the procedure in the nurse's record	To follow-up any fluctuations and continuity of care

SPONGE BATH

Definition

Sponge bath is the procedure of cleaning the body of the patient, who is in the bed (unable to take bath himself/herself).

Purposes

- To prevent bacteria spreading on skin
- To clean the patient's body
- To stimulate the circulation
- To improve general muscular tone and joint
- To make patient comfort and help to induce sleep
- To observe skin condition and objective symptom.

Equipments

- A pair of gloves
- Apron
- Emollient
- Soap with soap dish
- Jug
- Basin

- Bucket
- Sponge cloth
- Face towel
- Bath towel
- Gauze piece: 2–3
- Mackintosh
- Bottom sheet, top sheet, draw sheets
- Nail cutter.

Procedure

The procedure for sponge bath is detailed in Table 3.5.

Table 3.5: Procedure for sponge bath

Sl No	Care action	Rationale
1.	Explain the purpose and procedure to the patient; if he/she is alert or oriented, question the patient about personal hygiene preferences and ability to assist with the bath	Providing information to get cooperation; encourage the patient to assist with care and to promote independence
2.	Gather all required equipments near the patient bedside	Organization facilitates accurate skill performance
3.	Assess and plan care in action with the patient and family/friend, if needed	To plan care will support participation and independence
4.	Check the room temperature; switch off air cooler (AC)/fan if not needed	To make the patient comfortable, and prevent the chillness and cold
5.	Wash your hands and put on gloves	To prevent the spread of organisms
6.	Provide urinals, bedpan or commode to the patient	To avoid any disturbance during procedure and to prevent any discomfort
7.	Remove the gloves and wash hands, use disposable gloves and apron	To prevent the cross-contamination and to prevent soiling of uniforms
8.	Provide proper privacy to the patient	To maintain the self-esteem and to make patient more comfortable
9.	Assist to remove clothing without exposing the patient	To maintain privacy and dignity, and body temperature
10.	Remove the patient's cloth and cover the patient body with top sheet; if an intravenous (IV) tubing is present on the patient's upper extremity, thread the IV tubing and bag through the sleeve of the soiled cloth and rehang the IV solution; check the IV flow rate	Removing the cloth permits easier access when cleansing the patient body and be sure that IV delivery is uninterrupted and to maintain the sterile setup
11.	Fill two basins about two third full with warm water (43°C–46°C or 110°F–115°F)	Water at proper temperature relaxes the patient and provides warmthness
12.	Assist the patient to move toward the right side of the cot	Easy to do the procedure
13.	Lift the patient's head and shoulder, and put mackintosh and big towel under the patient's body from the head to shoulders; place face towel under the chin, which has also covered the top sheet	To prevent the bottom sheet from becoming wet Soap irritates the eyes

Contd...

Contd...

Sl No	Care action	Rationale
	Make a mitt with the sponge towel and moisten it with plain water Wash the patient's eyes; clean from inner to outer corner; use a different section of the mitt to wash each eye Wash the patient's face, neck and ears; use soap on these areas only if the patient prefers; rinse and dry carefully	Washing from inner to outer corner prevents sweeping debris into the patient's eyes Using a separate portion of the mitt for each eye prevents the spread of infection
14.	Wash, rinse and dry upper half of the body, starting with the side furthest away from your side; care needs to be taken not to wet drains/dressings and IV devices	To promote patient well-being and cleanliness, and reduce the risk of cross infection
15.	Wash, rinse and dry legs, starting with the side furthest away from your side; roll patient, wash back; then using disposable pads, wash sacral area, check pressure points and cover areas that are not being washed Return patient on to their back, ensuring they are covered; apply napkin as required	To prevent and treat pressure ulcer and make the patient comfortable
16.	Clear area of any obstacles, ensure the environment warm and draw curtains, close doors to guarantee privacy and dignity	To maintain comfort, a safe environment, and promote privacy and dignity
17.	Change the water and wash the genital area with patient's verbal consent, (if patient is willing to wash this area themself, provide enough water to wipe); using a separate wipe, wash around the area and then dry it	To decrease risk of infection
18.	If patient is on urinary catheter, wear the gloves and wash the tubing away from the genital area; avoid using soap in genital area	To avoid the irritancy and to reduce risk of infection
19.	Turn the patient one side and remove the soiled sheet, and advance the new bottom sheet and draw sheet, if they are to remain in bed; ensure that a minimum of two nurses are present during this procedure	To reduce unnecessary activity and ensure the safe of the patient
20.	Dry and comb patient's hair as desired	To improve patient's comfort and promote self-esteem
21.	Cover the patient with top sheet; position the patient comfortably	To improve the patient's comfort and reduce the risk of pressure ulcers
22.	Take away all used articles and linen from the patient side	To maintain a safe environment and promote patient independence
23.	Remove the aprons and gloves, and dispose it according to hospital policy and wash the hands thoroughly	To prevent cross infection

Points to Note

- Remember, when washing genital area of female patients, wash from perineum to rectum.
- For male patients, retract the foreskin if uncircumcised when washing the penis.

NAIL CARE

Definition

Nail care is one of the nursing cares for maintaining the personal hygiene and to prevent the infections.

Purposes

- To keep nails clean
- To make the nails look neat
- To prevent the patient's skin from scratching
- To avoid infection caused by dirty nail.

Equipments

- Nail cutter
- Bowl with water
- Cotton
- Kidney tray
- Sponge cloth
- Middle towel
- Mackintosh
- Plastic bowl of small size
- Soap with soapdish
- Warm water
- Body lotion
- Clean gloves
- Face towel.

Procedure

The procedure for nail care is detailed in Table 3.6.

Table 3.6: Procedure for nail care

Sl No	Care action	Rationale
1.	Explain the procedure to the patient	To reduce the anxiety and to get the cooperation
2.	Arrange all the articles near to the patient	To minimize the time
3.	Wash your hands and wear gloves	To prevent the infection
4.	If patient is in bed, raise the backrest and place a towel under the hand; if the patient is in a chair, place a table in front and place a towel on the table	To make the patient comfortable till end of the procedure
5.	By using cotton with remover, remove nail polish from the nail	To prevent the infection
6.	Fill up the wash basin with warm water; immerse hands into a bowl of warm water	Warm water shall soften the nails and thicken the epithelial cells; to decrease the inflammation of skin and promote the local circulation

Contd...

Contd...

Sl No	Care action	Rationale
7.	Soak the fingers in the warm water for 5–10 minutes; soak one hand at a time or soak both at the same time	Soaking helps to cleanse the nails and make it easy to remove dirt and debris
8.	Place towel under patient's dried hands; gently remove dirt around and under each fingernails	To reduce the infections
9.	Cut short the finger nails by using nail clipper; shape and smooth the nails with nail file; wipe each fingertip with cotton dipped in antiseptic solution	Cutting straight prevents splitting of nail margins. To prevent the irregularity of the nail and formation of sharp that can irritate lateral margins
10.	Dry the hands with towel	To make comfortable
11.	Remove and replace the articles from the patient care area	To make the patient comfortable with safety

Points to Note

• Before starting the nail care, examine the exterior part of fingers, toes, feet and nails, to give particular attention to areas of dryness, inflammation and cracking; also inspect areas between toes, heels and soles of feet.
• The integrity of feet and nails determines frequency and level of hygiene required.
• Heels, soles and sides of the feet are prone to irritation from ill-fitting shoes.

BACK CARE

Definition

Back care means cleaning and massaging the back, paying special attention to pressure points. Especially back massage provides comfort and relaxes the patient; thereby it facilitates the physical stimulation to the skin and the emotional relaxation.

Purposes

• To improve circulation to the back
• To refresh the mode and feeling
• To relieve from fatigue, pain and stress
• To induce sleep.

Equipments

• A clean gown
• Clean gloves
• Towels (face towels and bath towel)
• Basin with warm water

- Kidney tray
- Soap
- Oil/White paraffin/Emollient
- Mackintosh.

Procedure

The procedure for back care is detailed in Table 3.7.

Table 3.7: Procedure for back care

Sl No	Care action	Rationale
1.	Perform hand hygiene	To prevent spread of infection
2.	Assemble all equipments required	Organization facilitates accurate skill and performance
3.	Identify the patient, and his/her identification status and condition	To evaluate sufficient condition of the patient
4.	Explain the patient about the purpose of the procedure	Providing information and to get cooperation
5.	Put all required equipments to the bedside	Appropriate setting can make the time of the procedure minimum and effective
6.	Close all windows and doors, and put the screen or/and utilize the curtain, if it is there	To ensure that the room is warm; to maintain the privacy
7.	Expose the patient's back fully and observe whether there are any abnormalities	To find any abnormalities soon is important to prevent more complication and/or provide proper medication as soon as possible If you find out some redness, heat or sores, you cannot massage that place If the patient has already some red sore or broken down area, you need to report the senior staff and/or doctor
8.	Lather soap by sponge towel; wipe with soap and rinse with plain warm water	To maintain the self-esteem and to make patient more comfortable
9.	Provide a gentle massage over the patient's back by using emollients; the pattern for massage includes: • Using your palm, begin in sacral area with smooth, circular strokes • Move your hands up the center of the back and then over the both scapula • Massage in a circular motion over scapula • Move your hands down the sides of the back • Massage the areas over right and left iliac crest • Apply firm, continuous pressure without breaking contact with the patient's skin • Repeat the above steps for 3–5 minutes using more lotion as necessary • Pat dry excess lotion with the towel	To improve circulation and to provide sense of comfort for the patient

Contd...

Contd...

SI No	Care action	Rationale
10.	Help the patient to put on the clothes and in returning the patient to comfortable position	To keep the patient warm and comfortable
11.	Replace all equipments to their proper place	To prepare for the next procedure
12.	Perform hand hygiene	To prevent the spread of infection
13.	Document on the chart with your signature, including date, time and the skin condition; report any findings to senior staff	Documentation provides coordination of care; giving signature maintains professional accountability

Points to Note

♦ Back care must be provided during every shift for patients, who are admitted in the intensive care unit (ICU). For patient with pressure ulcers, back massage need to be provided every 2nd hourly.

Steps of Back Massage

Steps of back massage is given in Table 3.8.

Table 3.8: Steps of back massage

SI No	Steps	Rationale
1.	Effleurage/Stroking: Start with long gliding strokes; use your entire hand or thumb pad. Start from sacral region to scapular region and the shoulder (do not apply pressure on the spinal cord)	To improve the blood flow. To prevent injury
2.	Petrissage: Use gentle pressure to knead or squeeze the muscles; use thumb and distal phalanges	To relieve the deeper muscle tension and clear out toxins
3.	Friction: Use fingertips or thumb pads and do circulatory motion	To breakdown knots and to achieve muscles flexibility
4.	Cupping: Use cupped hands to strike either side of the back/spinal cord	To percuss the area
5.	Tapotement: Use edge of the palm and strike briskly on either side of the back	To stimulate circulation

FOOT CARE

Definition

Foot care involves all aspects of preventive and corrective care of the foot and ankle.

Purposes

1. To make the patient comfortable.
2. To prevent ingrown nails.

3. Help to reduce developing of foot ulcer in diabetes mellitus (DM) patients.
4. To assess the foot problems including foot pain, joint inflammation, plantar warts, fungal infections (e.g. athlete's foot), nerve disorders, torn ligaments, broken bones, bacterial infections and tissue injuries such as frostbite.

Equipments

- Nail cutter
- Kidney tray
- Sponge cloth
- Middle towel
- Mackintosh
- A basin with warm water
- Soap with soapdish, if needed
- Cream or lotion
- Clean gloves.

Procedure

The procedure for foot care is detailed in Table 3.9.

Table 3.9: Procedure for foot care

SI No	Care action	Rationale
1.	Explain the procedure to the patient	To reduce the anxiety and to get the cooperation
2.	Arrange all the articles near the patient	To easily access and to minimize the time
3.	Wash your hands and wear gloves	To prevent the infection
4.	If patient is in bed, raise the backrest; if not contraindicated, make the patient to sit in the chair comfortably	Make the patient comfortable till the end of the procedure
5.	Inspect the feet, observe for redness, edema, ulceration, callus formation or ingrown toenails and report promptly	To identify the early stage of infections and helping to teach the patient, the signs and symptoms of infection
6.	By using cotton with remover, remove nail polish from the nail	To prevent the infection
7.	Fill up the washbasin with warm water; immerse foot into a bowl of warm water	Warm water softens the hard skin, and calluses and thickens the epithelial cells to decrease the inflammation of skin and promote the local circulation
8.	Soak the foot in the warm water for 5–10 minutes; soak one foot at a time or soak both at the same time	Prolonged positioning may cause discomfort

Contd...

Contd...

SI No	Care action	Rationale
9.	Wash feet and legs with soap, unless their medical condition hinders access to the feet/legs	To avoid other complication
10.	Dry your feet and toes thoroughly after washing them, and apply a moisturizing foot cream	To remove the dirt and prevent the infection
11.	Gently remove hard skin and calluses with a pumice stone or foot file thoroughly	To prevent infection and complications, and promote the comfort
12.	Trim your toenails straight across, never at an angle or down the edges	To prevent ingrown toenails and inflammations
13.	Apply lotion generously to all areas below the knee; avoid putting lotion on broken skin, in between the toes or on nail beds	To prevent the dryness and cracks
14.	Position the patient on cot, if needed	To make the patient comfortable
15.	Remove and replace the articles from the patient care area and replace it	Remove and replace the articles from the patient care area and replace it
16.	Document the procedure in the nurse's record; if any signs and symptoms of infection report these signs promptly to the physician	To prevent the progress to worsen and to do the comparison study of the patient condition from present to future

Points to Note

- Educate the patient to wear footwear (non-skid socks included) at all times. Stress the importance of not going bare foot.
- Instruct the patient to not go to bed without washing the feet. If they leave dirt on the skin's surface, it can become irritated and infected. Wash the feet every evening with soap and water.

PERINEAL CARE

Definition

Perineal care is a aseptic procedure, which involves cleaning of the genitalia and surrounding area by using antiseptic solution. Proper assessment and care of the perineal area will need professional clinical judgment.

Purposes

- To keep the perineal area clean
- To prevent infection
- To make the patient comfortable.

Equipments

- Sterile perineal care pack containing cup with cotton balls
- Artery clamp and thumb forceps

- Antiseptic solution (Betadine)
- Extra cotton balls
- Mackintosh
- A pair of clean gloves.

Procedure

The procedure for perineal care is detailed in Table 3.10.

Table 3.10: Procedure for perineal care

SI No	Care action	Rationale
1.	Explain the procedure to the patient	To make sure that the patient understands the procedure
2.	Gather all the equipment near the bedside	To save time
3.	Provide privacy	To make the patient sense comfortable and treat patient with self-esteem
4.	Wash hands thoroughly	To minimize risk of cross infection
5.	Help out patient to lie down in dorsal recumbent position	Easy to do the procedure and make the patient comfortable
6.	Put the mackintosh; cover the patient with a draw sheet or sheet that is folded double	To prevent the staining of antiseptic solution in the top sheet
7.	Open the sterile perineal pack and pour antiseptic solution	To minimize risk of cross infection
8.	Wash hands again; wear a pair of clean gloves	To minimize risk of cross infection
9.	Clean thighs by using the cotton ball from the center to the peripheral area; use a separate cotton ball for each stroke	To minimize risk of cross infection
10.	Use non-dominant hand too gently and clean labia majora; retract labia from thigh with dominant hand, clean from perineum to rectum; give more attention in skin folds	Wiping from perineum to rectum reduces chance of transmitting fecal organisms to urinary meatus; skin folds may contain microorganisms
11.	Separate labia minora with non-dominant hand to expose urethral meatus and vaginal orifice; with dominant hand, clean downward from pubic area toward rectum in one smooth stroke	Reduces chance of transmitting microorganisms to urinary meatus
12.	Follow the front to back method, dry perineal area thoroughly (perineum to rectum)	To prevent the cross-contamination
13.	Position the patient as he/she desire	To make the patient comfortable
14.	Replace articles and wash hands	To arrange and keep it ready for next use, and minimize risk of cross infection
15.	Document procedure in the nurses record; if there is any foul-smelling discharge or any other abnormalities, inform the doctor	Help to identify the infection in early stage

---

/ **Points to Note**

For male catheter care:
* Gently grasp the patient's penis.
* In an uncircumcised male, carefully retract the foreskin prior to washing the penis.
* Cleanse in a circular motion, moving from the tip of the penis backwards toward the pubic area.
* Return the foreskin to its former position.
* Wash, rinse and dry the scrotum carefully.

PERFORMING PHYSICAL EXAMINATION

Definition

Physical examination is an important tool in assessing the client's health status. Approximately, 15% of the information used in the assessment, comes from the physical examination. It is performed to collect objective data and to correlate it with subjective data.

Purposes

* To collect objective data from the client
* To detect the abnormalities with systematic technique early
* To diagnose diseases
* To determine the status of present health in health checkup and refer the client for consultation, if needed.

Principles of Physical Examination

A systematic approach should be used, while doing physical examination. This helps avoiding any duplication or omission. Generally, a cephalocaudal approach (head to toe) is used, but in the case of infant, examination of heart and lung function should be done before the examination of other body parts, because when the infant starts crying, his/her breath and heart rate may change.

Methods of Physical Examination

* Inspection
* Palpation
* Percussion
* Auscultation.

Inspection

Inspection means looking at the client carefully to discover any signs of illness. Inspection gives more information than other method and is therefore the most useful method of physical examination.

Palpation

Palpation means using hands to touch and feel. Different parts of hands are used for different sensations such as temperature, texture of skin, vibration, tenderness, etc. For example, fingertips are used for fine tactile surfaces, the back of fingers for feeling temperature, and the flat of the palm and fingers for feeling vibrations.

Percussion

Percussion determines the density of various parts of the body from the sound produced by them, when they are tapped with fingers. Percussion helps to find out abnormal solid masses, fluid and gas in the body, and to map out the size and borders of certain organ like the heart.

Methods of percussion are:
1. Put the middle fingers of the patient's left hand against the body part to be percussed.
2. Tap the end joint of this finger with the middle finger of the right hand.
3. Give two or three taps at each area to be percussed.
4. Compare the sound produced at different areas.

Auscultation

Auscultation means listening the sounds transmitted by a stethoscope, which is used to listen to the heart, lungs and bowel sounds.

Equipments

- Tray: 1
- Watch with a seconds hand: 1
- Height scale: 1
- Weight scale: 1
- Thermometer: 1
- Stethoscope: 1
- Sphygmomanometer: 1
- Measuring tape: 1
- Scale: 1
- Torchlight or penlight: 1
- Spatula: 1
- Reflex hammer: 1
- Otoscope if available: 1 set
- Disposable gloves: 1 pair
- Cotton swabs and cotton gauze pad
- Examination table
- Record form
- Ballpoint pen, pencils.

Procedure

The procedure for performing physical examination is detailed in Table 3.11.

Table 3.11: Procedure for performing physical examination

Sl No	Action/Rationale	Normal finding	Abnormal finding
1.	**Explain the purpose and procedure** Providing information fosters patient's cooperation and allays anxiety	Preparation of the patient for physical examination	
2.	**Close doors and put screen** To provide privacy		
3.	**Encourage the client to empty bladder** A full bladder makes the patient uncomfortable		
4.	**Perform physical examination** *General examination* Assess overall body appearance and mental status *Inspection* a. Observe the client's ability to respond to verbal commands (responses indicate the client's speech and cognitive function)	Client responds appropriately to commands	Client has confused, disoriented or inappropriate responses
	b. Observe the client's level of consciousness (LOC) and orientation; ask the client to state his/her own name, current location and approximate day, month or year (responses indicate the client's brain function; LOC is the degree of awareness of environmental stimuli; it varies from full wakefulness and alertness to coma; orientation is a measure of cognitive function or the ability to think and reason)	The client is fully awake and alert; eyes are open and follow people or objects; the client is attentive to questions and responds promptly and accurately to commands If the patient is sleeping, he/she responds readily to verbal or physical stimuli and demonstrates wakefulness and alertness; the client is aware of who he/she is (orientation to person), where he/she is (orientation to place) and when it is (orientation to time)	Client has a lowered LOC and shows irritability, short attention span or dulled perceptions Client is uncooperative or unable to follow simple commands or answer simple questions At a lowered LOC, the client may respond to physical stimuli only; the lowest extreme is coma, when the eyes are closed and the client fails to respond to verbal or physical stimuli with no voluntary movement If LOC is between full awareness and coma, objectively note the client's eye movements; voluntary, withdrawal to stimuli or withdrawal to noxious stimuli (pain) only

Contd...

Contd...

Sl No	Action/Rationale	Normal finding	Abnormal finding
	c. Observe the client's ability to think, remember, process information and communicate (these processes indicate cognitive functioning) Inspect articulation on speech, style and contents of speaking	The client is able to follow commands, repeat and remember information Smooth, appropriate native language	Dysphasia, dysarthria, memory loss, disorientation, hallucination Not clear/not smooth/ inappropriate contents
	d. Observe the client's ability to see, hear, smell and distinguish tactile sensations	The client can hear even though the speaker turns away He/She can identify objects or reads a clock in the room and distinguish between sharp and soft objects	The client cannot hear tones and must look directly at the speaker He/She cannot read a clock or distinguish sharp from soft
	e. Observe signs of distress (alert the examiner to immediate concerns; if distress is noted, the client may require healthcare interventions before continuing the examination)		The client shows labored breathing, wheezing, coughing, wincing, sweating, guarding of body part (suggests pain), anxious facial expression or fidgety movements Posture is stopped or twisted Limb movements are uneven or unilateral
	f. Observe for facial expression and mood (these could be effected by disease or ill condition)	Eyes are alert and in contact with examiner The client is relaxed, smiles or frowns appropriately and has a calm demeanor	Eyes are closed or averted The client is frowning or grimacing and is unable to answer questions
	g. Observe general appearance: Posture, gait and movement (to identify obvious changes)	Posture is upright, gait is smooth and equal for the client's age and development; limb movements are bilateral	Posture is stopped or twisted; limb movements are uneven or unilateral
	h. Observe grooming, personal hygiene and dress (personal appearance can indicate self-comfort; grooming suggests his/her ability to perform self-care)	Clothing reflects gender, age, climate; hair, skin and clothing are clean, well-groomed and appropriate for the occasion	The client wears unusual clothing for gender, age or climate Hair is poor groomed, lack of cleanliness Excessive oil on the skin Body odor is present
5.	**Measurement** a. Height: i. Ask the client to remove shoes and stand with his/her back and heels touching the wall		

Contd...

Contd...

SI No	Action/Rationale	Normal finding	Abnormal finding
	ii. Place a pencil flat on client's head, so that it makes a mark on the wall iii. This shows his/her height measured with centimeter tape from the floor to the mark on the wall (or if available, measure the height with measuring scale) b. Weight: i. Weigh client without shoes and much clothing	> 140 cm (or 145 cm) in female Body mass index (BMI) is used to assess the status of nutrition using weight and height in the world Formula for BMI = weight (kg)/ height (m²) Normal BMI = 18.5–24.5	< 140 cm (or 145 cm) in female **Classification**　**BMI** • Under weight　< 18.5 • Healthy weight　18.5–24.5 • Over weight　25–29.9 • Obesity　> 30
6.	**Take vital signs** Vital signs provide baseline data a. Temperature b. Pulse (rate/minute) Take the pulse rate and check the beats c. Respiration Count the breaths without giving notice d. Blood pressure Take blood pressure under quiet and war	 36.5°C–37°C In adult, 60–80/min, regular and steady Breaths per minute: 16–20/min Clear sound of breaths, regular and steady 120/80 mm Hg	 • Hypothermia < 35°C • Pyrexia 38°C–40°C • Hyperpyrexia > 40°C • Bradycardia • Tachycardia • Pulse deficit, arrhythmia • Bradypnea < 10/min • Tachypnea > 20/min • Cheyne-Stokes • Kussmaul's respiration, wheeze, stridor • Hypotension: In normal adults, blood pressure (BP) < 95/60 mm Hg • Hypertension: BP > 140/90 mm Hg
7.	**Integumentary assessment** Assess integumentary structures (skin, hair, nails) and function ***Skin*** *Inspection and palpation* a. Inspect the back and palms of the client's hands for skin color; compare the right and	 The color varies from black brown or fair, depending upon the genetic factors	 Erythema, loss of pigmentation, cyanosis, pallor, jaundice

Contd...

SI No	Action/Rationale	Normal finding	Abnormal finding
	left sides make a similar inspection of the feet and toes	Color variations on dark pigmented skin may be best seen in the mucous membranes, nail beds, sclera or lips	
	b. Palpate the skin on the back and palms of the client's hands for moisture, texture: • Moisture • Texture	Slightly moist, no excessive moisture or dryness—firm, smooth, soft, elastic skin	Excessive dryness indicates hypothyroidism Oiliness in acne Roughness in hypothyroidism Velvety texture in hyperthyroidism
	c. Palpate the skin's temperature with the back of your hand	Warmth	Generalized warmth in fever and local warmth, coolness in hypothyroidism
	d. Pinch and release the skin on the back (this palpation indicates the skin's degree of hydration and turgor)	Pinched skin that promptly or gently returns to its previous state, when released signifies normal turgor	Pinched skin is very slow to return to normal position of the client's hand
	e. Press suspected edematous areas with the edge of fingers for 10 seconds and observe for the depression	Depression recovers quickly	Depression recovers slowly or remains Edema indicates fluid retention, a sign of circulatory disorders
	f. Inspect the skin for lesions; note the appearance, size, location, presence and appearance of drainage	Skin is intact, without reddened areas, but with variations in pigmentation and texture, depending on the area's location and its exposure to light and pressure; moles, warts are normal	Erythema, ecchymosis, lesions include rashes, macules, papules, vesicles, wheals, nodules, pustules, tumors or ulcers Wounds include incisions, abrasions, lacerations, pressure ulcers
	Nail a. Inspect the color, shape and lesions of the nails	Pink color and longitudinal bands may be seen in the nails of some people	Koilonychia (spoon-shaped nails) seen in protein deficiency anemia

Contd...

Contd...

Sl No	Action/Rationale	Normal finding	Abnormal finding
	b. Check capillary refill by pressing the nail to blanch; then quickly release pressure, note the return of color	Normally the color returns to pink within 3 seconds; absence of discoloration, cyanosis, clubbing, separation from the edge, etc.	Cyanosis and clubbing is present if there is poor oxygen saturation in the blood Sluggish color return indicates respiratory or cardiovascular dysfunction
	Hair and scalp Inspect the hair for color, distribution, growth and texture	Color may differ from gray to complete black Texture varies from straight to curly The scalp should be clean and absence of scales, lesions, etc.	Alopecia (excessive hair loss is seen in cancer patients) Pediculosis Dandruff Redness and scaling
8.	**Head and neck assessment** ***Face*** Inspect the client's facial expression, symmetry, movement, etc.	Relaxed facial expression without having any deviation and involuntary movement	Blunt expression indicates Parkinson disease Moon face, i.e. Cushing's syndrome Edema around the eyes—glomerulonephritis
	Eyes a. Eyebrows: Observe the eyebrow for color and distribution	Normal black- or brown-colored lashes with normal distribution	Scaliness in seborrheic dermatitis
	b. Eyelids: Inspect the eyelids for edema, lesions, distribution and direction of eyelashes	Eyelashes grow in a downward direction	Ptosis Sty Ectropion Entropion Failure of the eyelids to close
	c. Conjunctiva and sclera: Inspect the color of the sclera and conjunctiva	Transparent white color of the sclera and dark pink conjunctiva	A yellow sclera indicates jaundice and pale conjunctiva indicates anemia
	d. Cornea and lens: Inspect the cornea under good lighting; note any opacities of the lens	Transparent	Opacities in the lens due to cataract
	e. Pupils: Inspect the papillary size, shape, symmetry and reaction • Pupillary response to light:	Pupils are equal, round, symmetrical and equally reacting to light	Unequal pupils Miosis—constriction of the pupils Mydriasis—dilation of the pupils
	– Ask the client to look straight and focus the torchlight from the periphery to the center of the eye	The pupils constrict when the torch approaches the center and it dilates as it is removed	Unresponsive to light otitis media or otitis externa

Contd...

Contd...

Sl No	Action/Rationale	Normal finding	Abnormal finding

	− Remove it to the other side and observe how the pupils react
	f. Coordination of eye movements:
	   • **Ask the client to keep the head still and follow the object in the examiner's hand with the eyes only**
	   • **Move the object toward** right, left, up and down
	g. Visual acuity test:
	   • **Use Snellen chart to check the visual acuity**
	   • **Make the patient to sit** 20 feet away from the Snellen chart and ask to read the letters /numbers by closing one eye
	   • **Repeat the same in the other eye**
	   • **Compare visual acuity of** the client with normal vision
		Both eyes move together to follow the direction of the object without moving his head
		
		20/20 is normal
			Eyes do not move together when the object moves indicates paralysis of cranial nerves
			
			Myopia (near sightedness)
			Hypermetropia (far sightedness)

	Ears a. Inspect the shape, location of ears and measure the size b. External auditory meatus: Inspect the external auditory meatus using torchlight or otoscope to assess redness, foreign body, swelling, discharge and cerumen c. Hearing test: i. Whisper test: Stay 30–60 cm away from client's ear and whisper slowly some two syllable words	Equal size bilaterally The top of the pinnae meet the eye-occiput line Normally client repeats the word correctly	Microtica or macrotica The top of the pinnae do not meet the eye-occiput line; commonly seen in mentally retarded children Clear blood from the ear indicates brain hemorrhage Impacted cerumen causes conductive hearing loss A sticky yellow discharge indicates otitis media or otitis externa If the client does not repeat the words, it indicates hearing loss

Contd...

Contd...

Sl No	Action/Rationale	Normal finding	Abnormal finding
	ii. Rinne test: This test is performed by placing a high-frequency (512 Hz) vibrating tuning fork against the patient's mastoid bone and asking the patient to tell you, when the sound is no longer heard; once the client signal that cannot hear it, quickly position the still vibrating tuning fork 1–2 cm from the auditory canal and again ask the patient to tell you if they are able to hear the tuning fork	Air conduction should be greater than bone conduction and so the patient should be able to hear the tuning fork next to the pinna after they can no longer hear it, when held against the mastoid	If they are not able to hear the tuning fork after mastoid test, it means that their bone conduction is more than air conduction; this indicates conductive hearing loss Sensorineural hearing loss—patients usually can hear better on the mastoid process than air process, but indicate the sound has stopped much earlier than conductive loss patients
	iii. Weber test: Keep the vibrated tuning fork in the vertex of the head	The client will hear the sound equally in both the ears	If the client hears more sound in left ear than the right, it means the client has conductive hearing loss in left ear because the sound gets lateralized to the deafer ear
	Nose		
	a. Inspect the shape, size, symmetry of the nose	Nostrils are uniform in size, no flare, no deviation and no obstruction in both vestibule	Asymmetrical in size Deviated nasal septum Flaring nostrils Obstruction in the nose by polyps
	b. Inspect the interior aspect of the nose using pen/torchlight or rhinoscope	No polyps, inflammation, bleeding and foreign body	Nasal mucosa is red and swollen (rhinitis) Deviation of the lower septum is common
	c. Palpate for frontal and maxillary sinus tenderness	No tenderness and pain	Local pain, tenderness, nasal discharge and tenderness suggest acute sinusitis
	Mouth		
	a. Observe the color, moisture and cracking of the lips	No bluish discoloration, cracks and ulcers	Lips bluish (cyanosis) and pallor Cracks, ulcer
	b. Inspect the gums, teeth and tongue	No inflammation and infection in gums, tongue and teeth	Gingivitis Loose teeth Dental caries Coated tongue in typhoid
	Pharynx Ask the client to open the mouth and say 'aah', which helps to see	Pink throat No difficulty in swallowing	Tonsillitis Adenoiditis

Contd...

Contd...

SI No	Action/Rationale	Normal finding	Abnormal finding
	the pharynx well; if not, use spatula to press the tongue; inspect soft palate, tonsils, pharynx and uvula to detect symmetry, swelling or tonsillar enlargement	Pink and small tonsils	Difficulty in swallowing In cranial nerve X paralysis, the soft palate fails to rise and the uvula deviates to the opposite side
	Neck		
	a. Inspect the neck for its symmetry, enlargement of lymph nodes; observe the range of motion of the neck	Head positions centered in the midline and head should be held erect	Rigid neck occurs with arthritis
	b. Lymph nodes: Palpate the lymph nodes by using the pads of your index and middle fingers to detect any palpable nodes with size, shape, mobility, consistency and tenderness	Lymph nodes are neither visible nor becomes red Normal nodes feel movable, discrete, soft, nontender	Enlargement of lymph nodes Lymph adenopathy (> 1 cm) due to infection, allergy or neoplasm Diffuse lymphadenopathy may be seen in human immunodeficiency virus/ acquired immunodeficiency syndrome (HIV/AIDS)
	c. Trachea: • **Inspect the trachea to find out any deviation from its normal** • **Palpate for any tracheal shift; place the index finger on the trachea in the sternal notch and slip it off to each side**	Normally trachea is in midline No deviation from the midline	Tracheal push toward one side suggests mass in the neck Tracheal deviation suggests mediastinal mass, atelectasis, etc.
	d. Thyroid gland i. Inspect the thyroid gland and confirm that it rise with swallowing and then fall to their resting position	Normally thyroid gland cannot be palpable; no enlargement, presence of nodules and tenderness	Diffuse enlargement suggests goiter Firm suggests malignancy Soft in Graves' disease Tenderness in thyroiditis
	ii. Palpate the thyroid gland • **Stand behind the client** • **Ask the client to flex the neck slightly forward** • **Place the fingers of both hands on the client's neck and ask him/her to swallow water; feel for the thyroidisthmus rising up under your finger pads**		

Contd...

Contd...

SI No	Action/Rationale	Normal finding	Abnormal finding
9.	**Chest and lungs** a. Inspection: Make the patient in supine or sitting or semi-Fowler's position to examine the chest; observe the shape and movement of anterior and posterior chest	Anteroposterior (AP) diameter may increase with age Shoulders are even, spine is midline and straight Posterior chest slightly rises and falls on respiration	Barrel chest; AP diameter may increase in chronic obstructive pulmonary disease Structural deformities Scoliosis (lateral curvature) Lordosis (pronounced lumbar curvature) Kyphosis (abnormal spinal curvature and vertebral rotation deform the chest)
	b. Palpation: Palpate the posterior wall over areas to detect any tender masses, swelling or painful area	No tenderness, superficial lumps or masses, normal skin mobility and turgor	Tender pectoral muscles or costal cartilage Pain Masses
	c. Percussion: Percuss the posterior chest to identify any area with an abnormal percussion	Resonance is normal lung sound	Hyperresonance is found in chronic obstructive pulmonary disease (COPD) and asthma Dullness is found in pneumonia, pleural effusion and atelectasis
	d. Auscultation: Listen to the breath posteriorly with mouth open and more deeply than the normal, to note intensity; identify any variation and any adventitious sounds; repeat auscultation in the posterior chest	Breath sounds are usually louder in upper anterior lung fields Bronchial, bronchovesicular, vesicular sounds are the normal breath sounds	Decreased or absent breath sounds suggest atelectasis, pleural effusion, pneumothorax and COPD Increased breath sound suggests pneumonia
10.	**Heart/Pericardium** Make the patient to be in supine position with the head elevated 30°: a. Inspection: Inspect the anterior chest for apical pulsation	Normally seen in children and those with thinner chest	A heave or lift suggests ventricular hypertrophy
	b. Palpation: Palpate the apical pulse by using finger pad to detect some abnormal condition; ask the client to exhale and then hold it; aids the examiner in locating the pulsation in the fourth or fifth intercostal space	The apical pulse is palpable in about half of adult But not palpable in obese clients with thick chest walls	Not palpable in pulmonary emphysema due to overriding lungs

Contd...

Contd...

SI No	Action/Rationale	Normal finding	Abnormal finding
	c. Percussion: It is done to outline the heart's borders and detect cardiac enlargement: • Place your non-dominant hand's fingers on the client's fifth intercostal space over the left side of the chest near the anterior axillary line • Slide your non-dominant hand's finger toward yourself, percussing as you go • Note the change of sound from resonance over the lung to dull over the heart d. Auscultation: • Place the stethoscope on the chest and hear the sound in second right (aortic valve area) and left (pulmonic area) intercostal space • Then auscultate left lower sternal border (tricuspid valve area) and fifth intercostal space at left midclavicular line (mitral valve area) • Listen S1 and S2; note the rate and rhythm • Listen for murmurs	Percussion sound does not increase Rate ranges from 60 to 100 beats per minute S1 is loudest at the apex and S2, at the base; the rhythm should be regular	Cardiac enlargement is due to increased ventricular wall thickness Irregular rhythm suggests cardiac diseases Both heart sounds are diminished in emphysema, obesity and pericardial effusion Diastolic murmur suggests heart diseases
11.	**Breasts and axillae** a. Inspection: Observe for the size, shape and symmetry of the breasts; inspect color, dimpling, edema or skin lesions and discharge in the breast and nipple; and observe the axillary and subclavicular regions for lymphatic drainage; note any bulging, edema and discoloration	Symmetrical in shape Often the left breast is slightly larger than the right No edema and discoloration normally But fine blue vascular network is visible during pregnancy	Sudden enlargement of breast suggests inflammation or new growth Edema, hyperpigmentation, redness and heat with inflammation, unilateral superficial veins in a non-pregnant woman; recent nipple retraction signifies acquired disease

Contd...

Contd...

SI No	Action/Rationale	Normal finding	Abnormal finding
	b. Palpation: • **Help her to be in a supine position** • **Place a small pad or towel under the side to be palpated and raise her arm over the head** • **Use the pads of your three fingers and make a gentle rotary motion on the breast; start at the nipple and palpate out to the periphery** • **Move in a clockwise direction** • **Apply gentle pressure on the nipple from outside the areola toward the center and observe any discharge appears; note its color and consistency**	In nulliparous woman, normal breast tissue feels firm, smooth and elastic Premenstrual enlargement is normal During lactation, milk secretion is normal	Heat, redness and swelling in non-lactating woman suggests inflammation
12.	**Abdomen** Make the client to lie down in supine position after emptying the bladder: a. Inspection: • **Observe the contour and symmetry of the abdomen** • **Inspect symmetry of the abdomen** • **Observe the location, contour and bulges of umbilicus** • **Observe for peristalsis movement and aortic pulsation in the epigastric region** b. Auscultation: • **Listen to the abdomen before performing percussion or palpation**	Normally ranges from flat to round The abdomen should be symmetric bilaterally Normally it is in midline and inverted with no signs of inflammation Normally, peristalsis waves are visible in very thin persons and aortic pulsation is visible in epigastrium Normal sound consists of clicks and gurgles	Abdominal distension Scaphoid abdomen Hernia Enlarged and everted with umbilical hernia Increased peristalsis with the abdominal distension, suggests intestinal obstruction Marked pulsation of the aorta occurs with widened pulse pressure Hyperactive sound will be loud, rushing and high pitched, which suggests increased motility in gastrointestinal infections

Contd...

Contd...

Sl No	Action/Rationale	Normal finding	Abnormal finding
	• **Listen for the bowel sounds using stethoscope**		Hypoactive or absence of sound indicates paralytic ileus or peritonitis
	• **Listen for the vascular sounds or bruit with the stethoscope**	Normally no sound will be heard	Systolic bruit occurs with stenosis or occlusion of an artery
	c. Percussion: It is done to assess the presence of gas in the abdomen and to identify possible masses:		
	• **Percuss the abdomen lightly in all four quadrants** • **Note any large areas of dullness**	Tympany should dominate because of the presence of gas in the gastrointestinal tract Normal dullness in the liver and spleen	Absence of tympany
	d. Palpation: It is done to screen for organomegaly, mass or tenderness:		
	• **Place the client in supine position; keeping your finger pads on the abdominal surface, gently depress the surface about 1–5 cm** • **Move clockwise and explore the entire abdomen**	No abdominal mass Normally, liver edge, full bladder and right kidney can be palpable	Mass, tenderness, rigidity
	Liver • Stand on the client's right side • Place your left hand under the client's back parallel to the 11th and 12th ribs • Lift up to support the abdominal contents • Place your right hand on the right upper quadrant with fingers parallel to the midline • Push deeply down when the client takes deep breath • Feel for liver sliding over the fingers, as the client inspires • Note any enlargement or tenderness	Liver is normally not palpable	If the liver is palpable more than 1–2 cm below the right costal margin, it indicates enlargement

Contd...

Contd...

Sl No	Action/Rationale	Normal finding	Abnormal finding
	Spleen Make the patient to lie in supine position: • Stand on the client's right side • Place your left hand over the abdomen and behind the left side at the 11th and 12th ribs • Lift up, to support the abdominal contents • Place your right hand on the left upper quadrant with fingers pointing toward the left axilla • Push deeply down and under the left costal margin, when the client takes deep breath • Note any enlargement or tenderness	Normally spleen is not palpable No enlargement and tenderness	The enlarged spleen is palpable about 2 cm below the left costal margin on inspiration
	Kidneys • Place the client in supine position • Place your left hand between the client's lowest rib and pelvic bone • Place your right hand on the client's right flank region • As the client takes deep inspiration, press your right hand deeply just below the costal margin • Try to capture the kidney between two hands • Note the enlargement or tenderness	Normally both kidneys are not palpable	Enlarged kidney Tenderness Kidney mass Bilateral enlargement suggests polycystic kidney disease
	Percussion in the kidney It is performed to assess the tenderness in the kidney: • Place the ball of one hand in the costovertebral angle • Strike it with the ulnar surface of your fist	Normally painless	Pain with fist percussion suggests pyelonephritis Sometimes it may be due to musculoskeletal cause

Contd...

Contd...

Sl No	Action/Rationale	Normal finding	Abnormal finding
13.	**Genitalia and excretory system** *Female genitalia* • Place the patient in dorsal recumbent position; observe the skin color, hair distribution, labia majora, any lesions • Look for any discharge or bleeding from the vagina, prolapsed, etc.	No redness or swelling in labia Usually no discharge from the vagina No prolapsed and bleeding from the vagina, except during menstruation	Foul smelling; white, yellow discharge from the vagina Bleeding per vagina
	Male genitalia • Inspect the skin, glans and urethral meatus • Observe for urethral discharge • Inspect and palpate the scrotum and penis; palpate gently each scrotal half between thumb and first two fingers	The glans looks smooth without lesions and the foreskin easily retractable Asymmetry is normal, with the left scrotal half, lower than the right No lump, no tenderness Testes are equal in size	Phimosis—unable to retract the foreskin Purulent discharge from the urethra suggests urethritis Abnormalities in scrotum are varicocele, hydrocele, tumor, orchitis, hernia
	Anus Inspect the anal region for any irritation, cracks, fissure and dilated vessels using torchlight or proctoscope	No irritation, fissure, cracks No dilated vessels in anus	Hemorrhoids Fissures
14.	**Musculoskeletal system** • Ask the client to stand and then inspect neck, shoulder, arms, hands, hips, knees, legs, ankle and feet; compare the symmetry of both sides	No bone or joint deformities No swelling or redness of joints No muscle wasting	Presence of bone and joint deformities Redness or swelling suggests joint inflammation Muscle wasting suggests degenerative diseases
	• Check the range of motion and watch for signs of pain	Able to move joints freely and no signs of pain, while moving	Signs of pain, while moving the joint indicates dislocation or subluxation
15.	**Peripheral vascular examination** • Inspect the arms and legs for color, size, any lesion and skin changes • Palpate peripheral pulses	Symmetrical in shape No edema, no changes in skin color and normal pulse rate	Edema of upper extremities Varicose vein in lower extremities

Contd...

Contd...

Sl No	Action/Rationale	Normal finding	Abnormal finding
	• Press the skin gently and firmly at the tibia, ankles and feet for 5 seconds and then release; note whether the fingers leave an impression on the skin • Ask the client to stand and assess the venous system for dilated and tortuous veins	No impression left on the skin, when pressed Edema during pregnancy is common due to weight bearing	Pallor with vasoconstriction Cyanosis Bilateral pitting edema occurs with heart failure, diabetic neuropathy or hepatic cirrhosis
16.	**Nervous system** ***Assessing sensation*** • Ask the client to close the eyes • Select areas on face arms, hands, legs and feet • Give a superficial pain, light touch and vibration to each site by turn • Note the client's ability of sensation on each site	Feels pain sensation, light touch and vibration Equally in both sides	Decreased pain or touch sensation suggests paralysis or paresthesia; it is commonly seen in patients with hemiparesis
	Assessing motor function Ask the client to stand and walk across the room in his/her regular walk backward and turn toward you	Straight and balanced walk	Unbalanced walk, limping Uncoordinated or unsteady walk suggests cerebellar dysfunction

	Checking reflexes
	It is done to detect the intactness of the arc at specific spinal canal
	Deep tendon reflexes
	a. Biceps reflex (C5–C6):
	  • **Support the client's forearm**
	  • **Place your thumb on the biceps tendon and strike a blow on your thumb with the knee hammer**
	  • Observe the response
		Normal response is contraction of the biceps muscle and flexion of the forearm	Hyperreflexia
			Hyporeflexia

	b. Triceps reflex (C7–C8):
	  • **Tell the client to flex the arm toward the chest and keep it in a relaxed manner**
	  • **Strike the triceps tendon directly just above the elbow**
	  • Observe the response
		Normal response is extension of the forearm	

Contd...

Contd...

Sl No	Action/Rationale	Normal finding	Abnormal finding
	c. Brachioradialis reflex (C5–C6): • Hold the client's thumb to suspend the forearms in relaxation • Strike the forearm directly, about 2–3 cm above the radial styloid process • Observe the response	Normal response is flexion and supination of the forearm	
	d. Quadriceps reflex or 'knee jerk' (L2–L4): • Let the lower legs dangle freely to flex the knee and stretch the tendons • Strike the tendon directly just below the patella • Observe the response and palpate contraction of the quadriceps	Normal response is extension of the lower leg	
	e. Achilles reflex or 'ankle jerk' (L5 to S2): • Position the client with the knee flexed • Hold the foot in dorsiflexion • Strike the Achilles tendon directly • Feel the response	Normal response is the foot plantar flexion against your hand	
	Superficial reflex a. Plantar reflex (L4 to S2) • Position the thigh in slight external rotation • With the reflex hammer, draw a light stroke up the lateral side of the sole of the foot and inward across the ball of the foot • Observe the response	Normal response is plantar flexion of all the toes, extension of big toe and inversion, and flexion of the forefoot	Fanning of toes indicates upper motor neuron disease

NASOGASTRIC TUBE INSERTION

Definition

Nasogastric intubation refers to the process of placing a soft plastic nasogastric (NG) tube through a patient's nostril, past the pharynx and down the esophagus into a patient's stomach.

Purposes

1. To remove substances from the stomach or as a means of testing stomach function or contents.
2. To deliver tube feedings to a patient when they are unable to eat.
3. Other substances that are delivered through a NG tube may include ice water to stop bleeding in the stomach or medications to neutralize swallowed poisons.
4. To remove air that accumulates in the stomach during cardiopulmonary resuscitation (CPR).
5. To remove stomach contents after major trauma or surgery, to prevent aspiration of the stomach contents.
6. To prevent nausea and vomiting by removing stomach contents and preventing distention of the stomach when a patient has a bleeding ulcer, bowel obstruction or other gastrointestinal diseases.
7. For laboratory studies.

Equipments

- Sterile gloves
- Appropriate size of Ryle's tube
- Xylocaine jelly (2%)
- Stethoscope
- Disposable syringe
- A cup of water
- Adhesive plaster
- Appropriate size suction catheter (if needed)
- Laryngoscope (if needed)
- Mask.

Procedure

The procedure for nasogastric tube insertion is detailed in Table 3.12.

Table 3.12: Procedure for nasogastric tube insertion

Sl No	Care action	Rationale
1.	Explain the procedure to the patient/patient relatives	To get valid consent from the patient/patient relatives
2.	Arrange needed articles near the bedside	Easy to perform the procedure and to prevent unnecessary contamination
3.	Place the mackintosh and draw sheet under the head and neck	To prevent the soiling of the linen
4.	Position the patient; if possible, make the patient to sit in upright for optimal neck/stomach alignment	Easy to insert the tube into the gastrointestinal (GI) tract

Contd...

Contd...

Sl No	Care action	Rationale
5.	Examine nostrils for deformity/obstructions to determine the best side for insertion	To prevent bleeding, while doing the procedure
6.	Measure tubing from bridge of nose to earlobe, then to the point halfway between the end of the sternum and the navel; mark measured length with a marker or note the distance	To insert the appropriate size to prevent coiling of the tube inside the GI tract
7.	Lubricate 2–4 inches of tube with lubricant (preferably 2% Xylocaine); this procedure is very uncomfortable for many patients, so a squirt of Xylocaine jelly in the nostril not and a spray of Xylocaine to the back of the throat, will help alleviate the discomfort	For easy insertion of tube into the stomach
8.	• Pass tube via either nare posteriorly, past the pharynx into the esophagus and then the stomach • Instruct the patient to swallow (may offer ice chips/water) and advance the tube as the patient swallows; swallowing of small sips of water may enhance passage of tube into esophagus • If resistance is met, rotate tube slowly downward advancement toward ear; do not force	To ensure the cleanliness of the hair
9.	Withdraw tube immediately if changes occur in patient's respiratory status, if tube coils in mouth; if the patient begins to cough or turns pretty colors	To prevent the complication
10.	Advance tube until mark is reached	To place the tube into the stomach accurately
11.	Check for placement by attaching syringe to free end of the tube, aspirate sample of gastric contents; obtain an X-ray to verify placement before instilling any feedings/medications or if you have concerns about the placement of the tube	To prevent the misplacement of the tube
12.	Secure tube with tape or commercially prepared tube holder	To prevent the misplacement of the tube
13.	Monitor the vital signs of the patient	To identify the abnormalities immediately
14.	Remove the mackintosh form the patient side	To make the patient comfortable
15.	Wash and replace the equipments	To make it arrange for next use
16.	Document the procedure and patient's parameters (during and after the procedure) in the nurse's record	To follow-up care for the patient

NASOGASTRIC TUBE FEEDING

Definition

Ryle's tube feeding or nasogastric feeding is nourishing through the tube to stomach, when the patient is unable to eat or drink by mouth. It is called nasogastric tube because it passes through the nose, down the throat and into the stomach. It is also called NG tube.

Purposes

1. To provide sufficient nourishment and hydration support to the patient.
2. For therapeutic purposes.
3. Help to drain out the stomach content in case of gastric problem or postoperative, etc.
4. To assess acceptance level of feeds in postoperative patients who undergo surgery and have NG tube in situ.

Equipments

A tray containing:
- A 20 cc syringe
- Measured amount of feed
- Stethoscope
- Bowl with water
- Kidney tray
- Water
- Towel
- Adhesives and scissors, if needed.

Procedure

The procedure for nasogastric tube feeding is detailed in Table 3.13.

Table 3.13: Procedure for nasogastric tube feeding

Sl No	Care action	Rationale
1.	Explain procedure to patient	To get the cooperation from the patient
2.	Assist the patient to a Fowler's position in bed or sitting position on chair; if the sitting position is contraindicated, a slightly elevated right side lying position is acceptable	To enhance the gravitational flow of the solution and to prevent the aspiration
3.	Wash the hands with soap and water	To prevent cross infection
4.	Place towel around the neck	To prevent soiling of the patient cloth
5.	Assess the tube placement by attaching the syringe to open end of the tube and aspirate gastric secretion	To check the position of the tube as well as to assess the absorption of the last feeding

Contd...

Contd...

SI No	Care action	Rationale
6.	Before administering the feeding , check the temperature and texture of the feed	The excessive cold feeding may cause cramps and minimize the risk of contamination
7.	Pinch the loop and remove the syringe from the tube and rinse it	To prevent air entry into the stomach
8.	Connect the barrel of the syringe to a pinched or clamped nasogastric tube	To make sure the gravity flow of the fluid
9.	Allow the feeding to flow slowly at the prescribed rate and pinch or clamp the tube, stop the feed if the patient feels discomfort	Quickly administering the feed can cause the flatus, pain and reflex vomiting
10.	At the end of the feed, flush the tube with a measured amount of water	To keep the tube clean
11.	Pinch the loop of the tube and remove the syringe, and close the tube with plunger	To prevent air entry into the stomach
12.	Allow the patient in semi-Fowler's position for 5–10 minutes	To enhance the patient comfortable and prevent aspiration of the fluid
13.	Document in the nurse's record, and in intake and output chart	To maintain the accurate record
14.	Replace all the articles	To keep it ready for next use

ADMINISTRATION OF OXYGEN THERAPY

Definition

Method by which oxygen is supplemented at higher percentages than what is available in atmospheric air.

Purposes

- To relieve dyspnea
- To reduce or prevent hypoxemia and hypoxia
- To alleviate the struggle associated with breathing.

Sources of Oxygen

Therapeutic oxygen is available from two sources:
- Wall outlets (central supply)
- Oxygen cylinders.

Nursing Alert

1. Explain the client the dangers of lighting matches or smoking cigarettes, cigars, pipes, etc. Be sure the client has no matches, cigarettes or smoking materials on the bedside table.
2. Make sure that warning signs (Oxygen—No Smoking) are posted on the client's door and above the client's bed.

3. Do not use oil on oxygen equipment.
   Rationale: Oil can ignite if exposed to oxygen.
4. With all oxygen delivery systems, the oxygen is turned on before the mask is applied to the client.
5. Make sure the tubing is patented at all times and that the equipment is working properly.
6. Maintain a constant oxygen concentration for the client to breathe; monitor equipment at regular intervals.
7. Give pain medications as needed; prevent chilling and try to ensure that the client gets needed rest. Be alert to cues about hunger and elimination.
   Rationale: The client's physical comfort is important.
8. Watch for respiratory depression or distress.
9. Encourage or assist the client to move about in bed.
   Rationale: To prevent hypostatic pneumonia or circulatory difficulties. Many clients are reluctant to move because they are afraid of the oxygen apparatus.
10. Provide frequent mouth care. Make sure the oxygen contains proper humidification.
    Rationale: Oxygen can cause drying of mucous membrane.
11. Discontinue oxygen only after a physician has evaluated the client. Generally, you should not abruptly discontinue oxygen given in medium-to-high concentrations (above 30%). Gradually decrease it in stages and monitor the client's arterial blood gases or oxygen saturation level.
    Rationale: These steps determine whether the client needs continued support.
12. Always be careful when you give high levels of oxygen to a client with chronic obstructive pulmonary disease (COPD). The elevated levels of oxygen in the patient's body can depress their stimulus to breathe.
13. Never administer oxygen to a hyperventilating patient.
14. Wear gloves because any time you might come into contact with the client's respiratory secretions.
    Rationale: To prevent the spread of infection.

Equipments

- Client's chart and Kardex
- Oxygen connecting tube: 1
- Flowmeter: 1
- Humidifier filled with sterile water: 1
- Oxygen source: Wall outlets or oxygen cylinder
- Tray with nasal cannula of appropriate size or oxygen mask: 1
- Kidney tray: 1
- Adhesive tape
- Scissors: 1
- Oxygen stand: 1
- Gauze pieces, cotton swabs, if needed
- 'No Smoking' signboard
- Gloves: 1 pair (if available).

Characteristics of Oxygen Administration

The features of low flow system of oxygen administration is given in Table 3.14.

Table 3.14: Characteristics of low flow system of oxygen administration

Method	Flow rate (L/min)	Oxygen concentration delivered	Advantages	Disadvantages
Nasal cannula	1 2 3 4	22%–24% 26%–28% 28%–30% 32%–36%	Convenient Comfortable more than face mask Brings less anxiety Allows client to talk and eat	Assumes an adequate breathing pattern Unable to deliver concentrations above 44%
	5 6	36%–40% 40%–44%	Mouth breathing does not affect the concentration of delivered oxygen	
Simple face mask	5–6 6–7 7–8	40% 50% 60%	Can deliver high concentration of oxygen more than nasal cannula	May cause anxiety; can lead to hotness and claustrophobia may become dirty easily, so cleansing is needed frequently Should be removed, while eating and talking Tight seal or long wearing can cause skin irritation on face

Note: There are other high flow devices such as venture mask, oxygen hood and tracheostomy mask. You should choose appropriate method of oxygen administration with doctor's prescription and nursing assessment.

Procedure

Nasal Cannula Method

The procedure for nasal cannula method is detailed in Table 3.15.

Table 3.15: Procedure for nasal cannula method

Sl No	Care action	Rationale
1.	Check doctor's prescription including date, time, flow liter/minute and methods	To avoid medical error
2.	Perform hand hygiene and wear gloves if available	To prevent the spread of infection
3.	Explain the purpose and procedures to the patient	Providing information fosters the client's cooperation and allays his/her anxiety

Contd...

Contd...

SI No	Care action	Rationale
4.	Assemble equipments	Organization facilitates accurate skill performance
5.	Prepare the oxygen equipment: • Attach the flowmeter into the wall outlet or oxygen cylinder • Fill humidifier about one third with sterile water or boiled water • Blowout dusts from the oxygen cylinder • Attach the cannula with the connecting tubing to the adapter, on the humidifier	Humidification prevents drying of the nasal mucosa To prevent entering dust from exit of cylinder to the nostril
6.	Test flow by setting flowmeter at 2–3 L/min and check the flow on the hand	Testing flow before use is needed to provide prescribed oxygen to the client
7.	Adjust the flowmeter's setting to the ordered flow rate	The flow rate via the cannula should not exceed 6 L/min Higher rates may cause excess drying of nasal mucosa
8.	Insert the nasal cannula into client's nostrils, adjust the tubing behind the client's ears and slide the plastic adapter under the client's chin, until he/she is comfortable	Proper position allows unobstructed oxygen flow and eases the client's respirations
9.	Maintain sufficient slack in oxygen tubing	To prevent the tubing from getting out of place accidentally
10.	Encourage the client to breathe through the nose rather than the mouth and expire from the mouth	Breathing through the nose inhales more oxygen into the trachea, which is less likely to be exhaled through the mouth
11.	Initiate oxygen flow	To maintain doctor's prescription and avoid oxygen toxicity
12.	Assess the patient's response to oxygen and comfort level	Anxiety increases the demand for oxygen
13.	Dispose of gloves if worn and perform hand hygiene	To prevent the spread of infection
14.	Place 'No Smoking' signboard at entry into the room	The sign warns the client and visitors that smoking is prohibited because oxygen is combustible
15.	Document the following: Date, time, method, flow rate, respiratory condition and response to oxygen	Documentation provides coordination of care Sometimes oxygen inhalation can bring oxygen intoxication
16.	Sign the chart	To maintain professional accountability
17.	Check the oxygen setup including the water level in the humidifier; clean the cannula and assess the client's nares at least every 8 hours	Sterile water needs to be added when the level falls below the line on the humidification container Nares may become dry and irritated, and require the use of a water-soluble lubricant In long use cases, evaluate for pressure sores over ears, cheeks and nares

Simple Face Mask Method

The procedure of simple face mask method is detailed in Table 3.16.

Table 3.16: Procedure of simple face mask method

Sl No	Care action	Rationale
1.	Perform hands hygiene and put on gloves if available	To prevent the spread of infection
2.	Explain the procedure and the need for oxygen to the client	The client has a right to know what is happening and why Providing explanations allay client's anxiety
3.	Prepare the oxygen equipment: • Attach the humidifier to the threaded outlet of the flowmeter or regulator • Connect the tubing from the simple mask to the nipple outlet on the humidifier • Set the oxygen at the prescribed flow rate	To maintain the proper setting The oxygen must be flowing before the mask is applied to the client
4.	To apply the mask, guide the elastic strap over the top of the client's head; bring the strap down to just below the client's ears	This position will hold the mask most firmly
5.	Gently, but firmly pull the strap extensions to center the mask on the client's face with a tight seal	The seal prevents leaks as much as possible
6.	Make sure that the client is comfortable	Comfort helps relieve apprehension and lowers oxygen need
7.	Remove and properly dispose gloves; wash your hands	Respiratory secretions are considered contaminated
8.	Document the procedure and record the client's reactions	Documentation provides for coordination of care
9.	Sign the chart and report the senior staffs	To maintain professional accountability
10.	Check periodically for depressed respirations or increased pulse	To assess the respiratory condition and find out any abnormalities as soon as possible
11.	Check for reddened pressure areas under the straps	The straps, when snug, place pressure on the underlying skin areas

Nursing alert: The simple mask is a low-flow device that provides an oxygen concentration in the 40%–60% range, with a liter flow of 6–10 L/min. But, the simple mask requires a minimum oxygen flow rate of 6 L/min to prevent carbon dioxide build up.

SURGICAL DRESSING

Definition

Surgical dressing is a sterile procedure, which is a loosely woven cotton dressing for incisions made during surgery.

Purposes

- To prevent the infection
- To prevent further tissue damage
- To promote wound healing
- To absorb inflammatory exudates and to promote drainage
- To change the contaminated wound into a clean wound
- To absorb fluid and provide a dry environment
- To immobilize and support wound.

Equipments

- Sterile dressing tray
- Cleaning solution prescribed, Betadine/Normal saline
- Sterile gloves
- Adhesives/Bandages/Tegaderm
- Scissors
- Extra sterile packs of cotton balls and gauze
- A pair of clean gloves
- Mackintosh and draw sheet
- Disposable mask and apron
- Medication as per doctors order (if needed)
- Labeled specimen container (if needed)
- Roller bandage (if needed)
- Kidney tray.

Procedure

The procedure for surgical dressing is detailed in Table 3.17.

Table 3.17: Procedure for surgical dressing

SI No	Care action	Rationale
1.	Explain the procedure to the patient	Make sure the patient and the relatives understand importance of the dressing and to give valid consent
2.	Before starting the procedure, ensure that the sweeping and the mopping of the ward is completed	To allow dust and airborne organisms to settle, before the insertion site and sterile fields are exposed
3.	Arrange and keep the needed articles near the bedside	To minimize unnecessary contamination and to perform the procedure easily
4.	Wash the hands	To reduce the risk of cross-contamination
5.	Make sure that foot-controlled dustbins are present at the bedside with appropriate covers	To minimize airborne contamination
6.	Provide privacy to the patient	To ensure the patient's comfortableness

Contd...

Contd...

SI No	Care action	Rationale
7.	Position the patient comfortably and drape the patient appropriately	To make the patient feel comfortable and to perform the procedure easily
8.	Wear gloves, remove the adhesive tape and old dressing, and remove the glove and wash the hands	To minimize the infection and contamination
9.	Wash the hands and wear sterile gloves	To minimize the infection and contamination
10.	Open the tray and pour the normal saline into the bowl	To clean the wound
11.	Using thumb forceps, pick up cotton ball, wet with saline and using artery clamp, soak adherent gauze	To remove the adherent gauze without causing trauma to the wound
12.	Using the same artery clamp, remove gauze and cotton ball, and discard in appropriate waste bin	To prevent cross-contamination
13.	Clean the wound from less contaminated area to more contaminated area	To reduce the risk of transfer of microorganism from contaminated to non-contaminated area
14.	Use separate cotton ball for each stroke	To minimize the risk of contamination
15.	Move in progressive strokes away from the incision line to wound edge	To enable disinfection process to be completed; to prevent skin reaction in response to the application of a transparent dressing to moist skin
16.	Use dry gauze to clean the incision	To promote healing
17.	Apply antiseptic as prescribed, using the same technique as for cleaning; include drainage site	To prevent sepsis
18.	Apply the sterile dressing to incision/ wound/ drain site	Avoids infection
19.	If drain is present, use sterile gauze and wrap around drain incision site	To prevent infection at the drain site
20.	Avoid the application of bulky dressing that may disturb the patient's mobility; ensure proper coverage of entire wound If using a commercially available dressing such as Tegaderm with pad, make sure that the size is appropriate; when fixing the commercially available dressing, mold it into place so that there are no creases or folds	Provides esthetic sense
21.	Secure dressing with bandage or adhesive, if needed	To prevent dislodgement
22.	Remove the gloves and wash the hands	To minimize the cross-contamination
23.	Make the patient to sit in a comfortable position and wash, replace the articles	To make it ready for next usage
24.	Document the procedure in the nurse's record	Helps to do the continuous assessment for the patient

---

Points to Note

- Observe character and amount of drainage, and assess condition of wound using the REEDA assessment scale:
  - R: Redness.
  - E: Ecchymosis.
  - E: Edema.
  - D: Drainage.
  - A: Approximation of the skin.
- Removal of old dressing:
  - Clean and dry wound: Remove with gloved hand by pinching the pad.
  - Dry dressing, adherent to the wound: Soak with normal saline. After a while, remove with gloved hand. Remove the gloves.
  - Wet or infected dressing : Remove with gloved hand. Remove the gloves.
- Wound care:
  - Clean wound: Clean the wound from inside or from the center toward outside with each stroke.
  - Infected wound: Clean the wound from outside toward inside with each stroke.
  - Transverse or horizontal incision: Clean the wound from the center toward outside on either side with each stroke.
  - Vertical incision: Clean the wound from top to downwards with one stroke and toward outside on either side in the same vertical direction.
  - Circular wound: Clean from center toward outside with a circular stroke.

Specimen Collection

COLLECTION OF BLOOD SPECIMEN

Performing Venipuncture

Definition

Venipuncture is using a needle to withdraw blood from a vein, often from the inside surface of the forearm near the elbow.

Purposes

1. To examine the condition of client and assess the present treatment.
2. To diagnose disease.

Equipments

- Laboratory form
- Sterilized syringe
- Sterilized needles
- Tourniquet: 1
- Blood collection tubes or specimen vials as ordered
- Spirit swabs
- Dry gauze
- Disposable gloves if available: 1
- Adhesive tape or bandages
- Sharps disposal container: 1
- Steel tray: 1
- Ballpoint pen: 1.

Procedure

The procedure of venipuncture is given in Table 4.1.

Table 4.1: Procedure of venipuncture

Sl No	Care action	Rationale
1.	Identify the patient: • Outpatient are called into the phlebotomy area and asked their name and date of birth • Inpatient are identified by asking their name and date of birth	This information must match the requisition

Contd...

Contd...

Sl No	Care action	Rationale
2.	Reassure the client that the minimum amount of blood required for testing will be drawn	To perform once properly without any unnecessary venipuncture
3.	Assemble the necessary equipment appropriate to the client's physical characteristics	Organization facilitates accurate skill performance
4.	Explain to the client about the purpose and the procedure	Providing explanation fosters his/her cooperation and allays anxiety
5.	Perform hand hygiene and put on gloves if available	To prevent the infection of spreading
6.	Positioning: • Make the client to be seated comfortably or supine position • Assist the client with the arm extended to form a straight-line from shoulder to wrist • Place a protective sheet under the arm	To make the position safe and comfortable is helpful to success venipuncture at one try To prevent the spread of blood
7.	Check the client's requisition form, blood collection tubes or vials and make the syringe-needle ready	To assure the doctor's order with the correct client and to make the procedure smooth
8.	Select the appropriate vein for venipuncture	The larger median cubital, basilica and cephalic veins are most frequently used, but other may be necessary and will become more prominent if the client closes his/her fist tightly
9.	Applying the tourniquet: • Apply the tourniquet 3–4 inches (8–10 cm) above the collection site; never leave the tourniquet on for over 1 minute • If a tourniquet is used for preliminary vein selection, release it and reapply after 2 minutes	To prevent the venipuncture site from touching the tourniquet and keep clear vision Tightening of more than 1 minute may bring erroneous result due to the change of some blood composition
10.	Selection of the vein: • Feel the vein using the tip of the finger and detect the direction, depth and size of vein • Massage the arm from wrist to elbow; if the vein is not prominent, try the other arm	To assure venipuncture at one try
11.	Disinfect the selected site: • Clean the puncture site by making a smooth circular pass over the site with the spirit swab, moving in an outward spiral from the zone of penetration • Allow the skin to dry before proceeding • Do not touch the puncture site after cleaning • After blood is drawn the desired amount, release the tourniquet and ask the client to open his/her fist • Place a dry gauze over the puncture site and remove the needle • Immediately apply slight pressure; ask the client to apply pressure for at least 2 minutes	To prevent the infection from venipuncture site Disinfectant has the effect on drying To prevent the site from contaminating To avoid making ecchymoma The normal coagulation time is 2–5 minutes

Contd...

Contd...

Sl No	Care action	Rationale
	• When bleeding stops, apply a fresh bandage or gauze with tape	Rinsing removes loosened debris and make the mouth taste fresher
12.	• Transfer blood drawn into appropriate blood specimen bottles or tubes as soon as possible using a needless syringe • The container or tube containing an additive should be gently inverted five to eight times or shaking the specimen container by making figure of 8	• A delay could cause improper coagulation • Do not shake or mix vigorously
13.	Dispose of the syringe and needle as a unit into an appropriate sharps container	To prevent the spread of infection
14.	Label all tubes or specimen bottle with client name, age, sex, inpatient number, date and time	To prevent the blood tubes or bottles from misdealing
15.	Send the blood specimen to the laboratory immediately along with the laboratory order form	To avoid misdealing and taking erroneous results
16.	Replace equipments and disinfects materials if needed	To prepare for the next procedure and prevent the spread of infection
17.	Put off gloves and perform hand hygiene	To prevent the spread of infection

Collection of Blood for Culture

Definition

A blood culture is a collection and inoculation of blood into culture medium with the aim of growing pathogenic bacteria or fungi for diagnostic purposes.

Purposes

1. To identify the type of bacteria/fungi present and specific type of antibiotics to use to eradicate the microorganism.
2. To determine whether microorganisms have invaded the patient's bloodstream.

Equipments

A tray containing:
- A pair of sterile gloves
- Alcohol swabs
- Blood culture bottles (two bottles per set)
- Disposable syringe
- Tourniquet
- Sterile gauze pad
- Adhesive strip or tape.

Procedure

The procedure of blood collection for culture is given in Table 4.2.

Table 4.2: Procedure of blood collection for culture

SI No	Care action	Rationale
1.	Explain procedure to the patient	To get cooperation from the patient
2.	Arrange and keep the entire article near the patient side	To minimize the unnecessary contamination
3.	Position the patient comfortably	To do the procedure easily
4.	Select and keep the appropriate sample collection container and stick patient profile	To get accurate results and to avoid the specimen does not get missed
5.	Wash hands with soap and water with friction for 15 seconds or use alcohol based hand rub	To prevent infections
6.	Clean the rubber cap of the blood culture bottles with an alcohol pad in a circular motion; allow the alcohol to dry	To prepare the specimen container ready to receive the sample and to prevent the cross contamination
7.	Apply tourniquet 3–4 inches above intended site; palpate for a vein and select site, preferably in the antecubital fossa	To assess the patency of the vein, to get the adequate blood sample and to increase the venous pressure
8.	Wear sterile gloves	To minimize the contamination
9.	Site preparation to be done by: • Vigorously clean the venipuncture site with alcohol swabs and allow drying • Starting at the center of the site, swab concentrically with alcohol swab for 1 minute • Allow the site to dry • Do not touch the venipuncture site after preparation and prior to puncture	To minimize the contamination
10.	Hold the syringe with the bevel of needle facing upwards	To ensure the correct position of the needle
11.	Advance the needle into the patient vein, with patient's arm in a downward position and tube stopper uppermost	This reduces the risk of backflow of any anticoagulant into the patient's circulation
12.	As blood come into view in syringe, withdraw the plunger of syringe softly with steady suction until the required sample is obtained	To get accurate report; in sufficient sample may cause again repuncture for the patient
13.	Remove the tourniquet	To release the pressure
14.	Take out the needle from the punctured area and place the dry sterile cotton and apply gentle pressure	To prevent bleeding
15.	Do not recap the needle and remove the needle from the syringe, discard into sharps container as per institutional policy	To prevent the needle stick injury
16.	Distribute blood equally into aerobic and anaerobic labeled sample container	For investigation process

Contd...

Contd...

SI No	Care action	Rationale
17.	Gently rotate the bottles to mix the blood and the broth (do not shake vigorously) and send specimen to respective laboratories	To enhance the blood to mix with the liquid
18.	Make the patient comfortable; replace the equipment and wash hands	To make the patient feel comfortable and prevent cross infection
19.	Record the procedure with details and investigation as well as collection	Helps to assess the continuity of care

Arterial Blood Collection

Definition

Arterial blood gases (ABGs) are diagnostic tests performed on blood taken from an artery.

Purposes

1. Arterial blood gases or ABGs are done to evaluate oxygenation and acid-base balance in the body.
2. An ABG test measures the acidity (pH) and the levels of oxygen and carbon dioxide in the blood from an artery.
3. This test is used to check how well your lungs are able to move oxygen into the blood and remove carbon dioxide from the blood.

Equipments

A tray containing:
- A pair of gloves
- Dry cotton/gauze pieces
- Adhesive plaster
- Heparinized syringe and needle
- Alcohol swab
- Injection Xylocaine 2%.

Procedure

The procedure of arterial blood collection is given in Table 4.3.

Table 4.3: Procedure of arterial blood collection

SI No	Care action	Rationale
1.	Explain the procedure to the patient	To reduce the anxiety and to get the cooperation
2.	Prepare all the articles near the patient bedside	To ease to do the procedure

Contd...

Contd...

Sl No	Care action	Rationale
3.	Check the patient coagulation factors and platelet count before starting the procedure	To prevent bleeding
4.	Feel for radial pulses on both wrists to determine which will be the better site, from which to draw	To avoid to perform an arterial puncture on an extremity; it may cause an inadequate blood supply
5.	Perform the Allen's test on the hand, which has been selected for the puncture	To determine adequate collateral flow
6.	Prepare the puncture site aseptically	To prevent infection
7.	Put sterile gloves and anesthetize the puncture area with 2% Xylocaine, according to the physician order	The use of a local anesthetic is not required, but may relieve uneasiness or be useful in reducing arterial spasm, if any case with difficulty in obtaining an arterial sample
8.	The heparinized syringe should be used to withdraw the blood sample	To prevent clotting of blood
9.	Puncture the skin about 5–10 mm distal to the finger directly over the artery; the puncture angle should be approximately 45° toward the direction of the blood flow	To obtain the blood easily
10.	Slowly advance the needle and syringe with one hand, while continuing to palpate the artery with the other hand; when a flash of arterial blood is observed in the hub of the needle, do not advance the needle further	To prevent deep injury
11.	While holding the syringe and needle motionless with one hand, gently pull back on the plunger of the syringe with the other hand to allow the syringe to fill	To prevent damage of the artery
12.	If the needed amount of blood has been obtained, should remove the needle and syringe rapidly, and press down on the puncture site with sterile gauze	To prevent the bleeding
13.	If any air bubbles present in the syringe, it is to be removed immediately and recap the needle	To prevent the inaccuracy in results
14.	Send the specimen to the blood gas analyzer	To do the analysis
15.	The needle is advanced just slightly under the skin; once the needle is in the artery the syringe will readily fill Arterial blood will pulsate whereas blood from a vein will not; arterial blood is also brighter red (if oxygenation is adequate) than blood from a vein When the needle is withdrawn, a gauze should be placed over the punctured site and pressure applied for about 5 minutes (longer if the patient has bleeding tendencies), if any bleeding occurs at the end of this time, pressure should be maintained until no further bleeding occurs	To obtain the sample

Contd...

Contd...

Sl No	Care action	Rationale
16.	Once the sample is obtained, remove the visible gas bubbles; label the syringe with patient profile	Air bubbles can dissolve into the sample and cause inaccurate results
17.	The sealed syringe is taken to a blood gas analyzer	The sample cannot be immediately analyzed; it is chilled in an ice bath in a glass syringe to slow metabolic processes, which can cause inaccuracy Samples drawn in plastic syringes are not iced and are analyzed within 30 minutes
18.	Document the procedure; collect the arterial blood gas (ABG) report and paste it in the appropriate place in the clinical chart	To monitor differences and detect trends; any irregularities should be brought to the attention of the appropriate senior nursing and medical teams

Points to Note

- Allen test is used to test blood supply to the hand, specifically, the patency of the radial and ulnar arteries. It is performed prior to radial arterial blood sampling or cannulation.

Allen test procedure

1. The hand is elevated and the patient is asked to make a fist for about 30 seconds.
2. Pressure is applied over the ulnar and the radial arteries so as to occlude both of them.
3. Still elevated, the hand is then opened. It should appear blanched (pallor can be observed at the finger nails).
4. Ulnar pressure is released and the color should return in 7 seconds.
5. Inference: Ulnar artery supply to the hand is sufficient and it is safe to cannulate/prick the radial.
6. If color does not return or returns after 7–10 seconds, the test is considered negative and the ulnar artery supply to the hand is not sufficient. The radial artery therefore cannot be safely pricked/cannulated.

Measurement of Capillary Blood Glucose

Definition

The collection of capillary blood from a fingertip quickly evolved as the standard sampling methodology. It is performed in homes and in hospitals for monitoring purposes that require relatively small samples of blood. It is more cost-effective, less traumatic and more convenient to obtain a blood sample by lancing the skin capillaries than it is by using healthcare practitioners to draw a tube of venous blood.

Purposes

1. Helps to observe immediate and daily levels of blood glucose control and dose adjustments.
2. Helps to identify the value variation of the patient in continuous insulin infusion.
3. To identify hypoglycemia and hyperglycemia.
4. Help out in the safe management of hyperglycemia and hypoglycemia.
5. Determines the effect of daily activities such as physical activity and meals on blood glucose.

Equipments

- Blood glucose meter
- Test strips
- Control solution
- Single use lancets
- Cotton swabs
- Disposable gloves.

Procedure

The procedure of capillary blood glucose measurement is given in Table 4.4.

Table 4.4: Procedure of capillary blood glucose measurement

Sl No	Care action	Rationale
1.	Explain the procedure to the patient	The patient should be attentive of the procedure in order to relieve some of his/her anxiety and to be able to cooperate in the procedure
2.	Ask the patient to sit down or lie down	To ensure the patient's safety
3.	Wash your hands and put on gloves	To decrease the risk of cross infection and risk of contamination
4.	Clean the fingertip with the alcohol swab where has to prick	To minimize the risk of contamination
5.	Allow the area to dry and prick the fingertip with the help of single use lancet	To minimize the risk of cross infection and accidental needle stick injury
6.	Take a blood sample from the pricking side of the finger, ensuring the side of the piercing is rotated; avoid frequent use of the index finger and thumb The finger may bleed without assistance or may need assistance by 'exploiting' to form a droplet of blood, which is large enough to cover the test pad	The side of the finger is used as it is less painful and easier to obtain a hanging droplet of blood; the site is rotated to reduce the risk of infection from multiple stabbing, and to prevent the areas from becoming toughened and to reduce pain

Contd...

Contd...

SI No	Care action	Rationale
7.	Apply the blood to the testing strip; some test strips are hydrophilic and are dosed/filled from the side and are not dropped directly onto the strip	The window on the test strip allows verification of a correctly dosed strip
8.	Dispose of lancet into a puncture proof sharps container	To reduce the risk of needle stick injury
9.	Record value immediately after the test has been done	To ensure the accuracy of the result
10.	Dispose all the waste according to the hospital policy	To reduce the risk of cross infection
11.	Ensure the patient comfortable and watch for bleeding in the puncture side; if bleed, apply pressure with dry cotton balls	To ensure the patient's comfort and safety. To minimize the complication
12.	Wash and dry hands	To prevent cross infection
13.	Record the result in the nurses' notes and in appropriate record (diabetic chart); if any variations in the value are found, it should be intimated immediately to the medical team by the nurses	To prevent complications

Points to Note

Before taking the device to the patient, the monitor needs to be checked for the following:
- Opening date of the strip box.
- The test strip should not be left in the open environment.
- It should be kept in the strip box with closed lids.

Collection of Blood Sample from Arterial Cannula

Definition

Arterial blood sampling blood can be drawn from an indwelling arterial cannula.

Purposes

1. To evaluate the adequacy of ventilatory ($PaCO_2$) acid-base (pH and $PaCO_2$) and oxygenation (PaO_2 and SaO_2) status, and the oxygen-carrying capacity of blood (PaO_2, HbO_2, Hb total and dyshemoglobins).
2. To quantitate the patient's response to therapeutic intervention and/or diagnostic evaluation (e.g. oxygen therapy, exercise testing).
3. To monitor severity and progression of a documented disease process.

Equipments

- A pair of gloves
- Disposable syringe (5 mL, 10 mL)
- Heparinized syringe (5 mL, 10 mL)
- Labeled specimen container
- Gauze pieces
- Alcohol swab.

Procedure

The procedure of blood sampling from arterial cannula is detailed in Table 4.5.

Table 4.5: Procedure of blood sampling from arterial cannula

Sl No	Care action	Rationale
1.	Explain the procedure to the patient	To ensure that the patient understands the procedure
2.	Arrange and keep all the articles near the patient side	To minimize unnecessary contamination
3.	Wash hands with bactericidal soap and water or bactericidal alcohol hand rub	To minimize the risk of cross infection
4.	Turn stopcock off to patient	To prevent the blood backflow from the line
5.	Remove the bung from stopcock; wipe with alcohol swab and attach sterile syringe to stopcock	To obtain the first sample from the line and prevent the entry of microorganism
6.	Open stopcock to syringe and intra-arterial catheter; aspirate 3 mL of blood and discard it	To get the accurate report
7.	Turn stopcock to the half-closed position, quickly remove syringe and replace with heparinized syringe	To obtain blood sample
8.	Open stopcock to syringe and intra-arterial catheter and obtain arterial blood gas sample	To do the analysis
9.	Close stopcock to the syringe and remove syringe containing blood sample and gently rotate syringe, cover the syringe with an arterial blood gas (ABG) cap to prevent contamination with air	Send for analysis and ensure that the blood and heparin in the syringe are mixed
10.	Activate flush device to clear arterial line	To prevent the clotting of the tube
11.	Turn stopcock off to the patient and flush side port of stopcock into sterile syringe until all blood is cleared from stopcock	To prevent infection and clotting of the tube
12.	Close stopcock, clean with alcohol and replace sterile protective cap	To prevent entry of the microorganisms and direct contamination of the cannula
13.	Check whether pressure infuser cuff is inflated to 300 mm Hg	To prevent back flow of blood into circuit
14.	Analyze or send to nearest blood gas analyzer and document result	To obtain accurate results as soon as possible
15.	Document the procedure in the nurse's record	To perform the follow-up care for the patient

> **Points to Note**
>
> ◆ Before taking blood sample from arterial line, ensure that arterial line is patent, i.e. the pressure bag is pumped up to 300 mm Hg, the tubing from the arterial site to the 3-way tap is clear and the line flushes easily.

Collection of Blood Sample from Central Venous Catheter

Definition

Blood can be drawn from a central venous access device, where the catheter is threaded into the central vasculature.

Purposes

1. To provide fluid resuscitation.
2. To provide parenteral feeding.
3. To measure the central venous pressure.
4. To administer the irritant drugs.
5. To collect the blood sample.
6. To provide long-term access like transfusion of blood or blood products, administration of drugs such as cytotoxic and antibiotic therapy.

Equipments

- Sterile dressing pack
- Alcohol swab
- A pair of gloves
- Labeled specimen container
- Disposable syringe (5 mL, 10 mL)
- Sterile disposable syringes 10 mL
- Injection: Normal saline 0.9%
- Water for injection.

Procedure

The procedure of blood sampling from central venous catheter is given in Table 4.6.

Table 4.6: Procedure of blood sampling from central venous catheter

SI No	Care action	Rationale
1.	Explain the procedure to the patient	To get the cooperation and reduce the anxiety of the patient
2.	Arrange the articles near the bedside	To minimize unnecessary contamination
3.	Assess all medications and infusions before selecting a port for sampling	To avoid the dilated sample and to get the accurate results

Contd...

Contd...

SI No	Care action	Rationale
4.	Wash hands with soap and water or bactericidal hand rub	To reduce the risk of infection
5.	If intravenous (IV) fluid is on flow, switch it off	To get the accurate results
6.	Before removing bung from stopcock, check the clamp or adaptor of the CVP line whether it is locked or not	To prevent bleeding
7.	Remove the bung from the stopcock and clean the catheter with alcohol swab	To minimize the entry of microorganism into the catheter
8.	Connect 10 mL syringe to the stopcock Open the stopcock Release the clamp and withdraw 5–10 mL of blood, close the clamp and discard the blood sample	To prevent contamination and to prevent the mixing
9.	Connect another disposable syringe in the stopcock and release the clamp, and withdraw the required amount of blood	To do the analysis
10.	Once the blood is withdrawn, close the clamp and transfer the blood to labeled specimen container; flush the line with 0.9% normal saline (NS) or sterile water	To prevent blood clotting in the lines
11.	When required, disconnect the administration set from the catheter and cover the end of the set with sterile cap	To reduce the risk of contaminating the end of the administration set
12.	Reconnect the IV fluids or medication as per physician order	To continue the treatment of the patient
13.	Document the procedure in the nurse's record	To perform the follow-up care of the patient

COLLECTION OF URINE SPECIMEN

Definition

Urinalysis in which the components of urine are identified, is part of every client assessment at the beginning and during an illness.

Purposes

1. To diagnose illness.
2. To monitor the disease process.
3. To evaluate the efficacy of treatment.

Nursing Alert

1. Label specimen containers or bottles before the client voids.
   Rationale: Reduce handling after the container or bottle is contaminated.

2. Note on the specimen label if the female client is menstruating at that time.
   Rationale: One of the tests routinely performed is a test for blood in the urine. If the female client is menstruating at the time a urine specimen is taken, a false-positive reading for blood will be obtained.
3. To avoid contamination and necessity of collecting another specimen, soap and water cleansing of the genitals immediately preceding the collection of the specimen is supported.
   Rationale: Bacteria are normally present on the labia or penis and the perineum and in the anal area.
4. Maintain body substances precautions, when collecting all types of urine specimen.
   Rationale: To maintain safety.
5. Wake a client in the morning to obtain a routine specimen.
   Rationale: If all specimen are collected at the same time, the laboratory can establish a baseline. And also this voided specimen usually represents that was collecting in the bladder all night.
6. Be sure to document the procedure in the designated place and mark it off on the Kardex.
   Rationale: To avoid duplication.

Collection of Single-voided Specimen

Equipments

1. Laboratory form.
2. Clean container with lid or cover: 1 (wide-mouthed container is recommended).
3. Bedpan or urinal: 1 (as required).
4. Disposable gloves: 1 (if available).
5. Toilet paper as required.

Procedure

The procedure for collection of urine sample is given in Table 4.7.

Table 4.7: Procedure for collection of urine sample

SI No	Care action	Rationale
1.	Explain the procedure	Providing information fosters his/her cooperation
2.	Assemble equipments and check the specimen form with client's name, date and content of urinalysis	Organization facilitates accurate skill performance Ensure that the specimen collecting is correct
3.	Label the bottle or container with the date, client's name, department identification and doctor's name	Ensure correct identification and avoid mistakes

Contd...

Contd...

SI No	Care action	Rationale
4.	Perform hand hygiene and put on gloves	To prevent the spread of infection
5.	Instruct the client to void in a clean receptacle	To prevent cross contamination
6.	Remove the specimen immediately after the client has voided	Substances in urine decompose when exposed to air; decomposition may alter the test results
7.	Pour about 10–20 mL of urine into the labeled specimen bottle or container and cover the bottle or container	Ensure the client voids enough amount of urine for the required tests Covering the bottle retards decomposition and it prevents added contamination
8.	Dispose of used equipment or clean them; remove gloves and perform hand hygiene	To prevent the spread of infection
9.	Send the specimen bottle or container to the laboratory immediately with the specimen form	Organisms grow quickly at room temperature
10.	Document the procedure in the designated place and mark it off on the Kardex	To avoid duplication Documentation provides coordination of care

Collection of 24-hour Urine Specimen

Definition

Collection of 24-hour urine specimen is defined as the collection of all the urine voided in 24 hours without any spillage of wastage.

Purposes

1. To detect kidney and cardiac diseases or conditions.
2. To measure total urine component.

Equipments

- Laboratory form
- Bedpan or urinal: 1
- A 24 hours collection bottle with lid or cover
- Clean measuring jar: 1
- Disposable gloves: 1 (if available)
- Tissue paper (if available)
- Ballpoint pen: 1.

Procedure

The procedure for collection of 24-hour urine sample is given in Table 4.8.

Table 4.8: Procedure for collection of 24-hour urine sample

SI No	Care action	Rationale
1.	Explain the procedure	Providing information fosters his/her cooperation
2.	Assemble equipments and check the specimen form with client's name, date and content of urinalysis	Organization facilitates accurate skill performance Ensure that the specimen collecting is correct
3.	Label the bottle or container with the date, client's name, department identification and doctor's name	Ensure correct identification and avoid mistakes
4.	Instruct the client: • Before beginning 24-hour urine collection, ask the client to void completely • Document the starting time of 24-hour urine collection on the specimen form and nursing record • Instruct the client to collect all the urine into a large container for the next 24 hours • In the exact 24 hours later, ask the client to void and pour into the large container • Measure total amount of urine and record it on the specimen form and nursing record • Document the time when finished the collection	To measure urinal component and assess the function of kidney and cardiac function accuracy The entire collected urine should be stored in a covered container in a cool place
5.	Sending the specimen: • Perform hand hygiene and put on gloves if available • Mix the urine thoroughly • Collect some urine as required or all the urine in a clean bottle with lid • Transfer it to the laboratory with the specimen form immediately	To prevent contamination Ensure the client voids enough amount of the urine for the required tests Covering the bottle retards decomposition and it prevents added contamination. Substances in urine decompose, when exposed to air; decomposition may alter the test results
6.	Dispose of used equipment or clean them; remove gloves and perform hand hygiene	To prevent the spread of infection
7.	Document the procedure in the designated place and mark it off on the Kardex	To avoid duplication Documentation provides coordination of care

Collection of Urine for Culture

Definition

Collecting a urine culture is a process that it obtains specimen urine with sterile technique.

Purposes

1. To collect uncontaminated urine specimen for culture and sensitivity test.
2. To detect the microorganisms cause urinary tract infection (UTI).
3. To diagnose and treat with specific antibiotic.

Equipments

- Laboratory form
- Sterile gloves: 1
- Sterile culture bottle with label as required
- Sterile kidney tray or sterile container with wide mouthed if needed
- Bedpan (if needed): 1
- Tissue paper (if needed)
- Ballpoint pen: 1.

Procedure

The procedure of urine culture is given in Table 4.9.

Table 4.9: Procedure of urine culture

Sl No	Care action	Rationale
1.	Assemble equipments and check the specimen form with client's name, date and content of urinalysis	Organization facilitates accurate skill performance Ensure that the specimen collecting is correct
2.	Label the bottle or container with the date, client's name, department identification and doctor's name	Ensure correct identification and avoid mistakes
3.	Explain the procedure to the client	Providing information fosters his/her cooperation
4.	Instruct the client: • Instruct the client to clean perineum with soap and water • Open sterilized container and leave the cover facing inside up • Instruct the client to void into sterile kidney tray or sterilized container with wide mouth • If the client needs bedrest and needs to pass urine more, place bedpan after you collect sufficient amount of sterile specimen	To prevent the contamination of specimen from perineum area The cover should be kept the sterilized state To secure the specimen kept in sterilized container surely
5.	Remove the specimen immediately after the client has voided; obtain 30–50 mL at midstream point of voiding	Substances in urine decompose when exposed to air; decomposition may alter the test results Ensure the client voids enough amount of the urine for the required tests Emphasize first and last portions of voiding to be discarded
6.	Close the container securely without touching inside of cover or cap	Covering the bottle retards decomposition and it prevents added contamination
7.	Dispose of used equipment or clean them Remove gloves and perform hand hygiene	To prevent the spread of infection
8.	Send the specimen bottle or container to the laboratory immediately with the specimen form	Organisms grow quickly at room temperature
9.	Document the procedure in the designated place and mark it off on the Kardex	To avoid duplication Documentation provides coordination of care

Collection of Urine Specimen from Retention Catheter

Equipments

- Laboratory form
- Disposable gloves: 1 (if available)
- Container with label as required
- Spirit swabs or disinfectant swabs
- A 10–20 mL syringe with 21–25-gauge needle
- Clamp or rubber band: 1
- Ballpoint pen: 1.

Procedure

The procedure of urine specimen collection from retention catheter is given in Table 4.10.

Table 4.10: Procedure of urine specimen collection from retention catheter

Sl No	Care action	Rationale
1.	Assemble equipments; label the container	Organization facilitates accurate skill performance
2.	Explain the procedure to the client	Providing information fosters his/her cooperation
3.	Perform hand hygiene and put on gloves if available	To prevent the spread of infection
4.	Clamp the tubing: • Clamp the drainage tubing or bend the tubing • Allow adequate time for urine collection *Nursing alert:* You should not clamp longer than 15 minutes	Collecting urine from the tubing guarantees a fresh urine Long-time clamp can lead back flow of urine and is able to cause urinary tract infection
5.	Cleanse the aspiration port with a spirit swab or another disinfectant swab (e.g. Betadine swab)	Disinfecting the port prevent organisms from entering the catheter
6.	Withdrawing the urine: • Insert the needle into the aspiration port • Withdraw sufficient amount of urine gently into the syringe	This technique for uncontaminated urine specimen, preventing contamination of the client's bladder
7.	Transfer the urine to the labeled specimen container *Nursing alert:* The container should be clean for a routine urinalysis and be sterile for a culture	Careful labeling and transfer prevents contamination or confusion of the urine specimen Appropriate container brings accurate results of urinalysis
8.	Unclamp the catheter	The catheter must be unclamped to allow free urinary flow and to prevent urinary stasis
9.	Prepare and pour urine to the container for transport	Proper packaging ensures that the specimen is not an infection risk
10.	Dispose of used equipments and disinfect if needed; remove gloves and perform hand hygiene	To prevent the spread of infection

Contd...

Contd...

SI No	Care action	Rationale
11.	Send the container to the laboratory immediately	Organisms grow quickly at room temperature
12.	Document the procedure in the designated place and mark it off on the Kardex	To avoid duplication Documentation provides coordination of care

COLLECTION OF SPUTUM SPECIMEN

Sputum for Routine Test

Definition

Sputum specimen collection is a procedure to collect expectorated secretions from a patient's respiratory tract.

Purposes

1. To identify the type of pathogenic microorganism present in the respiratory tract.
2. To monitor the response to treatment.
3. Identification of antibiotics to which cultured organism is sensitive.
4. Suspected pulmonary tuberculosis.

Equipments

A clean tray containing:
• Specimen container
• Gloves
• Mask
• Kidney tray.

Procedure

The procedure of routine test for sputum is given in Table 4.11.

Table 4.11: Procedure of routine test for sputum

SI No	Care action	Rationale
1.	Explain the procedure to the patient	To understand the importance of the investigation
2.	Provide privacy to the patient	To make comfortable to the patient
3.	Wash the hands with soap and water, wear gloves	To reduce the infection
4.	Make the patient to sit straightly, if not contraindicated	To obtain the sample easily
5.	Gargle with water immediately prior to obtaining a sputum specimen	To reduce the number of oral bacteria; do not use a mouthwash or any other gargle

Contd...

Contd...

SI No	Care action	Rationale
6.	Educate the patient to take two or three deep breaths and cough deeply	Help to bring out the sputum easily
7.	If sputum is raised should be expectorated directly into the labeled sputum container	To obtain sterile specimen
8.	Close the lid securely and send the specimen to the laboratory	To do the analysis
9.	Document the procedure in the nurse's record	Help to follow continuity of care

Points to Note

If the patient is unable to produce the desired amount of sputum:
- Instruct the patient to drink two glasses of water.
- Position the patient for postural drainage.
- Provide support for effective coughing by placing the hands or a pillow over the diaphragmatic area and apply mild pressure.
- Perform chest percussion.

Collection of Sputum for Culture

Definition

Collection of coughed out sputum for culture is a process to identify respiratory pathogens.

Purposes

1. To detect abnormalities.
2. To diagnose disease condition.
3. To detect the microorganism causes respiratory tract infections.
4. To treat with specific antibiotics.

Equipments

- Laboratory form
- Disposable gloves: 1 (if available)
- Sterile covered sputum container: 1
- Label as required
- Kidney tray or plastic bag for dirt: 1
- Tissue paper as required
- Ballpoint pen: 1.

Nursing Alert

Nurse should give proper and understandable explanation to the client:

1. Give specimen container on the previous evening with instruction how to treat.
2. Instruct to raise sputum from lungs by coughing, not to collect only saliva.
3. Instruct the client to collect the sputum in the morning.
4. Instruct the client not to use any antiseptic mouthwashes to rinse his/her mouth before collecting specimen.

Procedure

The procedure of sputum collection for culture is given in Table 4.12.

Table 4.12: Procedure of sputum collection for culture

Sl No	Care action	Rationale
1.	Assemble equipments; label the container	Organization facilitates accurate skill performance Careful labeling ensures accuracy of the report and alerts the laboratory personnel to the presence of a contaminated specimen
2.	Explain the procedure to the client	Providing information fosters his/her cooperation
3.	Perform hand hygiene and put on gloves if available	To prevent the spread of infection; the sputum specimen is considered highly contaminated, so you should treat it with caution
4.	Instruct the client: • Instruct the client to collect specimen early morning before brushing teeth • Instruct the client to remove and place lid facing upward • Instruct the client to cough deeply and expectorate directly into specimen container • Instruct the client to expectorate until you collect at least 10 mL of sputum • Close the container immediately when sputum is collected • Instruct the client to wipe around mouth if needed; discard it properly	To obtain overnight accumulated secretions To maintain the inside of lid as well as inside of container A sputum specimen should be from the lungs and bronchi; it should be sputum rather than mucous To obtain accurate results To prevent contamination Tissue papers used by any client are considered contaminated
5.	Remove and discard gloves; perform hand hygiene	To prevent contamination of other objects, including the label
6.	Send specimen to the laboratory immediately	To prevent the increase of organisms
7.	Document the procedure in the designated place and mark it off on the Kardex	To avoid duplication Documentation provides coordination of care

Collection of Throat Swab

Purpose

• To identify the type of pathogenic microorganism present in the throat.

Equipments

A clean tray containing:
- Throat swab culture container
- A pair of gloves
- Towel
- Mackintosh
- Torch/Spotlight
- Wooden spatula/tongue depressor
- Gauze pieces
- Kidney tray.

Procedure

The procedure of sample collection from throat swab is given in Table 4.13.

Table 4.13: Procedure of sample collection from throat swab

SI No	Care action	Rationale
1.	Explain the procedure to the patient	To get the cooperation
2.	Provide privacy to the patient	To make comfortable to the patient
3.	Make the patient to sit straight in the bed or raise the head end of the bed, if not contraindicated	To obtain the sample correctly
4.	Put the Mackintosh and towel around the neck or below the chin	To prevent the soil
5.	Ask the patient to tilt head backward and open mouth, stretch the tongue out	To ease to take the sample
6.	Visualize the tongue and throat by using the spotlight or torch	To assess any problems like ulceration, bleeding, etc.
7.	Use tongue spatula to press the tongue downward to the floor of the mouth	To ease to take the sample
8.	Use sterile cotton swab to wipe down both of the tonsillar arches and the posterior nasopharynx, without touching the sides of the mouth	To prevent the contamination
9.	Place the swab in labeled culture tube and close the tube	To prevent misusage
10.	Remove the Mackintosh and towel, and place the patient in comfort position	To make the patient comfortable
11.	Send the specimen to the laboratory	To do the analysis
12.	Document the procedure in the nurse's record	Help to follow continuity of care
13.	Document the procedure in the nurse's record in details	To follow-up the continuity of care

Points to Note
- If the patient is unconscious, use tongue depressor to access the peritonsillary region.

STOOL SAMPLE COLLECTION

Definition

Stool specimen collection is the process of obtaining a sample of a patient's feces for diagnostic purposes.

Purposes

1. The purpose of a stool culture (STC) is either to identify the causative agent of diarrhea or to detect the bacterial carrier state in a patient.
2. To identify the abnormal elements in the stool.

Equipments

A clean tray containing:
- Specimen container
- A pair of gloves
- Wooden tongue depressor
- Clean bedpan if needed.

Procedure

The stool sample collection procedure is given in Table 4.14.

Table 4.14: Procedure of stool sample collection

SI No	Care action	Rationale
1.	Explain the procedure to the patient	To understand about the importance of the test
2.	Provide privacy to the patient	To make patient feel comfortable
3.	Urinate before collecting the stool, so that you do not get any urine in the stool sample; do not urinate while passing the stool	To get the accurate results
4.	If the patient collect the specimen himself/herself, the following steps need to be explained to the patient: • Clean the genitalia with water • Pass the motion in the clean bedpan • Avoid contaminating the stool specimen with urine or water during collection • A small amount of stool is removed with stick and placed in the labeled container	To obtain the stool specimen completely
5.	To collect a stool specimen from a child in diapers, line the diaper with plastic wrap and transfer a portion of the stool to the collection specimen container	To prevent the contamination and to get the accurate result
6.	Wash the hands with soap and water	Wash the hands with soap and water

Contd...

Contd...

SI No	Care action	Rationale
7.	Send the specimen container to the laboratory	To do the analysis
8.	Document the procedure in the nurse's record	To do the follow-up care for the patient

Points to Note
- Avoid using antacids, barium, bismuth, antibiotics, antiamebics, antidiarrheal medication or oily laxative 1 week prior to collection of the specimen.
- Do not refrigerate the specimen containers.

VAGINAL SWAB COLLECTION

Purpose

The vaginal swab test is done to identify the infections in vaginal area, as well as other abnormalities of vaginal wall and cervical cells.

Equipments

A clean tray containing:
- Specimen container with swab stick
- A pair of gloves
- A gauze pieces
- Kidney tray.

Procedure

The procedure of vaginal swab collection is given in Table 4.15.

Table 4.15: Procedure of vaginal swab collection

SI No	Care action	Rationale
1.	Explain the procedure to the patient	To get the valid consent
2.	Provide privacy to the patient	To make patient feel comfortable
3.	Arrange all the articles near the bedside	To minimize the unnecessary contamination
4.	Wash the hands with soap and water	To prevent infection
5.	Make the patient in lithotomy position in the bed and tell the patient to be relaxed	To make the patient comfortable and easy to perform the procedure
6.	Wear gloves	To avoid the infection
7.	Remove the swab stick from the collection kit or the tube and do not touch the soft tip or lay the swab down	To avoid the infection

Contd...

Contd...

SI No	Care action	Rationale
8.	Insert the swab into the vagina about 2 inches; gently rotate the swab for 10–30 seconds and withdraw the swab without touching the skin	To prevent the contamination
9.	Place the swab into the labeled test tube and the tip of the swab is visible below the tube label; recap the container	For the easy visualization of the sample and to identify any abnormalities
10.	Clean the genital area with clean gauze pieces	To feel the patient comfortable
11.	Remove the gloves and discard as per the hospital policy and perform handwashing	To prevent cross infection
12.	Send the sample to laboratory	To do the analysis
13.	Document the procedure in the nurses record	To perform the follow-up care for the patient

WOUND SWAB COLLECTION

Purpose

The wound swab test is to help identify microorganisms causing wound infection.

Equipments

A clean tray containing:
- Dressing tray
- Adhesive plaster
- Specimen container with swab stick
- A pair of gloves
- Gauze pieces
- Kidney tray.

Procedure

The procedure of wound swab collection is given in Table 4.16.

Table 4.16: Procedure of wound swab collection

SI No	Care action	Rationale
1.	Explain the procedure to the patient	To get the valid consent
2.	Provide privacy to the patient	To make patient feel comfortable
3.	Arrange all the articles near the bedside	To minimize the unnecessary contamination
4.	Wash hands with soap and water	To prevent infection
5.	Make the patient in comfortable position according to the wound site	To make the patient comfortable and easy to perform the procedure

Contd...

Contd...

Sl No	Care action	Rationale
6.	Wear the gloves	To avoid the infection
7.	Remove the solid dressing materials with artery forceps	To prevent the contamination
8.	Wash the hands and wear another pair of gloves	To minimize the contamination
9.	Remove the swab stick from the collection kit or the tube and do not touch the soft tip or lay the swab down	To avoid the infection
10.	Take the swab before cleaning the wound	To collect the maximum number of organisms
11.	Use a 'zig-zag' motion whilst simultaneously rotating between the fingers	Ensure all the swab will contain sufficient amounts of bacteria
12.	Place the swab into the labeled test tube and the tip of the swab is visible below the tube label; recap the container	Easy to visualize the sample and to identify any abnormalities
13.	Perform the dressing in an aseptic manner according to the physician order	To prevent the infection
14.	Remove the gloves, discard as per hospital policy and perform handwashing	To prevent cross infection
15.	Wash the articles and replace it	To keep it ready for next usage
16.	Send the sample to laboratory	To do the analysis
17.	Document the procedure in the nurse's record	To perform the follow-up care for the patient

Administration of Medications

ADMINISTRATION OF ORAL DRUGS

Definition

Oral medication is administration of drugs by mouth via the alimentary tract.

Purpose

Drugs are taken by this route because of convenience, absorption of drug, ease of use and cost containment. It is the most common method used.

Equipments

- Clean tray to keep all the equipments needed
- Medication container to keep the opened tablets to be administered
- Ounce glass
- Clean bowl with gauze piece
- Scissors
- Small kidney basin
- Spoon.

Procedure

The procedure of administration of oral drugs is given in Table 5.1.

Table 5.1: Procedure of administration of oral drugs

Sl No	Care action	Rationale
1.	Wash hands	To prevent cross infection
2.	Identify the patient	To prevent error
3.	Check for the physician's order; follow the six rights of the medication administration	To prevent medication error
4.	Empty the required dose into the medicine container; avoid touching the preparation	To minimize the cross infection and contamination of the drug
5.	Explain the action, dose and expected adverse effect of the drug to the patient	Patient has the rights to know the treatment
6.	Administer the drug as prescribed orally through mouth with a spoon	No self-administration of drug according to policy

Contd...

Contd...

SI No	Care action	Rationale
7.	Offer a glass of water	To swallow the medication
8.	Documentation to be done in medication administration record (MAR)	To ensure that patient has received the treatment properly

PREPARATION OF INJECTIONS

Definition

The parenteral route refers to medications that are given by injection or infusion ('para' meaning besides, 'enteron' meaning intestine). It is the forcing of drug in the form of fluid into cavity, a blood vessel or intestine.

Purposes

1. To get a rapid and systematic effect of the drug.
2. To provide the needed effect even when the patient is unconscious or unable to swallow.
3. Assures that the total dosage will be administered and the same will be absorbed for the systematic actions of the drug.
4. Provides the only means of administration for medications that cannot be given orally.
5. To obtain a local effect at the site of injection.
6. To restore blood volume by replacing the fluid (in cases of bolus).
7. To give nourishment when it cannot be taken by mouth (in case of total parenteral nutrition).

Equipments

- Clean tray or receiver in which to place drug and equipment
- Use 21 G needle(s) to ease reconstitution and drawing up; 23 G if from a glass ampule
- Use 21, 23 or 25 G needle, size dependent on route of administration
- Syringe(s) of appropriate size for amount of drug to be given
- Swabs saturated with 70% isopropyl alcohol
- Sterile topical swab, if drug is presented in ampule form
- Drug(s) to be administered
- Patient's prescription chart, to check dose, route, etc.
- Recording sheet or book as required by law or hospital policy
- Any protective clothing required by hospital policy for specified drugs such as antibiotics or cytotoxic drugs.

Procedure

Single-dose Ampule

Solution preparation: Single-dose ampule solution preparation is detailed in Table 5.2.

Table 5.2: Protocol for single-dose ampule solution preparation

SI No	Care action	Rationale
1.	Inspect the solution for cloudiness or particulate matter; if this is present, discard and follow hospital guidelines on what action to take, e.g. return drug to pharmacy	To prevent the patient from receiving an unstable or contaminated drug
2.	Tap the neck of the ampule gently	To ensure that all the solution is in the bottom of the ampule
3.	Cover the neck of the ampule with a sterile topical swab and snap it open; if there is any difficulty a file may be required	To minimize the risk of contamination To prevent aerosol formation or contact with the drug, this could lead to a sensitivity reaction To reduce the risk of injury to the nurse
4.	Inspect the solution for glass fragments; if present, discard	To minimize the risk of injection of foreign matter into the patient
5.	Withdraw the required amount of solution, tilting the ampule if necessary	To avoid drawing in any air
6.	Replace the sheath on the needle and tap the syringe to dislodge any air bubbles; expel air	To prevent aerosol formation To ensure that the correct amount of drug is in the syringe

Powder preparation: Single-dose ampule powder preparation is detailed in the Table 5.3.

Table 5.3: Single-dose ampule powder preparation for injection

SI No	Care action	Rationale
1.	Tap the neck of the ampule	To ensure that any powder lodged here falls to the bottom of the ampule
2.	Cover the neck of the ampule with a sterile topical swab and snap it open; if there is any difficulty a file may be required	To minimize the risk of contamination To prevent contact with the drug this could cause a sensitivity reaction To prevent injury to the nurse
3.	Inject the correct diluents slowly into the powder within the ampule	To ensure that the powder is thoroughly wet before agitation and is not released into the atmosphere
4.	Agitate the ampule	To dissolve the drug
5.	Inspect the contents	To detect any glass fragments or any other particulate matter; if present, continue agitation or discard as appropriate

Contd...

Contd...

SI No	Care action	Rationale
6.	When the solution is clear withdraw the prescribed amount, tilting the ampule if necessary	To ensure the powder is dissolved and has formed a solution with the diluents To avoid drawing in air
7.	Replace the sheath on the needle and tap the syringe to dislodge any air bubbles; expel air	To prevent aerosol formation To ensure that the correct amount of drug is in the syringe
8.	Attach a new needle if required (and discard used needle into appropriate sharps container) or attach a plastic end cap	To reduce the risk of infection To avoid tracking medications though superficial tissues To ensure that the correct size of needle is used for the injection To reduce the risk of injury to the nurse

Multidose Vial

Powder preparation: The procedure is described in the Table 5.4.

Table 5.4: Powder preparation from multidose vial

SI No	Care action	Rationale
1.	Remove the tamper evident seal and clean the rubber septum with the chosen antiseptic and let the air dry for at least 30 seconds	To prevent bacterial contamination of the drug, as the plastic lid prevents damage and does not ensure sterility
2.	**Restitution method** Insert a 21 G needle into the cap to vent the bottle	To prevent pressure differentials, this can cause separation of needle and syringe
3.	Inject the correct diluent slowly into the powder within the vial	To ensure that the powder is thoroughly wet before it is shaken and is not into the atmosphere
4.	Remove the needle and the syringe	To enable adequate mixing of the solution
5.	Place a sterile topical swab over the venting needle and shake to dissolve the powder	To prevent contamination of the drug or the atmosphere To mix the diluents with the powder and dissolve the drug
6.	Inspect the solution for cloudiness or particulate matter, if this is present, discard; follow hospital guidelines on what action to take, e.g. return to pharmacy	To prevent patient from receiving an unstable or contaminated drug
7.	**Reconstitution method** With the needle sheathed draw into the syringe a volume if air equivalent to the required volume of solution to be drawn up	To prevent bacterial contamination of the drug
8.	Remove the needle cover and insert the needle into the vial through the rubber septum	To gain access to the vial
9.	Invert the vial; keep the needle in the solution slowly depress the plunger to push the air into the vial	To create an equilibrium in the vial

Contd...

Contd...

Sl No	Care action	Rationale
10.	Release the plunger, so that the solution flows back into the syringe (if a large volume of solution is to be withdrawn use a push pull technique)	To create an equilibrium in the vial
11.	Inject the diluents into the vial; keeping the tip of the needle above the level of the solution in the vial, release the plunger; the syringe will fill with the air, which has been displaced by the solution	This 'equilibrium method' helps to minimize the build up of pressure in the vial
12.	With the needle and syringe in place, gently swirl the vials to dissolve all the powder	To mix the diluents with the powder and dissolve the drug
13.	Inspect the solution for cloudiness or particulate matter; if this is present, discard and follow hospital guidelines on what action to take, e.g. return drug to pharmacy	To prevent patient from receiving an unstable or contaminated drug
14.	**Withdrawal of medication from vial** Withdraw the prescribed amount of solution and inspect for pieces of rubber, which may have 'cored out' of the cap	To ensure that the correct amount of drug is in the syringe To prevent the injection of foreign matter into the patient
15.	Remove air from syringe without spraying into the atmosphere by injecting air back into the vial or replace the sheath on the needle and tap the syringe to dislodge any air bubbles; expel air	To reduce risk of contamination of practitioner To prevent aerosol formation To avoid complication
16.	Attach a new needle if required (and discard used needle into appropriate sharps container) or attach a plastic end cap	To reduce the risk of infection To avoid possible trauma to the patient if the needle has barbed To avoid tracking medications through superficial tissues To ensure that the correct size of needle is used for the injection

Aftercare

- Inspection of the site for bleeding and abscess; if bleeding, apply pressure
- Watch for signs and symptoms of allergic reactions
- If the patient develops numbness or weakness on walking it may be due to nerve injury; ask patient take rest and inform the doctor
- Apply warmth if the patient develops pain redness and induration
- Clean all articles and replace them
- Wash hands.

ADMINISTRATION OF INTRAMUSCULAR INJECTION

Definition

Administration of injection (medication) with an angle of 90° into the muscle.

Purpose

Provides faster medication absorption than the subcutaneous because of a greater muscular vascularity.

Equipments

- Clean tray or receiver in which to place drug and equipment
- Syringe(s) of appropriate size for amount of drug to be given
- Swabs saturated with 70% isopropyl alcohol
- Sterile topical swab, if drug is presented in ampule form
- Drug(s) to be administered
- Patient's prescription chart, to check dose, route, etc.
- Recording sheet or book as required by law or hospital policy
- Any protective clothing required by hospital policy for specified drugs such as antibiotics or cytotoxic drugs.

Sites

- Vastus lateralis
- Ventrogluteal
- Deltoid
- Dorsogluteal.

Procedure

Follow the procedure for administration of intramuscular injection is given in the Table 5.5.

Table 5.5: Procedure for administration of intramuscular injection

SI No	Care action	Rationale
1.	Cleanse hands with alcoholic hand rub	Hands to be cleansed before and after each patient contact
2.	Explain and discuss the procedure with the patient	To ensure the patient understands the procedure and gives his/her valid consent
3.	Consult the patient's prescription sheet: • Drug • Dose • Date and time of administration • Route and method of administration • Dilute as appropriate • Validity of prescription	To ensure that the patient is given the correct drug in the prescribed dose using the appropriate diluents and by the correct route
4.	Assist the patient into the required position	To access to the injection site and to ensure the designated muscle is flexed and therefore relaxed
5.	Remove the appropriate garment to expose the injection site	To gain access for injection

Contd...

Contd...

SI No	Care action	Rationale
6.	Assess the injection site for signs of inflammation, edema, infection and skin lesions	To promote effectiveness of administration To reduce the risk of infection To avoid skin lesions and avoid possible trauma to the patient
7.	Clean the injection sites with a swab saturated with 70% isopropyl alcohol for 30 seconds and allow it to dry for 30 seconds	To reduce the number of pathogens introduced into the skin by the needle at the time of insertion, to prevent stinging sensation if alcohol is taken into the tissues upon needle entry
8.	Stretch the skin around the injection site	To facilitate insertion of the needle and to reduce the sensitivity of nerve endings
9.	Holding the needle at an angle of 90°, quickly plunge into the skin	To ensure that the needle penetrates the muscle
10.	Pull back the plunger; if no blood is aspirated, depress the plunger at approximately 1 mL every 10 seconds and inject the drug slowly; if blood appears, withdraw the needle completely, replace it and begin again; explain to the patient what has occurred	To confirm that the needle is in the correct position and not in a vein; this allows time for the muscle fibers to expand and absorb the solution To prevent pain and ensure even distribution of the drug
11.	Wait 10 seconds before withdrawing needle	To allow the medication to spread into the tissue
12.	Withdraw the needle rapidly; apply pressure to any bleeding point	To prevent hematoma
13.	Record the administration on appropriate charts	To maintain accurate records, provide point of reference in the event of any queries and prevent any duplication of treatment
14.	Ensure that all sharps and non-sharp waste are disposed safely and in accordance with locally approved procedures (sharps in the sharps bin and syringes into yellow clinical waste bag)	To ensure safe disposal and to avoid laceration or other injury to staff

ADMINISTRATION OF SUBCUTANEOUS INJECTIONS

Definition

A subcutaneous (SC) injection is a method of drug administration into the subcutaneous tissue. Up to 2 mL of a drug solution can be injected directly beneath the skin. The drug becomes effective within 20 minutes.

Purposes

1. Subcutaneous injection is the method used to administer drugs when a small amount of fluid is to be injected, when the patient is unable to take the drug orally, or the drug is destroyed by intestinal secretions.
2. Administration prevents complication because:

- The skin and underlying tissues are free of abnormalities
- Not over bony prominences
- Free of large blood vessels and nerves.
    3. Self-administration is possible.

Equipments

- Clean tray or receiver in which to place drug and equipment
- Use 23 G needle if from a glass ampule
- Use 1–2 mL syringes appropriate for the amount of drugs to be given
- Swabs saturated with 70% isopropyl alcohol
- Sterile topical swabs, if drug is presented in ampule form
- Drugs to be administered
- Patient's prescription chart, to check dose, route, etc.
- Recording sheet (MAR) as required by law policy.

Sites

- Outer aspect of the upper arm
- Posterior chest wall below the scapula
- Anterior abdominal wall from below the breast to the iliac crest
- The anterior and lateral aspect of the thigh.

Procedure

The procedure to be followed in the administration of the subcutaneous injections is explained in the Table 5.6.

Table 5.6: Procedure for administration of subcutaneous injection

Sl No	Care action	Rationale
1.	Explain and discuss the procedure with the patient	To ensure that the patient understands the procedure and gives his/her valid consent
2.	Consult the patient's prescription chart and ascertain the following: • Drug • Dose • Date and time of administration • Route and method of administration • Dilute as appropriate • Validity of prescription • Signature of doctor	To ensure that the patient is given the correct drug in the prescribed dose using the appropriate diluent and the correct route
3.	Assist the patient into the required position	Allow to access to the appropriate injection site
4.	Remove appropriate garments to expose the injection site	To gain access for injection

Contd...

Contd...

SI No	Care action	Rationale
5.	Assess the injection site for signs of inflammation, edema, infection and skin lesions	To promote effectiveness of administration To reduce the risk of infection To avoid skin lesions and avoid possible trauma to the patients
6.	Choose the correct needle size	To minimize the risk of missing the subcutaneous tissue and any ensuing pain
7.	Clean the injection site with a swab saturated with 70% isopropyl alcohol	To reduce the number of pathogens introduced into the skin by the needle at the time of insertion
8.	Gently pinch the skin up into a fold	To elevate the subcutaneous tissue and lift the adipose tissue away from the underlying muscle
9.	Insert the needle into the skin at an angle of 45° and release the grasped skin; inject the drug slowly	Injection mediation into compressed tissue irritated nerve fibers and causes the patient discomfort
10.	Withdraw the needle rapidly; apply pressure to any bleeding point; do not rub	To prevent hematoma formation Interferes with absorption
11.	Ensure that all sharps and non-sharp waste are disposed safely and in accordance with locally approved procedures such as needle into white puncture proof container and syringes into red waste bag	To ensure safe disposal and to avoid laceration or other injury to staff
12.	Record the administration on appropriate sheets	To maintain accurate records, provide a point of reference in the event of any queries and prevent any duplication of treatment

Nursing Alert

With the subcutaneous route, a small thin needle is inserted beneath the skin and the drug injected slowly. The drug moves from the small blood vessels into the bloodstream.

ADMINISTRATION OF INSULIN INJECTIONS

Definition

Insulin is a hormone used to control glycemia. It must be administered by injection because it is a protein and therefore would be broken down and destroyed in the gastrointestinal tract.

Purposes

1. To provide sufficient insulin throughout 24 hours to cover basal requirements.
2. To deliver higher boluses of insulin in an attempt to match the glycemic effect of meals.

3. To control diabetes mellitus.
4. To treat hyperglycemia.

Blood Glucose Monitoring

Blood glucose (BG) levels are often checked qac (30 min before meals), qhs (at bedtime) or prn (as needed):
- Preprandial (fasting or before a meal) 70–130 mg/dL
- Postprandial (1–2 h after the start of a meal) less than 180 mg/dL
- These ranges may vary depending on institution and physician protocols.

Insulin Administration According to the Classification

Rapid Onset-fast Acting Insulin

Rapid onset-fast acting insulin is fast acting. It starts working within1–15 minutes. It is clear in appearance and its peak time is about 1 hour later, and lasts for 3–5 hours. When you inject rapid onset-fast acting type of insulin, patient must eat immediately after the inject. The two rapid onset-fast acting insulin types currently available are:
- NovoRapid (insulin aspart)
- Humalog (Lispro)
- Glulisine (apidra).

Short-acting Insulin

Short-acting insulin looks clear and begins to lower blood glucose levels within 30 minutes, so patient need to take the injection half an hour before eating. Short-acting insulin has peak effect of 4 hours and works for about 6 hours. Short-acting insulin types, currently available include:
- Actrapid
- Humulin
- Hypurin Neutral (highly purified bovine insulin).

Intermediate-acting Insulin

Intermediate-acting insulin looks cloudy. They have either protamine or zinc added to delay their action. This insulin starts to show its effect about 90 minutes after the inject, peak at 4–12 hours and lasts for 16–24 hours.
      Intermediate-acting insulins presently available with protamine:
- Protaphane
- Humulin NPH
- Hypurin Isophane (bovine).

Mixed Insulin

Mixed insulin is cloudy in appearance. It is a combination of either a rapid onset-fast acting or a short-acting insulin and intermediate-acting insulin. Advantage of it is that, two types of insulin can be given in one injection.

When it shows 30/70 then it means 30% of short acting is mixed with 70% of intermediate-acting insulin. The mixed insulins currently available include:
- NovoMix 30
- Humalog Mix 25/75
- Mixtard 30/70
- Mixtard 20/80.

Points to Note

+ Roll well the vial of insulin in order to mixed them evenly.

Long-acting Insulin

There are two kinds of long-acting insulin available in market, both with clear appearance:
1. Lantus (glargine): It has no peak period as it works constantly when released into your bloodstream at a relatively constant rate (full 24 hour).
2. Levemir (detemir): It has a relatively flat action, can last up to 24 hours and may be given once or twice during the day.

Frequently Used Regimens

1. Two injections daily of a mixture of short- and intermediate-acting insulins (before breakfast and the main evening meal).
2. Three injections daily using a mixture of short- and intermediate-acting insulins before breakfast; short-acting insulin alone before an afternoon snack or main evening meal; intermediate-acting insulin before bed or variations of this:
   - Basal-bolus regimen of short-acting insulin 20–30 minutes before main meals (e.g. breakfast, lunch and the main evening meal); intermediate- or long-acting insulin at bedtime
   - Basal-bolus regimen of rapid-acting insulin analog immediately before main meals (e.g. breakfast, lunch and main evening meal); intermediate- or long-acting insulins at bedtime, probably before breakfast and occasionally at lunchtime
   - Insulin pump regimes are regaining popularity with a fixed or variable basal dose and bolus doses with meal.

None of these regimens can be optimized without frequent assessment by BG monitoring.

Daily Insulin Dosage

Daily insulin dosage varies greatly between individuals and changes over time. It therefore requires regular review and reassessment. Dosage depends on many factors includes the following:
- Age
- Weight

- Stage of puberty
- Duration and phase of diabetes
- State of injection sites
- Nutritional intake and distribution
- Exercise patterns
- Daily routine
- Results of BG monitoring (and glycosylated hemoglobin)
- Concurrent illness.

The 'correct' dose of insulin is that which achieves the best attainable glycemic control for an individual child or adolescent.

> **Points to Note**
>
> ✦ Healthcare professionals have the responsibility to advice patients, other care providers and young people on adjusting insulin therapy safely and effectively. This training requires regular review, reassessment and reinforcement.

Route of Administration

Subcutaneous or Hypodermic (into the Subcutaneous Tissue)

Needles: 25–27 G, 5/8–1/2 inch.

Syringes: Includes the following:
- 1 mL for 100 unit of insulin
- 1 mL for 40 units of insulin.

Position: 45°–90° angle.

Advantages
- Allows slower, more sustained drug administration than IM injection
- Injected into the adipose tissues beneath the skin, a drug moves into the bloodstream more rapidly than if given by mouth
- Minimal tissue risk
- Allows slower absorption
- Minimal risk of hitting blood vessel.

Cautions
- Do not give in scarred areas, in moles, inflamed or edematous areas
- Do not massage after administration
- Outer aspect of the upper arm
- Anterior thigh
- Loose tissue of the lower abdomen
- Upper hips
- Buttock
- Upper back.

Procedure

The procedure for the insulin administration is described in Table 5.7.

Table 5.7: Procedure for insulin injection administration

Sl No	Care action	Rationale
1.	Wash hands	To prevent infection
2.	Check the medicine order and make sure that the solution in the vial matches the ordered solution	Avoids medication error
3.	Obtain an insulin syringe	
4.	Pick up the vial and verify the type of insulin, which is prescribed	Avoids medication error
5.	Check the patient's most recent blood glucose, if in case of doubt or assessment changes always recheck and reassess	To avoid overdosage
6.	If applicable, verify the blood glucose and use sliding scale insulin administration dosage on the patient's medication administration record (MAR)	To avoid overdosage
7.	Wipe the insulin vial with a sterile gauze alcohol pad, if the insulin is cloudy roll between palms of your hands	Rotating the vial between both hands resuspend the modified insulin preparation and help to warm the medication; shaking insulin vial causes bubbles to form, which take up space and alters the dose
8.	Withdraw the appropriate type and amount of insulin	To achieve the therapeutic effect
9.	Pull back on barrel of syringe to draw in a volume of the ordered medication dose; holding the vial between the thumb and fingers of the non-dominant hand, insert the needle through the rubber stopper into the air space, not the solution	Enhances easy withdrawal of medication
10.	Invert the vial and withdraw the ordered dose of medication by pulling back on the plunger; make sure the needle is in the solution to be withdrawn	Prevents the entry of air
11.	Expel air bubbles and adjust dose if necessary	To prevent complication
12.	Remove needle from vial and cover the needle with guard using one hand or scoop method	Avoids needle stick injury
13.	Take medication into patient's room and verify, administer the subcutaneous (SC) injection; remember to never massage the insulin injection site (Figs 5.1A and B)	
14.	Record the administration on appropriate sheets	To maintain accurate records, provide a point of reference in the event of any queries and prevent any duplication of treatment

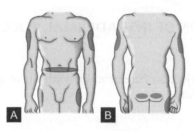

FIGURES 8.1A and B: Insulin injection sites. **A.** Anterior sites; **B.** Posterior sites.

Insulin Pen

Preparation, dosing and rationale of insulin pen is explained in Table 5.8.

Table 5.8: Nursing intervention in insulin pen usage

SI No	Care action	Rationale
1.	Gather supplies; verify insulin type: • Pen device (with cartridge) • Pen needle • Alcohol wipe • Sharps container	To save time
2.	Wash hands	To prevent infection
3.	Choose injection site	To administer medication
4.	Clean injection site	To prevent infection
5.	Screw pen needle firmly onto pen	Ensures the needle from dislodging form the pen
6.	Prime: Dial '2' units	To remove the primary medicine, which is lodged in the pocket of cartridge
7.	Hold upright; remove air by pressing the plunger; repeat 'prime' if no insulin shows at end of needle	To avoid air embolism
8.	Dial number of units to be administered as per order	To avoid medication error
9.	Pinch up the skin	Ensures the correct size of the needle
10.	Push the needle into the skin at 90°	Avoids injury
11.	Release pinched skin	Causes pain
12.	Leave needle in skin and keep pressing the button for 5–10 seconds	To ensure to deliver the required dose completely
13.	Remove and dispose of pen needle	Avoids needle stick injury
14.	Document time, dose, site and blood glucose value	To maintain accurate records, provide a point of reference in the event of any queries and prevent any duplication of treatment

Points to Note

- Check site for leakage, lipoatrophy, lipohypertrophy.
- Check for signs and symptoms of hypoglycemia.
- Meal/Snack dose.
- Timeliness in relation to eating.
- Supervision of food amount.

ADMINISTRATION OF INTRADERMAL INJECTIONS

Definition

Administration of injection (medication) with an angle of 5°–15° into the dermal layer of the skin.

Purpose

Certain medications may be injected intradermally to test the allergy.

Equipments

- Clean tray or receiver in which to place drug and equipment
- Syringe(s) of appropriate size for amount of drug to be given
- Swabs saturated with 70% isopropyl alcohol
- Sterile topical swab, if drug is presented in ampule form
- Drug(s) to be administered
- Patient's prescription chart, to check dose, route, etc.
- Recording sheet or book as required by law or hospital policy
- Any protective clothing required by hospital policy for specified drugs such as antibiotics or cytotoxic drugs.

Site

- Forearm.

Procedure

The procedure for intradermal injection is described in Table 5.9.

Table 5.9: Procedure for administration of intradermal injection

Sl No	Care action	Rationale
1.	Cleanse hands with alcoholic hand rub	Hands to be cleansed before and after each patient contact
2.	Explain and discuss the procedure with the patient	To ensure the patient understands the procedure and gives his/her valid consent
3.	Consult the patient's prescription sheet: • Drug • Dose • Date and time of administration • Route and method of administration • Dilute as appropriate • Validity of prescription	To ensure that the patient is given the correct drug in the prescribed dose using the appropriate diluents and by the correct route
4.	Assist the patient into the required position	Assist the patient into the required position
5.	Remove the appropriate garment to expose the injection site	To gain access for injection
6.	Assess the injection site for signs of inflammation, edema and infection and skin lesions	To promote effectiveness of administration To reduce the risk of infection To avoid skin lesions and avoid possible trauma to the patient
7.	Clean the injection sites with a swab saturated with 70% isopropyl alcohol for 30 seconds and allow it to dry for 30 seconds	To reduce the number of pathogens introduced into the skin by the needle at the time of insertion, to prevent stinging sensation if alcohol is taken into the tissues upon needle entry
8.	Stretch the skin around the injection site	To facilitate insertion of the needle and to reduce the sensitivity of nerve endings

Contd...

Contd...

SI No	Care action	Rationale
9.	Holding the needle level up at an angle of 5°–15°, slowly plunge into the skin and administer the drug	To ensure that the needle penetrates the dermis
10.	Notice that, while injecting the medication, small bleb approximately 6 mm in diameter appears on the skin surface	Bleb indicates medication is deposited in dermis
11.	Withdraw the needle, while applying alcohol swab or gauze gently over site rapidly	To minimize discomfort
12.	Apply gentle pressure; do not massage site	Massaging damages underlying tissues, it may disperse medication into underlying tissue layers and alter test results
13.	Stay with the patient 3–5 minutes and observe for any allergic reactions	Severe anaphylactic reaction is characterized by dyspnea, wheezing and circulatory collapse
14.	Record the administration on appropriate charts	To maintain accurate records, provide point of reference in the event of any queries and prevent any duplication of treatment
15.	Ensure that all sharps and non-sharp waste are disposed off safely and in accordance with locally approved procedures (sharps in the sharps bin and syringes into yellow clinical waste bag)	To ensure safe disposal and to avoid laceration or other injury to staff

Points to Note

◆ For intradermal injections, use blue ink pen and draw circle around perimeter of injection site.
◆ Do not use red ink pen.

ADMINISTRATION OF INTRAVENOUS INJECTIONS

Definition

Intravenous (IV) injection is defined as the parenteral administration of bolus medication directly into the vein through the existing IV line.

Methods of Infusion

In intravenous injection administration there are three methods:
1. Continuous infusion.
2. Intermittent infusion.
3. Direct intermittent injection.

Continuous Infusion

Continuous infusion may be defined as the intravenous delivery of medication or fluid at a constant rate over a prescribed time period, ranging from 24 hours to days, to achieve a controlled therapeutic response.

Intermittent Infusion

Intermittent infusion is the administration of a small volume infusion, i.e. 50–250 mL over a period of between 20 minutes and 2 hours. This may be given as a specified dose at one time or at repeated intervals during 24 hours.

Direct Intermittent Injection

Direct intermittent injection involves the injection of a drug from a syringe into the injection port of the administration set or directly into a vascular access device.

Purposes

1. To administer large volume of fluid.
2. Rapid absorption is achieved.
3. In emergencies, fast-acting medications can be delivered quickly.
4. Establishes continuous fluid infusions.
5. To establish constant therapeutic blood levels.
6. Medications that are highly alkaline and irritating to subcutaneous tissue are given intravenously.
7. Intravenous therapy is used primarily for fluid replacement in patients unable to take oral fluids.

Equipments

- Clean tray or receiver in which to place drug and equipment
- To ease reconstitution 21 G needle(s) and drawing up, 23 G if from a glass ampule
- Needles of 21, 23 or 25 G can be used, size dependent on route of administration
- Syringes of appropriate size for amount of drugs to be given
- Swabs saturated with 70% isopropyl alcohol
- Drugs to be administered
- Patient's prescription chart, to check dose, route, etc.
- Medication administration record (MAR), recording sheets as required by hospital policy
- Any personal protective devices required by hospital policy for specified drugs such as cytotoxic drugs
- Three-way connectors with stopper
- Gloves
- Kidney basin
- Spread sheet to prevent soiling of bedsheet.

Procedure

Procedure for intravenous injection administration is described in the Table 5.10.

Table 5.10: Procedure for administrating intravenous injection

Sl No	Care action	Rationale
1.	Collect and check all equipments	To prevent delays and enable full concentration on the procedure
2.	Check that the packing of all equipment is intact	To ensure sterility, if the seal is damage, discard
3.	Wash hands with bactericidal soap and water or bactericidal alcohol hand rub	To prevent contamination of medication and equipment
4.	Prepare needle(s), syringe(s) and other supplies by placing on a tray or receiver	To contain all items in a clean area
5.	Inspect all equipment	To check that none is damaged; if so, discard or report
6.	Consult the patient's prescription chart and ascertain the following: • Drug • Dose • Date and time of administration • Route and method of administration • Dilute as appropriate • Validity of prescription • Signature of doctor	To ensure that the patient is given the correct drug in the prescribed dose using the appropriate
7.	Check all details with another nurse if required by hospital policy	To minimize any risk of error
8.	Select the drug in the appropriate volume, dilution or dosage and check the expiry date	To reduce wastage; treatment with medication that is outside the expiry is dangerous The expiry date indicates when a particular drug is no longer pharmacologically efficacious
9.	Proceed with the preparation of the drug, using protective clothing if advisable	To protect practitioner during preparation
10.	Take the prepared dose to the patient, whose identity is checked	To prevent error and confirm patient's identity
11.	Evaluate the patient's knowledge of the medication being offered; if this knowledge appears to be faulty or incorrect, offer an explanation of the use, action, dose and potential side-effects of the drug or drugs involved	A patient has a right to know the information about the treatment
12.	Close room door or curtains if appropriate	To ensure patient privacy and dignity
13.	Administer the drug as prescribed	To ensure patient receives treatment
14.	Do not recap; follow biomedical waste management (BWM) policy	To minimize risk of contamination and prevent risk of injury to nurses
15.	Record the administration on appropriate chart; documentation must include date, time, amount, route, name of the drug and reaction of patient; follow-up observation also must be recorded	To maintain accurate records, provide a point of reference in the event of any queries and prevent any duplication of treatment

> **Points to Note**
>
> * The rate and the flow of solution.
> * Complications like infection, phlebitis (venous inflammation), thrombophlebitis (clot formation), air embolism, local infiltration and allergic reactions.
> * Accuracy of flow is very important.

ADMINISTERING MEDICATIONS BY HEPARIN LOCK

Definition

A heparin lock is an IV catheter that is inserted into a vein and left in place either for intermittent administration of medication or as open line in the case of an emergency.

Administering medications by heparin lock is defined as one of IV therapy, which can allow to be freedom clients while he/she has not received IV therapy.

Purposes

* To provide intermittent administration of medication
* To administer medication under the urgent condition.

Equipments

General

* Client's chart and Kardex
* Prescribed medication
* Spirit swabs
* Disposable gloves, if available: 1
* Kidney tray: 1
* Steel tray: 1.

For Flush

* Saline vial or saline in the syringe: 1
* Heparin flush solution: 1
* Syringe (3–5 mL) with 21–25 gauge needle: 1.

For Intermittent Infusion

* Bottle or IV bag with 50–100 mL solution: 1
* Intravenous tubing set: 1
* Intravenous stand: 1
* Needle of 21–23 gauge: 1
* Adhesive tape.

Nursing Alert

- A heparin lock has an adapter, which is attached to the hub (end) of the catheter
- An anticoagulant, approximately 2 mL heparin, is injected into the heparin lock
- To reduce the possibility of clotting, flush the heparin lock with 2–3 mL of saline 8 hourly (or once a every duty); saline lock
- Choose heparin lock or saline lock to decrease the possibility of making coagulation according to your facility's policy or doctor's order.

Procedure

Procedure for administration of medication by heparin lock is described in Table 5.11.

Table 5.11: Procedure for administration of medication by heparin lock

Sl No	Care action	Rationale
1.	Perform hand hygiene	To prevent the spread of infection
2.	Assemble all equipments	Organization facilities accurate skill performance
3.	Verify the medication order	To reduce the chances of medication errors
4.	Check the medication's expiration date	Out dated medication may be ineffective
5.	**For bolus injection** Prepare the medication; if necessary, withdraw from an ampule or a vial	Preparing the medication before entering the client's room facilitates administration
6.	Explain the procedure to the client	Providing information fosters his/her cooperation
7.	Identify the client before giving the medication	Abiding by the 'five rights' prevents medication errors
8.	Put on gloves	Gloves act as a barrier
9.	Cleanse the heparin lock port with a spirit swab	Spirit swab removes surface contaminants and decreases the potential for introducing pathogens into the system
10.	• Steady the heparin lock with your dominant hand • Insert the needle of the syringe containing 1 mL of saline into the center of the port • Aspirate for blood return • Inject the saline • Remove the needle and discard the syringe in the sharps container without recapping it	Blood return on aspiration generally indicates that the catheter is positioned in the vein Saline clears the tubing of any heparin flush or previous medication Most accidental needle-sticks occur during recapping Proper disposal prevents injury

Contd...

Contd...

Sl No	Care action	Rationale
11.	• Cleanse the port again with a spirit swab • Insert the needle of the syringe containing the medication • Inject the medication slowly • Withdraw the syringe and dispose of it properly	Rapid injection of medication can lead to speed shock
12.	• Cleanse the port with a spirit swab • Flush the lock with 1 mL heparin flush solution according to hospital/agency policy	To remove contaminants and prevents infection via the port Flush clears the lock of medication and keeps it open Some agencies recommend only a saline flush to clear the lock
13.	**For intermittent infusion** • Use premixed solution in the bag • Connect the tubing and add the needle or needless component • Prepare the tubing with solution	Preparing the medication before enter the client's room facilitates administration
14.	Follow the former action given in step 6–10	Because the preparation is same like bolus injection
15.	• Cleanse the port again with a spirit swab • Insert the needle or needleless component attached to the intravenous (IV) set up into the port • Attach it to the IV infusion pump or calculate the flow rate • Regulate drip according to the prescribed delivery time • Clamp the tubing and withdraw the needle when all solution has been infused • Discard the equipments used safely according to hospital/agency's policy	To remove contaminants and prevents infection via the port Infusing more than required amount of solution will cause fluid overload Clamping prevents air entry Proper disposal prevents injury
16.	• Cleanse the port with a spirit swab • Flush the lock with 1 mL heparin flush solution according to hospital/agency policy	To remove contaminants and prevents infection via the port Flush clears the lock of medication and keeps it open Some agencies recommend only a saline flush to clear the lock
17.	Remove gloves and perform hand hygiene	To prevent the spread of infection
18.	Record: • Record the IV medication administration on the appropriate form • Record the fluid volume on the client's balance sheet	Documentation provides coordination of care
19.	Check the client's response to the medication within the appropriate time	Drugs administered parenterally have rapid onsets of action

ADMINISTRATION OF EYE MEDICATIONS

Eye Ointment Application

Definition

An eye ointment is a semisolid preparation applied to the eye.

Purpose

Eye ointment is used to treat conditions like, keratitis, scleritis, postexternal and internal ocular surgeries, postglaucoma surgeries, ocular injuries.

Equipments

- Clean tray to keep all the required materials
- Sterile dressing pack
- Sterile water for irrigation
- Sterile swab
- Prescribed eye ointment.

Procedure

The procedure of eye ointment application is listed in Table 5.12.

Table 5.12: Procedure for eye ointment application

SI No	Care action	Rationale
1.	Explain the procedure to the patient	To get the consent
2.	Follow the six rights of the drug administration	To prevent medication error
3.	Make the patient to lie down in supine position	To ensure the ointment gone into the inferior fornix of the eye
4.	Wash hands	To prevent cross infection
5.	Clean the eyes with sterile water	To remove any discharges
6.	Hold the nozzle of the tube approximately 2.5 cm above the eye; apply a line of ointment to the inner edge of the lower lid from the nasal corner outwards	To reduce the risk of cross infection, contamination of the tube and trauma to the eye
7.	Ask the patient to close the eyes for 1 minute	To ensure the adequate absorption of the drops
8.	Document in medication administration record (MAR); special notes to be documented in the nurse's record	To maintain the accurate record

Instillation of Eyedrops

Definition

Eyedrop instillation is the instillation of sterile ophthalmic medication into the patient eyes.

Purpose

Eyedrops are used to treat the eye disorders like glaucoma, allergies and infections, and it is used to dilate the pupil for ophthalmic examination.

Equipments

- Clean tray to keep all the required materials
- Sterile dressing pack
- Sterile water for irrigation
- Sterile swab
- Prescribed eyedrops.

Procedure

Nursing action and rationale in the instillation of eyedrops is described in the Table 5.13.

Table 5.13: Nursing intervention and rationale in the instillation of eyedrops

Sl No	Care action	Rationale
1.	Explain the procedure to the patient	To get the consent
2.	Follow the six rights of the drug administration	To prevent medication error
3.	Make the patient to lie down in supine position	To ensure the drops instilled into the inferior fornix of the eye
4.	Wash hands	To prevent cross infection
5.	Clean the eyes with sterile water	To remove any discharges
6.	Ask the patient to look up, simultaneously pull down the lower eyelid and instill the prescribed eye drops	To ensure the drops are instilled into the inferior fornix of the eye
7.	Ask the patient to close the eyes for 1 minute	To ensure the adequate absorption of the drops
8.	Document in medication administration record (MAR); special notes to be documented in the nurses record	To maintain the accurate record

INSTILLATION OF EAR MEDICATION

Definition

Administration of medicine into the ear canal.

Purpose

Eardrops is used to treat or prevent ear infections.

Equipments

- Clean tray to keep all the required materials
- Sterile swab
- Prescribed eardrops.

Procedure

Action and rationale related to ear the medicine instillation is listed in the Table 5.14.

Table 5.14: Nursing intervention and rationale in eardrops instillation

Sl No	Care action	Rationale
1.	Explain the procedure to the patient	To get the consent and cooperation from the patient
2.	Follow the six rights of the drug administration	To prevent medication error
3.	Make the patient to lie on the lateral position with the affected side uppermost	To ensure the best position for instillation of the drops
4.	Wash hands	To prevent cross infection
5.	Pull the cartilaginous part of the pinna backwards and upwards; instill the drops	To ensure the proper instillation of the ear drops
6.	Advise the patient to be in same position for 1–2 minutes	For the proper absorption of the ear drops
7.	Document in medication administration record (MAR)	To maintain the accurate record

INSTILLATION OF NASAL MEDICATION

Definition

A nasal instillation is a medicine solution prepared for administration into the nasal canal. Nasal medicine is given in the form of nasal drops or nasal sprays.

Purpose

The purpose of a nasal instillation is to deliver medicine directly into the nose and onto the nasal membranes, where it will be absorbed into the body. The most common nasal medicines are decongestant, antihistamine and steroid nasal sprays used to relieve nasal congestion.

Equipments

- Clean tray to keep the equipments needed
- Prescribed nasal drops
- Clean gauze or tissue paper
- Clean kidney basin.

Procedure

Nasal medication instillation procedure is described in Table 5.15.

Table 5.15: Nursing intervention and rationale in nasal medication instillation

Sl No	Care action	Rationale
1.	Wash hands	To prevent cross infection
2.	Explain the procedure to the patient and get the consent	Patient has the rights to know the treatment
3.	Follow the six rights of drug administration	To prevent medication error
4.	Ask the patient to blow the nose (unless clinically contraindicated)	To clear the passage for easy penetration
5.	Extend the patient neck (unless clinically contraindicated), e.g. cervical spondylosis	To get a safe position for instillation of medication
6.	Avoid touching external nostrils and instill the prescribed strength	To prevent cross infection
7.	Instruct the patient to be in the same position for 1–2 minutes	To ensure the absorption of the medicine
8.	Record in medication administration record (MAR)	To maintain the record of treatment

ADMINISTRATION OF RECTAL MEDICATIONS

Definition

Administration of medicine into the rectum.

Purpose

Rectal medicine application method is preferred to administer laxatives, to obtain localized therapeutic effect or for diagnostic purpose. Also it used when the patient has nausea, vomiting, uncooperative patients or before surgeries.

Equipments

- Clean tray to keep all the equipments
- Prescribed medicine
- Clean gloves
- Clean gauze
- Clean kidney tray.

Procedure

Nursing action and rationale in rectal medicine application is listed in Table 5.16.

Table 5.16: Rectal medicine application

Sl No	Care action	Rationale
1.	Explain the procedure to the patient	To get the patient consent and for the cooperation
2.	Make the patient to lie down in left lateral position with right leg flexed	For the proper administration of the medication

Contd...

Contd...

Sl No	Care action	Rationale
3.	Wash hands and wear the clean gloves	To prevent cross infection
4.	Ask the patient to relax and to take a deep breath and insert the medicine	For easy administration of the medication and to prevent pain
5.	Advise the patient to lie down for 1 minute	For the good absorption of medication
6.	Document in medication administration record (MAR)	To keep accurate record

ADMINISTRATION OF VAGINAL MEDICATIONS

Definition

Administration of medicine (pessaries) into the vaginal orifice.

Purpose

Pessaries are used to have a therapeutic action.

Equipments

- Clean tray to keep all the equipments
- Prescribed medicine
- Clean glove
- Clean gauze
- Clean kidney tray.

Procedure

Procedure to be followed in the application of vaginal medicine is described in the Table 5.17.

Table 5.17: Nursing intervention and rationale in vaginal medication

Sl No	Care action	Rationale
1.	Explain the procedure to the patient	To get the patient consent and for the cooperation
2.	Follow the six rights of drug administration	To prevent medication error
3.	Make the patient to lie down in supine position with knees up	For the correct insertion of the pessaries
4.	Wash hands	To prevent cross infection
5.	Wear gloves and insert the prescribed pessary along the posterior wall of the vagina; ask the patient to lie down on left lateral for 1–2 minutes	To ensure that the pessary should retained
6.	Document in medication administration record (MAR)	To maintain the accurate record

PREPARATION AND ADMINISTRATION OF CHEMOTHERAPY DRUG

Handling, preparation, administration and disposal of cytotoxic agents may constitute an occupational hazard. While it has not been established that handling cytotoxic agents is consistently linked with adverse health risks, handlers must be aware of the possibility. The implementation of suitable safety precautions reduces the possibility of adverse health effects to hospital employees.

Definition

Other medical terms often used to describe cancer chemotherapy are antineoplastic (anticancer) and cytotoxic (cell killing).

Purposes

- To kill cancer cells
- Can be used as a primary form of treatment or as a supplement to other treatments
- Can be used in metastasis
- Can be used as adjuvant therapy
- Can ease the symptoms of cancer (palliative), helping some patients have a better quality life.

Side Effects of Chemotherapy

- Nausea, vomiting
- Myelosuppression
- Mucositis
- Diarrhea
- Constipation
- Cardiotoxicity
- Pulmonary toxicity
- Fever
- Nephrotoxicity
- Bladder toxicity
- Neurotoxicity
- Allergic reactions (i.e. rashes, petechiae, ecchymosis)
- Alopecia
- Hyperpigmentation
- Immunosuppression.

Terminology

Cytotoxic agents: Substances used in the treatment of malignant and other diseases. They are designed to destroys rapidly growing cancer cells. They have been shown to be mutagenic, carcinogenic and/or teratogenic, either in treatment doses or animal and bacterial assays.

Cytotoxic: An agent or process that is toxic to cells.

Chemotherapy: The use of any chemical agents to treat or control disease. Most often used to describe treatment of malignant and other diseases with cytotoxic agent.

Mutagenic: Capable of causing alterations/damage to genes.

Carcinogenic: Capable of causing cancer.

Teratogenic: Capable of causing fetal defects, either anatomic or functional.

Classification of Cytotoxic Drugs

- Cell cycle specific
- Non-cell cycle specific.

Complications of Unsafe Administration of Cytotoxic Drugs

Chemotherapy drugs are divided into several categories based on how they affect specific chemical substances within cancer cells (Table 5.18).

Table 5.18: Different categories of cytotoxic drugs

Vesicants	Irritants	Non-vesicants
Associated with severe local necrosis	May be associated with local necrosis	Uncommonly associated with local necrosis
Amsacrine	Carboplatin	L-asparaginase
Carmustine (BCNU)	Cisplatin	Bleomycin
Dactinomycin	Dacarbazine (DTIC)	Cyclophosphamide
Daunorubicin	Etoposide	Cytarabine
Doxorubicin	Methotrexate	Ifosfamide
Epirubicin	Mitozantrone	Mephalan
Idarubicin	Teniposide	Thiotepa
Vincristin		
Vinblastine		

Types of Drugs

Vesicants: Drugs, which are capable of causing pain, inflammation and blistering of the local skin, underlying flesh and structures, leading to tissue death and necrosis.

Exfoliants: Drugs, which are capable of causing inflammation and shedding of the skin, but less likely to cause tissue death.

Irritants: Drugs, which are capable of causing inflammation, irritation or pain at site of extravasation, but rarely cause tissue breakdown.

Inflammitants: Drugs, which are capable of causing mild to moderate inflammation and flare in local tissues.

Neutrals: Inert or neutral compounds that do not cause inflammation or damage.

Hazardous Cytotoxic Drugs

Drugs that meet one or more of the following criteria should be handled as hazardous:
- Carcinogenicity
- Teratogenicity or developmental toxicity
- Reproductive toxicity
- Organ toxicity at low doses
- Genotoxicity
- Structure or toxicity similar to drugs classified as hazardous using the above criteria.

Routes of Exposure

- Inhalation of aerosolized drug
- Dermal absorption
- Ingestion
- Injection
- Intrathecal.

Responsibilities of Healthcare Worker

- Participating in training before handling hazardous drugs and updating knowledge based on new information
- Referring to guidance documents and hospital policy as necessary for information regarding hazardous drugs
- Pregnant staff or those who are expecting to become pregnant should not handle cytotoxic drugs (Table 5.19)

Table 5.19: Phases of pregnancy and the effects of biohazards

Phase	Duration	Effect
Embryogenesis	Day 0–14	Repair or spontaneous abortion
Organogenesis	Day 15–84	Spontaneous abortion or irreparable malformation
Fetal development	Day 85 to birth	Functional defects

- Utilizing biological safety cabinets (BSCs) in drug preparation or laminar hood
- Follow universal precaution
- Washing hands after drug handling activities
- Disposing of materials contaminated with hazardous drugs separately from other waste in designated containers (black cover)
- Cleaning up hazardous drug spills immediately according to recommended procedures

- Follow institutional procedures for reporting and following up on accidental exposure to hazardous drugs (Table 5.20).

Table 5.20: Guidelines to be followed in the accidental exposure to hazardous drugs

Type of exposure	Immediate care
Skin exposure	Remove contaminated clothing and/or personal protective equipment (PPE) Wash affected area thoroughly with soap and water
Eye exposure	Flush eye(s) with water/isotonic eye wash for 15 minutes; do not rub the eyes
Exposure by inhalation or ingestion	Acute symptoms may require emergency intervention

Section
2

Advanced and Other Nursing Procedures

- ❑ Advanced Nursing Procedures
- ❑ Assisting Procedures
- ❑ Infection Control Procedures

Advanced Nursing Procedures

INTRAVENOUS CANNULATION

Definition

Intravenous (IV) cannulation is the procedure, where the insertion of a cannula into vessels for the purposes of administration of medication and IV fluids, etc.

Purposes

- For fluid and electrolyte replacement
- To administer the medicines
- To administer the blood/blood products
- To administer the total parenteral nutrition
- To assess the hemodynamic levels
- To collect the blood sampling.

Equipments

- Appropriate size of IV cannula
- Alcohol wipe
- A 2 mL syringe
- A 25 G needle
- A 5 mL ampule of 1% lignocaine solution
- Adhesive dressing for fixation of cannula
- Tourniquet
- Sharps container
- Gloves
- Isopropyl alcohol 70% solution (hand rub solution).

Procedure

Procedure for IV cannulation is provided in Table 6.1.

Table 6.1: Nursing intervention and rationale for intravenous cannulation

Sl No	Care action	Rationale
1.	Explain the procedure to the patient	To obtain the consent from patient
2.	Assess the condition of the patient	To determine reason for intravenous (IV) cannulation

Contd...

Contd...

Sl No	Care action	Rationale
3.	Position the patient with the arm extended to form a straight line from shoulder to wrist	Easy to perform the procedure and make the patient comfortable
4.	Provide privacy to the patient	To make the patient feel comfortable
5.	Wash the hands with soap and water	To minimize the infection
6.	Select the appropriate vein for IV cannulation; it should be straight and more prominent, e.g. the vein in the forearm or dorsum of the hand	Easy to access the line and to prevent the complication
7.	Palpate the vessel; apply a tourniquet 7–10 cm above site gently and it should not be too tight	To prevent the blood obstruction
8.	Put on gloves and clean skin (selected site) with alcohol wipe	To minimize and prevent the entry of the microorganism
9.	Infiltrate skin over proposed puncture site with 1% lignocaine solution (if the doctor prescribed)	To give anesthetic effect to the patient
10.	Hold patient's hand with your non-dominant hand, using your thumb to keep skin taut and anchor vein	To prevent the rolling of the hand
11.	Remove the protective sleeve from the needle taking care not to touch it at any time	To minimize the contamination
12.	Hold the cannula in your dominant hand, stretch the skin over the vein to anchor the vein with your non-dominant hand (do not repalpate the vein)	To prevent the rolling of the vein and to prevent the contamination
13.	The needle is inserted bevel up; the initial angle of entry should be approximately 15°–30°	Easy to capture and prick the vein correctly
14.	Observe for blood in the flashback chamber	Successful entry into the vessel is indicated by return of blood into the flash chamber
15.	Lower the cannula slightly to ensure the enters of lumen in the vessels and does not	To prevent the puncture of exterior wall of the vessel
16.	Gently advance the cannula over the needle whilst withdrawing the guide, noting secondary flashback along the cannula	To prevent the damage of the vein
17.	Release the tourniquet and apply gentle pressure over the vein (beyond the cannula tip) remove the white cap from the needle	To prevent bleeding
18.	Remove the needle from the cannula; attach the white lock cap and dispose of it into a sharps container	Needle is used only for introducing the cannula into the vein. White lock cap prevents leakage of blood from cannula
19.	Secure the cannula with an appropriate dressing and flush the cannula with 2–5 mL of 0.9% sodium chloride or attach an IV giving set and fluid	To prevent the clot
20.	Document the procedure in the nurses record	To provide a point of reference or comparison in the event of later queries

Points to Note

• Do not attempt a venipuncture more than twice. Notify your supervisor or patient's physician if unsuccessful.

INTRAVENOUS INFUSION

Definition

Intravenous infusion is a process that gives insertion of IV catheter for IV therapy.

Purposes

• To give nutrient instead of oral route
• To provide medication by vein continuously.

Equipments

• Prescribed IV solution
• Intravenous infusion set/IV tubing: 1
• Intravenous catheter or butterfly needle in appropriate size: 1
• Spirit swabs
• Adhesive tape
• Disposable gloves, if available: 1
• Intravenous stand: 1
• Arm board, if needed, especially for infant
• Steel tray: 1
• Kidney tray: 1.

Procedure

Procedure for starting an IV infusion is detailed in Table 6.2.

Table 6.2: Procedure for starting an intravenous infusion

Sl No	Care action	Rationale
1.	Assemble all equipments and bring to bedside	To save the time and do the procedure easily
2.	Check intravenous (IV) solution and medication additives with doctor's order	To prevent medication error
3.	Explain procedure to the client	To obtain consent from the patient
4.	Perform hand hygiene	To prevent cross infection
5.	Prepare IV solution and tubing: • Maintain aseptic technique when opening sterile packages and IV solution • Clamp tubing, uncap spike and insert into entry site on bag as manufacturer directs	This prevents spread of microorganisms This punctures the seal in the IV bag Suction effects cause to move into drip chamber also prevents air from moving down the tubing

Contd...

Contd...

SI No	Care action	Rationale
	• Squeeze drip chamber and allow it to fill at least one third to halfway • Remove cap at end of tubing, release clamp, allow fluid to move through tubing; allow fluid to flow until all air bubbles have disappeared • Close clamp and recap end of tubing, maintaining sterility of set up • If an electric device is to be used, follow manufacturer's instructions for inserting tubing and setting infusion rate • Apply label if medication was added to container • Place timetape (or adhesive tape) on container as necessary and hang on IV stand	This removes air from tubing in larger amounts that can act as an air embolus To maintain sterility This ensures correct flow rate and proper use of equipment This provides for administration of correct solution with prescribed medication or additive Pharmacy may have added medication and applied label This permits immediate evaluation of IV according to schedule
6.	Preparation the position: • Have the client in supine position or comfortable position in bed • Place protective pad under the client's arm	Mostly the supine position permits either arm to be used and allows for good body alignment
7.	Selection the site for venipuncture: • Select an appropriate site and palpate accessible veins • Apply a tourniquet 5–6 inches above the venipuncture site to obstruct venous blood flow and distend the vein • Direct the ends of the tourniquet away from the site of injection • Check to be sure that the radial pulse is still present	The selection of an appropriate site decreases discomfort for the client and possible damage to body tissues Interrupting the blood flow to the heart causes the vein to distend Distended veins are easy to see The end of the tourniquet could contaminate the area of injection, if directed toward the site of injection Too much tight the arm makes the client discomfort Interruption of the arterial flow impedes venous filling

8.	Palpation the vein
	• Ask the client to open and close the fist
	• Observe and palpate for a suitable vein
	• If a vein cannot be felt and seen, do the following:
	  – Release the tourniquet and have the client lower his/her arm below the level of the heart to fill the veins; reapply tourniquet and gently over the intended vein to help distend it
	  – Tap the vein gently
	  – Remove tourniquet and place warm, moist compress over the intended vein for 10–15 minutes
		Contraction of the muscle of the forearm forces blood into the veins, thereby distending them further
		To reduce several puncturing
		Lowering the arm below the level of the heart, tapping the vein and applying warmth help distend veins by filling them with blood

9.	Put on clean gloves, if available	Care must be used when handling any blood or body fluids to prevent transmission of human immunodeficiency virus (HIV) and other blood-borne infectious disease

Contd...

Contd...

Sl No	Care action	Rationale
10.	Cleanse the entry site with an antiseptic solution (such as spirit) according to hospital policy: • Use a circular motion to move from the center to outward for several inches • Use several motions with same direction as from the upward to the downward around injection site, approximate 5–6 inches	Cleansing that begins at the site of entry and moves outward in a circular motion carries organisms away from the site of entry Organisms on the skin can be introduced into the tissues or bloodstream with the needle
11.	Holding the arm with non-dominant hand: • Place an non-dominant hand about 1 or 2 inches below entry site to hold the skin taut against the vein • Place an non-dominant hand to support the forearm from the backside *Nursing alert:* Avoid touching the prepared site	Pressure on the vein and surrounding tissues helps prevent movement of the vein as the needle or catheter is being inserted The needle entry site and catheter must remain free of contamination from unsterile hands
12.	Puncturing the vein and withdrawing blood: • Enter the skin gently with the catheter held by the hub in the dominant hand, bevel side up, at a 15°–30° angle • The catheter may be inserted from directly over the vein or the side of the vein • While following the course of the vein, advance the needle or catheter into the vein • A sensation can be felt when the needle enters the vein • When the blood returns through the lumen of the needle or the flashback chamber of the catheter, advance either device 1/8–1/4 inch further into the vein • A catheter needs to be advanced until hub is at the venipuncture site	This technique allows needle or catheter to enter the vein with minimum trauma and deters passage of the needle through the vein The tourniquet causes increased venous pressure resulting in automatic backflow Having the catheter placed well into the vein helps to prevent dislodgement
13.	Connecting to the tube and stabilizing the catheter on the skin: • Release the tourniquet • Quickly remove protective cap from the IV tubing • Attach the tubing to the catheter or needle • Stabilize the catheter or needle with non-dominant hand	The catheter, which immediately is connected to the tube, causes minimum bleeding and patency of the vein is maintained
14.	Starting flow: • Release the clamp on the tubing • Start flow of solution promptly • Examine the drip of solution and the issue around the entry site for sign of infiltration	Blood clots readily if IV flow is not maintained If catheter accidentally slips out of vein, solution will accumulate and infiltrate into surrounding tissue
15.	Fasten the catheter and applying the dressing: • Secure the catheter with narrow non-allergenic tape	Non-allergenic tape is less likely to tear fragile skin

Contd...

Contd...

Sl No	Care action	Rationale
	• Place strictly sided-up under the hub and crossed over the top of the hub • Loop the tubing near the site of entry	The weight of tubing is enough to pull it out of the vein if it is not well anchored There are various ways to anchor the hub You should follow agency/hospital policy To prevent the catheter from removing accidentally
16.	Bring back all equipments and dispose in proper manner	To prepare for the next procedure
17.	Remove gloves and perform hand hygiene	To prevent the spread of infection
18.	If necessary, anchor arm to an arm board for support	An arm board helps to prevent change in the position of the catheter in the vein Site protectors also will be used to protect the IV site
19.	Adjust the rate of IV solution flow according to doctor's order	Doctor prescribed the rate of flow or the amount of solution in day as required to the client's condition Some medications are given very less amount Doctor may use infusion pump to maintain the flow rate
20.	Document the procedure including the time, site, catheter size and the client's response	This ensures continuity of care
21.	Return to check the flow rate and observe for infiltration	To find any abnormalities immediately

Nursing Alert

Nurse should have special consideration for the elderly and infant:

1. To older adults: Avoid vigorous friction at the insertion site and using too much alcohol.

   Rationale: Both can traumatize fragile skin and veins in the elderly.

2. To infant and children: Hand insertion sites should not be the first choice for children.

   Rationale: Nerve endings are more very close to the surface of the skin and it is more painful.

URINARY CATHETERIZATION

Definition

Urinary catheterization or Foley catheterization commonly referred to be an invasive procedure. It involves introducing a plastic or rubber tube into the urethra then advancing the tube into the bladder. Once in the bladder, the catheter provides for a continuous flow of urine.

Indications

Intermittent Catheterization

1. Collection of sterile urine sample.
2. Provide relief from discomfort of bladder distention.
3. Decompression of the bladder.
4. Measure residual urine.
5. Management of patients with spinal cord injury, neuromuscular degeneration or incompetent bladders.

Short-term Indwelling Catheterization

1. Postsurgery and in critically ill patients to monitor urinary output.
2. Surgical procedures involving pelvic or abdominal surgery repair of the bladder, urethra and surrounding structures.
3. Urinary obstruction (e.g. enlarged prostate), acute urinary retention.
4. Prevention of urethral obstruction from blood clots with continuous or intermittent bladder irrigations.
5. Instillation of medication into the bladder.

Long-term Indwelling Catheterization

1. Refractory bladder outlet obstruction and neurogenic bladder with urinary retention.
2. Prolonged and chronic urinary retention.
3. To promote healing of perineal ulcers, where urine may cause further skin breakdown.

Equipments

- Sterile catheterization pack
- Underpad or mackintosh
- Sterile gloves
- Appropriate size of urinary catheters
- Anesthetic lubricating jelly
- Sodium chloride (0.9%) or water for injection
- Adhesive plaster
- Syringe and needle
- Disposable plastic apron
- Sterile drainage bag set.

Procedure

Procedure to set urinary catheterization in females and males is detailed in Tables 6.3 and 6.4.

Table 6.3: Procedure of urinary catheterization in female

SI No	Care action	Rationale
1.	Explain the procedure to the patient	To obtain the consent from patient
2.	Assess the condition of the patient	To determine reason for catheterization
3.	Collect the history from the patient whether she has any latex allergy	To ensure no latex/coated latex products are used
4.	Provide privacy to the patient	To make the patient feel comfortable
5.	Do not expose the patient and assist into supine position with legs extended and cover patient's genital area	To maintain patient's dignity and comfort
6.	Prior to commencement for procedure, if applicable ensure patient has washed genital area using soap and water and assist, if necessary, wearing non-sterile gloves	To reduce presence of bacteria
7.	Arrange needed equipment near the bedside	To avoid the unnecessary contamination as well as easy to perform the procedure
8.	Place the mackintosh or underpad under the patient's buttocks	To prevent the soiling of the linen
9.	Wash hands using bactericidal soap and water or bactericidal alcohol hand rub	To decrease the risk of infection
10.	Wear sterile gloves (both pairs)	To reduce risk of cross infection
11.	Place sterile towels in patient's thighs and under buttocks in transversely and expose genital area	To create a secondary sterile field
12.	With thumb and one finger of your non-dominant hand, spread labia and identify meatus; be prepared to maintain separation of labia with one hand until urine is flowing well and continuously	Easy to identify and clean the meatus and insert the catheter
13.	Using cotton balls held with forceps, clean around the urethral orifice with 0.9% sodium chloride or an antiseptic solution by using single downward stokes	To reduce the cross-contamination
14.	Instil (3–6 mL) anesthetic gel into urethral meatus; allow sufficient time for 5 minutes (time for anesthetic gel to take effect)	Sufficient lubrication helps to prevent urethral trauma; use of a local anesthetic reduce the discomfort experienced by the patient
15.	Pick up sterile catheter with dominant hand, holding it by its inner wrapper and expose tip of catheter, the remaining length should lie in the container, which should be placed between the patients legs	To maintain sterility
16.	Gently insert the catheter into the meatus and pass along the urethra until urine flows	While inserting the catheter ensures that the balloon is positioned correctly in the bladder
17.	Inflate the balloon with sterile according to the manufacture's direction and ensured that the catheter is draining properly before hand; attach	To prevent urethral trauma

Contd...

Contd...

SI No	Care action	Rationale
	the catheter to the drainage system and tie the bag below and secure the catheter to the thigh	
18.	Make the patient comfortable; ensure the area is dry	To prevent infection and skin irritation
19.	Measure the amount of urine and record drainage	To assess the bladder capacity or to monitor renal capacity/fluid balance It is not necessary to measure the amount of urine if the patient is having routine catheter drainage
20.	Dispose all the used items as per institutional policy	To ensure a safe disposal of biomedical waste
21.	Record the procedure in nurse's record	To be aware of continuity of patient care

Table 6.4: Procedure of urinary catheterization in male

SI No	Care action	Rationale
1.	Explain the procedure to the patient	To obtain the consent from patient
2.	Assess the condition of the patient	To determine reason for catheterization
3.	Collect the history from the patient whether he has any latex allergy	To ensure no latex/coated latex products are used
4.	Provide privacy to the patient	To make the patient feel comfortable
5.	Do not expose the patient and assist into supine position with legs extended and cover patient's genital area	To maintain patient's dignity and comfort
6.	Prior to commencement for procedure, if applicable ensure patient has washed genital area using soap and water and assist, if necessary, wearing non-sterile gloves	To reduce presence of bacteria
7.	Arrange needed equipment near the bedside	To avoid the unnecessary contamination as well as easy to perform the procedure
8.	Place the mackintosh or underpad under the patient's buttocks	To prevent the soiling of the linen
9.	Wash hands using bactericidal soap and water or bactericidal alcohol hand rub	To decrease the risk of infection
10.	Wear sterile gloves (both pairs)	To reduce risk of cross infection
11.	If patient is uncircumcised, it will be necessary to retract the prepuce with non-dominant hand, holding penis with a gauze swab; clean penis with sterile normal saline 0.9% or antiseptic solution with dominant hand	To reduce risk of introducing infection to the urinary tract during the procedure
12.	Instil 11 mL of anesthetic gel into urethral meatus, still holding penis with non-dominant hand gently compress penis behind glans to retain gel and massage gel along urethra; allow 5 minutes for anesthetic gel to take effect	Adequate lubrication helps to prevent urethral trauma Use of a local anesthetic minimizes the discomfort experienced by the patient
13.	Pick up sterile catheter with dominant hand, holding it by its inner wrapper and expose tip of catheter, the remaining	To maintain sterility

Contd...

Contd...

Sl No	Care action	Rationale
	length should lie in the container, which should be placed between the patient's legs	
14.	Pick up catheter by holding inner wrapper and expose tip of catheter 1–2 inches (5 cm)	To prevent introduction of infection
15.	Holding penis at angle of 60°–90° to body, gently insert catheter into meatus and pass along urethra maintaining gentle pressure	To get the cooperation and reduce the anxiety
16.	Advance the catheter 6–8 cm and inflate the balloon according to the manufacturer's directions, having ensured that the catheter is draining adequately	Involuntary inflation of the balloon within the urethra is painful and causes urethral trauma
17.	Make the patient comfortable and ensure that the area is dry	If the area is left wet or moist, secondary infection and skin irritation may occur
18.	Record the procedure in details in the nurse's record	To provide a point of reference or comparison in the event of later queries

Points to Note

♦ While inserting the urinary catheter for male patients, if resistance is encountered getting the patient to cough may reduce spasm on the external sphincter and ease the passage of the catheter. Force should not be used and medical advice should be sought if further resistance is felt.

CARE OF URINARY CATHETER

Definition

Catheter care is the sterile procedure, where cleaning of the urinary catheter and perineal area by using the antiseptic solution. A Foley catheter is a tube that is put into the bladder to drain urine out of the body. A Foley catheter can stay in the bladder for hours or weeks.

Purposes

- To prevent infection
- To provide comfort
- To assess the placement of the catheter.

Equipments

A tray containing:
- A sterile dressing tray (thumb forceps and artery forceps, a bowel with sterile gauze and cotton)
- Mackintosh
- A pair of sterile gloves
- Micropore (adhesive tape)
- Mask
- Scissors.

Procedure

Urinary catheter care procedure is given in Table 6.5.

Table 6.5: Procedure of urinary catheter care

Sl No	Care action	Rationale
1.	Explain the procedure to the patient	To get the cooperation and reduce the anxiety
2.	Gather all the equipment, which needed for the catheter care	To save the time and do the procedure easily
3.	Provide privacy	To create the patient comfortable sense and treat patient with self-esteem
4.	Wash hands thoroughly	To minimize risk of cross infection
5.	Place the patient in lying down position	To make the comfortable and ease to perform the work
6.	Place the mackintosh under the perineal region	To prevent soiling of the sheets
7.	Wear mask and sterile gloves	To prevent the infection
8.	Clean the skin near the catheter by using wet cotton or gauze, if possible; gently wash around urinary opening with warm water	To minimize the contamination and prevent the infection
9.	Clean the external meatus for males and introitus for female patients with help of artery forceps by using the antiseptic solutions	To prevent the infection
10.	Hold the end of the catheter and clean around the catheter to remove any blood, crust or mucus; avoid the pulling of catheter	To prevent injury and traction of the tubing
11.	Cover the junction of the penis and the catheter by using sterile gauze, which is soaked with antiseptic solutions	To prevent the infection
12.	Tape the catheter by using the adhesive tape; make sure there is enough tubing left, so the catheter will not be pulled when patient moves his/her leg: • For women tape the catheter to the upper or lateral part of thighs • For men tape the catheter to the lower abdomen, so the catheter does not pull the penis downward	To prevent injury and traction of the tubing
13.	Remove the mackintosh and place the patient as they desire	To feel the comfortable
14.	Replace articles and wash hands	To arrange and keep it ready for next use and minimize risk of cross infection
15.	Document procedure in the nurse's record, if there is any foul smelling discharge or any other abnormalities inform to the concerned doctor	Help to identify the infection in early stage

Points to Note

Clean the skin around the catheter everyday and after every bowel movement:
• For females, always wash from their front to the back.
• For males, always wash from the tip of the penis to down.

BLADDER IRRIGATION

Definition

Bladder irrigation is the procedure in which instillation of a solution into the bladder to provide cleansing or to medication.

Purposes

1. To maintain patency of the retention catheter by removing bladder sediment or blood clots.
2. To instill medications/fluids as ordered.
3. To clean the bladder and maintain the patency of the urinary catheter.
4. To relieve congestion, swelling and pain in the bladder.
5. To arrest hemorrhage and to prevent clot formation after surgery.
6. To prepare the patient for bladder surgeries.
7. To promote healing.

Equipments

- Catheterization set
- Dressing pack
- Pair of sterile gloves
- Irrigation solution
- Asepto syringe
- Double lumen Foley catheter with drainage tubing bag
- Three-way adaptor
- Alcohol swab
- Antiseptic solution
- Kidney tray
- Mackintosh/Underpad
- Adhesive plaster and scissors.

Procedure

Procedure for bladder irrigation is detailed in Table 6.6.

Table 6.6: Procedure for bladder irrigation

Sl No	Care action	Rationale
Closed method		
1.	Explain the procedure to the patient	Explanations make easy to get cooperation and provide comfort for the patient
2.	Arrange all the articles and keep near the patient's bedside	To minimize the unnecessary consultation
3.	Provide privacy for the patient	To feel comfortable

Contd...

Contd...

Sl No	Care action	Rationale
4.	Check the physician's order before administering the solution	To know the type and amount of solution to be used
5.	Place the mackintosh/underpad under the patient buttocks	To prevent the soiling of the linen
6.	Position the patient in modified dorsal recumbent position	Easy to perform the position
7.	Drape the patient well	To make the patient comfortable
8.	Wash hands	To prevent the spread of infection
9.	Open the bladder irrigation set and keep additional dressing materials and pour the solution required	To carry out the procedure in an easy way
10.	Wear sterile gloves	To maintain the sterile environment while doing the procedure
11.	Follow the sterile catheterization procedure to insert the catheter	To prevent the infection
12.	If the patient is on urinary catheter, detach the uro sac or uro bag and cover the tip with sterile gauze pieces	To prevent the entry of the microorganisms
13.	Load the bladder wash syringe with solution prescribed and expel the air, attach the tip of the syringe into the catheter	To prevent positive pressure within the asepto syringe
14.	Install the solution slowly into the bladder usually not more than, 80–100 cc at a time	To prevent trauma to the bladder mucosa
15.	Remove the syringe and allow the urine to drain into the kidney tray	
16.	Repeat installing and emptying till the return flow is clean	To ensure proper removal of the block
17.	Connect the catheter to the uro sac and measure the return flow	To drain the urine continuously and follow-up care
18.	Remove the mackintosh and make the patient to lie down comfortably	To make the patient feel comfortable
19.	Remove the gloves; wash all the articles and replace properly	To prevent the cross-contamination and make the articles ready for further usage
20.	Document the procedure in the nurse's record	To assess the condition of the patient and perform the continuity of care
Continuous method		
1.	Prepare the bladder irrigation solution as prepared for intravenous (IV) infusion, hang the solution bottle on irrigation stand at a height of about 6–8 inches above the level of meatus and allow expelling air from the irrigating set	It helps to increase the flow rate of solution. Expelling air in the irrigating set prevents air embolism

Contd...

Contd...

Sl No	Care action	Rationale
2.	Place the mackintosh under the patient buttocks	To prevent the soiling of the linen
3.	Place the patient in dorsal recumbent position	To perform the procedure in an easy way
4.	Clean the catheter and uro bag junction with alcohol swab	To minimize the entry of microorganisms
5.	Wear gloves	To prevent the contamination
6.	Connect the tubing to the 3-way urinary catheter and allow about 500–800 mL of fluid at a time	To ensure that proper amount of solution flows into the bladder to wash out the bladder completely
7.	Do not clamp the irrigation tubing	To allow the free flow of fluids
8.	Assess the color of the return flow and measure the return flow for each 500 mL bottle	To assess for any abnormalities
9.	Continue irrigation till the return flow is clear	To ensure proper removal of the block from the bladder
10.	If the patient is post-transurethral resection of the prostate (TURP), the procedure is continued for 24 hours	To wash out the blood clot from the bladder
11.	Remove the mackintosh	To make the patient comfortable
12.	Remove the glove and wash hands	To prevent the cross-contamination
13.	Record time, amount and kind of solution used, character of return flow and response of the patient	To identify any abnormalities and report immediately

---

Points to Note

- For continuous irrigation: Unclamp the irrigating tube and adjust the flow rate similar to an IV infusion. The solution along with urine will continuously flow out of catheter into the drainage bag.
- For intermittent irrigation: Clamp the drainage tubing and unclamp the irrigating tube, adjust the flow rate and allow a specified amount of solution to flow.

EAR IRRIGATION

Definition

The ear irrigation is the procedure to remove the discharge of the ear canal, to soften and remove impacted cerumen or to dislodge a foreign object.

Purposes

- To relieve congestion, inflammation and pain in the ear
- To administer antiseptics
- To remove foreign bodies, earwax or discharges
- To evaluate the vestibular functions.

Equipments

A tray containing the following articles:
- Prescribed irrigating solution warmed to 37°C (98.6°F)
- Irrigation set (container and irrigating or bulb syringe)
- Basin
- Cotton-tipped applicator and cotton balls
- Mackintosh or underpad
- Kidney tray
- Otoscope, if needed.

Procedure

Procedure for ear irrigation is given in Table 6.7.

Table 6.7: Procedure for ear irrigation

Sl No	Care action	Rationale
1.	Explain the procedure to the patient	Explanations make easy to get cooperation and provide comfort for the patient
2.	Arrange and keep the needed articles near the patient bedside	For the planned approach to the work
3.	Provide privacy	To reduces unease of the patient
4.	Wash your hands	To prevent the spread of microorganisms
5.	Spread the mackintosh/underpads under the patient	To protect the linen soiling
6.	Make the patient sit up or lie with the head tilted toward the side of the affected ear and support a basin under the ear to receive the irrigating solution	Gravity causes the irrigating solution to flow from the ear to the basin
7.	Wear the sterile gloves	To keep up sterile technique while doing the procedure
8.	Clean the pinna and the meatus at the auditory canal, as necessary, with the normal saline or the irrigating solution	Materials lodged on the pinna and the meatus may be washed into the ear
9.	Fill the bulb syringe with solution, if an irrigating container is used, check for air bubbles	Air forced into the ear canal is noisy and therefore unpleasant for the patient
10.	Straightening the auditory canal by pulling the pinna down and back for an infant and up and back for an adult patient	Straightening the ear canal aids in allowing solution to reach all areas of the ears easily
11.	Direct a steady, slow stream of solution against the roof of the auditory canal, using only sufficient force to remove secretions; do not occlude the auditory canal with the irrigating nozzle and allow solution to flow out unimpeded	Solution directed at the roof of the canal aids in preventing injury to the tympanic membrane; continuous in- and out-flow of the irrigating solution helps prevent pressure in the canal
12.	Continue to irrigate till the ear is clear of discharge	To ensure that ear is cleaned completely
13.	Dry the ear with sterile cotton applicator	To ensure clean and dry surface

Contd...

Contd...

Sl No	Care action	Rationale
14.	Remove all wet mackintosh/underpad from the patient side	To make the patient comfortable
15.	When the irrigation is completed, place a dry cotton ball loosely in the auditory meatus and have the patient lie on the side of the affected ear on a an towel/underpad	The cotton ball absorbs excess fluid; gravity allows the remaining solution in the canal to escape from the ear
16.	Wash your hands; clean and replace the articles	Keep it ready for next use and to deters the spread of microorganisms
17.	Document the irrigation, the appearance of the drainage and the patient's response	To provide accurate documentation and help to provide follow-up care for the patient

> **Points to Note**
> - Avoid dropping or squirting on the eardrum.
> - Never use more than 500 mL of solution.
> - If the tympanic membrane is ruptured, check with the doctor before irrigation.
> - Monitor temperature of solution carefully.
> - Forceful instillation of the solution can rupture the tympanic membrane.
> - If pain or dizziness occurs, stop the procedure.
> - If irrigation is done to dislodge the wax, it is better to soften it by putting soda glycerin or hydrogen peroxide 3–4 days prior to the procedure.
> - If syringe is used for irrigation, do not use a large syringe as it is difficult to control and may exert undue pressure in forcing the fluid into the auditory canal.

EYE IRRIGATION

Definition

Eye irrigation is the procedure, where to flush eye(s) with solution to remove secretion and foreign bodies or to dilute chemicals.

Purposes

- Remove secretions from the conjunctival site
- Irrigate following the instillation of certain diagnostic drugs
- To relieve congestion, inflammation and pain in the eye
- To administer medications
- To remove foreign bodies, chemicals or discharge
- To prepare the patient for eye surgery.

Equipments

A tray containing the following articles:
- Sterile irrigating solution warmed to 37°C (98.6°F)
- Disposable gloves

- Sterile irrigating set (sterile container and irrigating or bulb syringe)
- Basin or irrigation basin
- Disposable syringe
- Solution container
- Cotton swabs
- Gauze pieces
- Warm sterile solution in a sterile jug
- Eye medicine, if needed
- Towel
- Kidney tray.

Procedure

The procedure of eye irrigation is detailed in the Table 6.8.

Table 6.8: Procedure for eye irrigation

SI No	Care action	Rationale
1.	Explain the procedure to the patient	Explanations make easy to get cooperation and provide comfort for the patient
2.	Arrange and keep the needed articles near the patient bedside	For a planned approach to the work
3.	Provide privacy	To reduces unease of the patient
4.	Wash your hands	To prevent the spread of microorganisms
5.	Spread the mackintosh/underpads under the patient	To protect the linen soiling
6.	Make the patient sit or lie with the head tilted toward the side of the affected eye; protect the patient and the bed with waterproof pad	Gravity will aid the flow of solution away from the unaffected eye and from the inner canthus of the affected eye toward the outer canthus
7.	Wear disposable gloves, clean the lids and the lashes with a cotton ball moistened with normal saline or the solution ordered for the irrigation; wipe from the inner canthus to the outer canthus and discard the cotton ball after each wipe	Materials lodged on the lids or in the lashes may be washed into the eye\nThis cleansing motion protects the nasolacrimal duct and the other eye
8.	Place the curved basin at the cheek on the side of the affected eye to receive the irrigating solution; if sitting up, ask the patient to support the basin	Gravity will aid the flow of solution
9.	Expose the lower conjunctival sac and hold the upper lid open with your non-dominant hand	The solution is directed on to the lower conjunctival sac because the cornea is very sensitive and easily injured\nThis also prevents reflex blinking
10.	Hold the irrigator about 2.5 cm (1 inch) from the eye; direct the flow of the solution from the inner canthus to the outer canthus along the conjunctival sac	This minimizes the risk of injury to the cornea; solution directed toward the outer canthus helps prevent the spread of contamination from the eye to the lacrimal sac, the lacrimal duct and the nose

Contd...

Contd...

Sl No	Care action	Rationale
11.	Irrigate until the solution is clear or all the solution has been used; use only sufficient force gently to remove secretions from the conjunctiva; avoid touching any part of the eye with the irrigating tip	Directing solutions with force may cause injury to the tissues of the eyes as well as to the conjunctiva. Touching the eye is uncomfortable for the patient
12.	Make the patient close the eye periodically during the procedure	It helps to move secretions from the upper conjunctival sac to the lower
13.	Dry the area after the irrigation with cotton balls or a gauze sponge; offer a towel to the patient if the face and neck are wet	Leaving the skin moist after irrigation is uncomfortable for the patient
14.	Wash the hands, clean and replace the equipments	To prevent the risk of cross infection and make it ready for next usage
15.	Document the irrigation, the appearance of the eye, drainage and the patient's response	To provide accurate documentation and to provide follow-up care for the patient

Points to Note

- When irrigating both eyes, have the patient tilt his/her head toward the side being irrigated to avoid cross-contamination.
- For chemical burns, irrigate each eye with at least 1,000 mL of normal saline solutions.
- In case of chemical burn, irrigation could last 10–15 minutes.

ENDOTRACHEAL/TRACHEAL SUCTIONING

Definition

Oropharyngeal, tracheal and endotracheal suction are methods of clearing secretions by the application of negative pressure via either a Yankauer sucker (oropharyngeal) or an appropriately sized tracheal suction catheter (tracheal/endotracheal).

Indications

- To remove thick mucus secretions from the trachea and lower respiratory tract
- Maintain a patent airway to ensure adequate oxygenation and ventilation
- To prevent or treat pulmonary infection
- To prevent hypoxia.

Equipments

- Appropriate size of suction catheters
- Sterile water for rinsing catheter
- Normal saline (0.9%)
- Suction apparatus (portable or wall suction) with tubing

- A pair of sterile gloves
- Kidney tray
- Disposable face mask
- Goggles
- Clean gloves
- Disposable apron
- Syringe to instill normal saline.

Procedure

Endotracheal/Tracheal suctioning is given in Table 6.9.

Table 6.9: Procedure for endotracheal/tracheal suctioning

Sl No	Care action	Rationale
1.	Confirm the patient's identity, explain the procedure	To identify the patient correctly and gain informed consent
2.	Assess the patient to ensure that suction is necessary (including the effectiveness of their cough)	To reduce potential complications from endotracheal suction and avoid unnecessary interventions
3.	Collect the needed equipments on a trolley and take to the bedside	Easy to perform the procedure
4.	Assist the patient into an upright position (if possible)	To allow optimum lung expansion and effective cough
5.	Check the saturation level (SpO$_2$) of the patient by using pulse oximeter	To enable evaluation of patient's oxygenation prior to and following the suction procedure to prevent the complication
6.	Wash hands	To reduce the risk of cross infection
7.	Put on disposable apron and protective visor/eyewear, according to institutional policy	To reduce risk of cross infection and to protect yourself from droplets/sputum contamination
8.	Connect suction catheter to suction tubing and turn suction machine on	To allow suction to begin
9.	Use sterile/clean glove	To reduce risk of cross infection
10.	Withdraw suction catheter from sleeve with clean gloved hand and grasp catheter with sterile/clean gloved hand away from catheter tip	To reduce risk of cross infection
11.	Advance catheter gently until a cough is stimulated or resistance is felt; do not apply suction during catheter insertion	To minimize risk of mucosal trauma
12.	When a cough is initiated or resistance is felt, withdraw the catheter approximately 1 cm and apply suction by occluding suction control port on catheter with thumb; withdraw gently and procedure should last not more than 15 seconds	To reduce potential complications from suctioning

Contd...

Contd...

Sl No	Care action	Rationale
13.	Rinse the suction tubing by dipping its end into the sterile water bottle and applying suction until the solution has rinsed the tubing through	To ensure sputum is removed from suction tubing
14.	Dispose of suction catheter and gloves in clinical waste disposable bin, as per institutional policy	To reduce risk of cross infection and ensure clinical waste is correctly disposed of
15.	Clear patient's oral secretions, if required	To maintain patient comfort
16.	Wash hands with soap and water	To reduce the risk of cross infection
17.	Record the procedure in the nurse's record	To assess the continuity of care

PERCUTANEOUS ENDOSCOPIC GASTROSTOMY FEEDING

Definition

Percutaneous endoscopic gastrostomy (PEG) is a procedure for placing a feeding tube directly into the stomach through a small incision in the abdominal wall using an instrument known as an endoscope.

Purposes

1. To provide sufficient nourishment and hydration support to the patient.
2. For therapeutic purposes.
3. Help to drain out the stomach content in case of gastric problem or postoperative, etc.
4. To assess acceptance level of feeds in postoperative patients, who undergone surgery and have nasogastric (NG) tube in situ.

Equipments

Clean tray containing:
- A 50 mL syringe
- Tissue paper
- Towel
- Measuring cup
- A cup of feed
- A cup of water
- Gloves (if needed)
- Disposable feeding bag
- Stethoscope
- Intravenous stand
- Administration set
- Infusion pump.

Procedure

Percutaneous endoscopic gastrostomy feeding and jejunostomy feeding are detailed in Table 6.10.

Table 6.10: Procedure of percutaneous endoscopic gastrostomy and jejunostomy feeding

SI No	Care action	Rationale
1.	Make clear the procedure to the patient	To get the patient's cooperation and consent
2.	Ensure rate, frequency and formula of the feed as per consultant order	To prevent the overload of the feed and complications
3.	Check the dressing site of the percutaneous endoscopic gastrostomy (PEG) tube for any redness, edema or oozing	Help to identify the infection in early stage
4.	Ensure the patient to lie down in Fowler's position or in supine with 30° of head end elevation	To avoid aspiration
5.	Arrange the entire needed article near the right side of the patient	Easy to perform the procedure
6.	Wash hands with soap and water	To prevent cross infection
7.	Check the tube potion by using the syringe, aspirate the gastric secretion or auscultate over the left upper quadrant with stethoscope and push 10–20 mL of air into the tube using syringe	To ensure the write position of tube that is placed in the stomach
8.	Connect the barrel of the syringe in the PEG tube connector	To make sure the gravity flow of the fluid
9.	Pore the measured amount of feed into the feeding tube, in case of 2-way tube, one way has to be used for feeding and another way for water to flush after the use	To keep the feeding tube clean
10.	In case of bag feed method: • Connect the tube to the bag • Fill the bag with feed • Expel the air in the connecting tube • Hang the bag to intravenous (IV) stand • Raise the bag up to 18 inches above the patient's abdomen • Fix the bag to the infusion pump and set the rate • Connect the proximal end of the tube to the feeding bag • Allow the feed to go off into the stomach	To ensure the proper amount and technique of feeding and to prevent complications
11.	Push measured amount of water into the tube after the feed	To prevent the obstruction of feed in the feeding tube and keep the tube clean
12.	Once the feed is over, wash the feeding bag with warm water	To avoid feed steamy over the bag and to ensure the bag is ready for next use
13.	Make the patient to continue the same Fowler's position for 5–10 minutes	To prevent aspiration
14.	Replace the articles and wash hands	To make it ready for next use and to prevent the contamination
15.	Document the procedure in the nurse's chart in detail and maintain the intake and output chart	To continue the perfect record of the patient

JEJUNOSTOMY FEEDING

Definition

The administration of nutritionally balanced liquefied foods or nutrients through a tube inserted into jejunum.

Purposes

To provide adequate nutrition to the patient, who has undergone gastrointestinal tract bypass surgery.

Equipments

- Clean tray to collect all the things
- Disposable feeding bag
- Stethoscope
- Measured amount of feed
- Intravenous stand
- Administration set
- Infusion pump.

Procedure

For jejunostomy procedure refer Table 6.10.

ADMINISTRATION OF TOTAL PARENTERAL NUTRITION

Definition

Total parenteral nutrition (TPN) is a solution, which contains all the required nutrients including protein, fat, calories, vitamins and minerals is injected over the course of several hours through intravenously into the body. TPN provides a complete and balanced source of nutrients for patients, who cannot consume a normal diet.

Purposes

1. Total parenteral nutrition is the intravenous administration of essential nutrients and is initiated when the gastrointestinal (GI) tract does not provide for adequate ingestion, digestion and absorption.
2. A general indication is anticipation of undernutrition (< 50% of metabolic needs) for more than 7 days.
3. Total parenteral nutrition is given before and after treatment to severely undernourished patients, who cannot ingest large volumes of oral feeding and are being prepared for surgery, radiation therapy or chemotherapy.

Equipments

Clean tray containing:
- Total parenteral nutrition solution
- Administration set or IV set
- Hand care gloves
- Alcohol swab
- Kidney tray.

Procedure

Procedure for administration of total parenteral nutrition is given in Table 6.11.

Table 6.11: Procedure for administration of total parenteral nutrition

Sl No	Care action	Rationale
1.	Explain the procedure to the patient	To get the consent and cooperation from the patient
2.	Arrange all the articles to keep in the medicine preparation trolley	To reduce the cross-contamination
3.	Wash hands with soap and water and dry the hands thoroughly	To prevent cross infection
4.	Wear hand care gloves	To prevent the infection
5.	Clean the intravenous (IV) port insertion site with alcohol swab for at least 15 seconds	To prevent bacterial growth and contamination
6.	Insert the sterile IV set into the port and let out the air in the set by flushing the set with the solution	To prevent the growth of bacteria and entry of air in the vein
7.	Label the bag with the started date and time or the drug name, which is added in the fluid	To prevent the continuous usage of total parenteral nutrition (TPN)
8.	Connect TPN to the infusion pump; set the pump on prescribed drops	To make sure the accurate flow rate
9.	Check the patency of IV line or central venous pressure (CVP) line before starting the TPN; using aseptic technique, attach tubing to appropriate IV line	To prevent the complication like extravasations and to prevent the entry of the microorganisms
10.	Start the infusion as per consultant prescription	To avoid the over usage of drugs
11.	Document in medication administration record (MAR)	To maintain an accurate record
12.	Record the procedure clearly in the nurse's notes	To assess the patient condition periodically

Points to Note

- In case of continuous infusion, the total parenteral nutrition solution should be changed every 24 hours.
- Before starting the infusion, the pump should be checked thoroughly to prevent hypo- or hyper-glycemia.
- Sugar level shall be checked every 2nd hourly or as per consultant's order.
- Frequent monitoring of the patient is very essential.

BLOOD TRANSFUSION

Definition

Blood transfusion is the process of transferring blood or blood-based products from one person into the circulatory system of another.

Purposes

- To treat a severe anemia or thrombocytopenia
- To raise the blood pressure
- To treat the critically ill patient like massive blood loss, major surgery, trauma, etc.
- To provide selected cellular components as a replacement therapy (e.g. clotting factors, platelets and albumin).

Equipments

- Appropriate blood administration set
- Intravenous stand
- Infusion pump (if needed)
- Equipment for patient's intravenous access requirements (if necessary)
- Blood pressure (BP) apparatus
- Stethoscope
- Intravenous cannulation tray (if needed).

Procedure

Procedure for blood transfusion is detailed in Table 6.12.

Table 6.12: Procedure for blood transfusion

Sl No	Care action	Rationale
1.	Explain the procedure to the patient/patient relatives	To understand importance of the transfusion and get the valid consent from patient/patient relatives
2.	Check the doctor's order for premedication	To prevent the allergic reaction
3.	Confirm the blood grouping and typing and crossmatching details	To prevent incorrect blood component transfused error
4.	Check the patient vital signs [blood pressure (BP), pulse, respiration, temperature]	Help to identify any abnormal reaction immediately
5.	The blood component should be cross-checked by duty medical officer (DMO)/consultant and nursing supervisor/senior staff nurse	To prevent the administration of outdated/expired blood products
6.	The following details to be checked in the blood component: • Blood group and crossmatch • Donor's name, patient's name	To ensure the safe delivery of blood components

Contd...

Contd...

Sl No	Care action	Rationale
	• The date of blood drawn • Date of expiry • Consent is obtained from the duty doctor for verification in the record • Checks for any clots or any other abnormality is present, if found the blood/blood product is return to blood bank	
7.	Intravenous (IV) cannula is checked for the patency before staring the transfusion	To prevent the extravasations
8.	Blood infusion started slowly for first 20 minutes; if no allergic reaction the transfusion can be continued by set up infusion via a volumetric infusion pump, if appropriate	To observe for the allergic reaction and to maintain the accurate transfusion rate
9.	Check and record the patient's temperature, pulse, BP and respiratory rate every 15 minutes during the 1st hour, followed by every 30 minutes till the transfusion is completed	Help to identify any abnormalities (allergic reaction) in an early stage itself
10.	As per the doctor's order the infusion rate should be followed; infusion should be finished within 4 hours of started	To prevent the risk of transfusion reaction and complications
11.	Record the procedure in the nurse's record in details	Help to assess the continuous progress of the patient
12.	Once the blood transfusion over, disconnect the blood transfusion set and discard as per institutional policy	To prevent the contamination

Points to Note

If any reaction occurs:
- Immediately blood transfusion is stopped and duty doctor is informed.
- Carry out the doctor's orders.
- The remains blood and blood sets send to the blood bank and documentation to be done.
- Recording and reporting of reactions if any, shall be done by the staff and consultant and then analyzed.
- The transfusion details will be recorded in the patient record.

INSERTION OF ENEMA AND SUPPOSITORIES

Definition

Enema is the procedure, which is used to refer to the process of instilling fluid through the anal sphincter into the rectum and lower intestine for a therapeutic purpose.

Purposes

- To stimulate peristalsis (involuntary contraction) and to evacuate stool from the rectum
- To administer medication
- To relive gaseous distention
- For diagnostic purposes
- To clean the bowl before some specific investigation or procedure
- To provoke anesthesia
- To reduce the temperature.

Equipments

A clean tray containing:
- Enema can with tubing's and clamp
- Suppositories or enema
- A pair of clean gloves
- Apron
- Mask
- Lubricant jelly
- Mackintosh
- Tissue paper
- Towels
- Bedpan.

Procedure

Procedure for enema and suppositories insertion is provided in Table 6.13.

Table 6.13: Procedure for enema and suppositories insertion

SI No	Care action	Rationale
1.	Explain the procedure and its importance	To get acceptance from the patient
2.	Wash the hands and wear the gloves, apron and mask	To prevent the infection and unnecessary mess
3.	Before start the procedure ask the patient to void and collect the history from the patient about previous ano/rectal surgery or abnormalities	To prevent any add up to assault
4.	Arrange all the equipments in the procedure room	For the easy use and to minimize the contamination
5.	Adjust the intravenous (IV) stand height to hang the enema can at the required height	To ensure the free flow of water
6.	Connect all the tubing and clamp in the enema can and hung the can in the IV stand	To prevent any obstruction of fluid flow during the procedure
7.	Loose the pyjama and place the patient in the mackintosh	To prevent mess in the procedural area

Contd...

Contd...

Sl No	Care action	Rationale
8.	Position the patient on the bed on his or her left side with the top knee bent and pulled slightly upward toward the chin	To aid relaxation and minimize resistance, and discomfort on insertion
9.	Allow the small amount of fluid to run into the kidney tray by releasing the clamp	To check any leakage of the tube and let out the air from the tube
10.	Apply the lubricant jelly in the distal part of the enema tube (3–4 inch)	Easy to advance the tube into the rectal area
11.	Ask the patient take deep breath and advance the tube 3–4 inches in to the rectal area	To aid relaxation and minimize resistance and discomfort on insertion
12.	Release the clamp and allow the solution to go inside and the solution should be in room temperature	To minimize shock and prevent bowel spasms
13.	Ensure the prescribed amount of fluid has passed, once it does over clamp the tube	To prevent the air entry
14.	Gently remove the tube by using the adequate gauze pieces and hold the patient's buttocks together	To avoid the splashing the excretion of fluid
15.	Remove and discard the gauzes and other items, which are used for the procedure as per institutional policy	To minimize the risk of contamination
16.	Instruct the patient to hold the fluid 5–10 minutes until there is a strong urge to defecate	To facilitate the fecal matter soft and peristalsis movement
17.	If the patient wants to pass motion immediately, give bedpan or assess the patient to the toilet	To provide comfortable to the patients
18.	In case of suppositories administration: • Insert suppositories about 4 cm into the rectum, usually using the index finger • Clean the patient perianal area; ask the patient to retain the suppository • Ensure that assistance is available if patient is unable to walk to the toilet • A suppository will take about 20 minutes to dissolve	To prevent cross infection Some patient may prefer to insert the suppository themselves, if so the nurse should explain the procedure and be available to offer assistance, if necessary
19.	Document that the suppository has been given; monitor the patient and record the effects of the rectal enema	Easy to assess the patient condition

COLOSTOMY CARE

Definition

Colostomy care is the procedure, where the colostomy bag is emptying and cleaning regularly.

Indications

- To prevent tissue damage and skin excoriation
- To prevent infection and promote healing
- To check for the patency of the ostomy
- To assess the stoma and the surrounding regions
- Help to identify the complication in early stage
- To maintain personal hygiene
- To prevent odor and leakage from the ostomy bag.

Equipments

- Dressing tray
- Disposable gloves
- Mask
- Cleaning solution
- Ostomy pouch with clamp
- Tape or belt
- Skin barrier (powder or paste)
- Mackintosh
- Sponge cloth or tissue paper
- Towel
- Basin with warm water
- Kidney tray.

Procedure

Colostomy care is detailed in Table 6.14.

Table 6.14: Procedure for colostomy care

SI No	Care action	Rationale
1.	Explain the procedure to the patient	To get the cooperation from the patient
2.	Provide privacy	To make comfortable to the patient
3.	Gather all the equipment near the bedside	To prevent unnecessary contamination and easy to perform the procedure
4.	Place the mackintosh under the patient site of the stoma	To prevent soiling of the linen
5.	Place the patient in supine position and cover the patient appropriately	To make the patient feel comfortable and to prevent the contamination
6.	Wash the hands; wear gloves and mask	To reduce the risk of cross infection
7.	Release the clamp and empty the motion content from the bag to the bedpan	To prevent splashing of the fecal matter
8.	Remove the pouch and keep it aside	

Contd...

Contd...

Sl No	Care action	Rationale
9.	Wash the skin around the stoma with water or normal saline and dry the area	Skin must be dry, pouch does not adhere to wet skin
10.	Observe the skin condition around the stoma side	Help to identify the complication in early stages
11.	Apply the skin barrier around the stoma site (paste or powder); allow 1–2 minutes for dry	It creates a flatter surface for pouch placement
12.	Measure the stoma size by measuring guide or stoma pattern according to that cut the Karaya sheet and prepares the pouch	To prevent the leakage from side of the stoma
13.	Peal the paper around the opening of the pouch; apply it to the non-covered shiny side of the Karaya sheet	Easy to stick over the area
14.	Remove the transparent layer from the Karaya sheet and apply it with the pouch as one unit, to the skin	Easy to attach around the stoma site
15.	Apply the belt as needed, to the edge of the faceplate over the Karaya sheet	Ensure the proper position for the bag
16.	Fold bottom edge of the pouch to fit clamp or devices	To prevent the leakage
17.	Dispose the waste material as per institutional policy	To prevent the contamination
18.	Remove the mackintosh and articles near the bedside	Make the environment clean and comfortable for the patient
19.	Remove the gloves and wash the hands	To reduce the risk of cross infection
20.	Make the patient comfortable	Ensure the patient comfortable
21.	Document the procedure in the nurse's record	Help to do the follow-up care for the patient

EXTRAVASATIONS

Definition

1. Extravasation is the inadvertent administration of drugs (vesicant solution or medication) into the surrounding tissues rather than into the intended vein, which can lead to tissue necrosis.
2. Extravasation is a complication of intravenous chemotherapy administration but in general condition that is often underdiagnosed, undertreated and under-reported.

Prevention of Extravasation

Focus

Safe intravenous technique and implementing appropriate strategies to minimize the risk. Forethought, planning and improved prevention measures can minimize the risk of extravasation:

1. Careful assessment of the most appropriate cannulation site should be undertaken before insertion. Siting the cannula over joints should be avoided, as tissue damage in these areas has serious consequences. If venous access proves difficult, the opinion of an experienced practitioner should be sought as placement of a central venous access device (CVAD) may be necessary.
2. Extravasations can occur in CVADs, often with delayed onset and can be recognized by the patient complaining of sudden pain, discomfort, inflammation or swelling around the extravasations site.
3. Some patient groups are at increased risk of extravasations. These include obese, elderly, pediatric patients, thrombocytopenic patients, diabetics with peripheral neuropathy and patients who have had previous chemotherapy/radiotherapy. Extra care should be taken with all these patient groups.
4. Vesicant drugs in a chemotherapy regimen must be given before the other cytotoxic agents.
5. When given peripherally, bolus doses (in syringes) of vesicants must be given via a fast running infusion of a compatible fluid. Continually assess the cannulation site throughout the administration for signs of swelling, pain or inflammation and monitor the fast running infusion for change in rate.
6. Only the following vesicant cytotoxics may be given by peripheral infusion (in bags), i.e. paclitaxel, vinca alkaloids, dacarbazine, streptozocin, treosulfan. However, the central venous route minimizes the extravasations risk and should be considered on an individual patient basis. Any other cytotoxic vesicant infusions (in bags) should be administered via CVAD.

Management of Extravasations of Cytotoxic Drugs

Administration of the vesicant drugs: It should be administered first since:
- The vascular integrity increases over time
- The vein is most stable and least irritated at the start of the treatment
- The initial assessment of vein patency is most accurate
- The vesicant drugs are irritant, increase the vein fragility and cause venous spasm masking the signs of extravasation, when administered last.

Signs and Symptoms

Extravasations should be suspected if one or more of the following symptoms have occurred:
1. The patient complains of burning, stinging or any discomfort/pain at the injection site.

2. This should be distinguished from a feeling of cold that may occur with some drugs.
3. Observation of swelling, redness or blistering at the injection site. This should be distinguished from the 'nettle rash' effect seen with anthracyclines.
4. No blood return is obtained. This is not a sign of extravasations, if found in isolation.
5. A resistance is felt on the plunger of the syringe of a bolus drug.
6. There is absence of free flow of the infusion.
7. If in any doubt, treat as extravasation.

Management of Extravasations

- Stop the chemotherapeutic drug infusion immediately
- Aspirate any residual drug and blood in IV tubing, needle and suspected infiltration site
- The peripheral access device can be left in situ or removed according to the physician order
- Apply hot or cold packs as indicated
- Administer antidote subcutaneously clockwise into the infiltrated area
- Elevate the limb to minimize the swelling
- Monitor the site frequently for pain, erythema, induration and necrosis
- Plastic surgeon consultation to remove the tissue containing the drug
- Surgical recommendation is required especially, when the lesion is greater than 2 cm
- There is significant residual pain 1-2 weeks after extravasations
- There is minimal healing 2-3 weeks after injury despite local therapeutic measures
- Document the extravasations management.

Documentation and Reporting

Purposes

- To provide an accurate account of what happened (in the event that there is litigation)
- To protect the healthcare professionals involved (showing they followed procedure)
- To gather information on extravasations, how and when they occurs—for audit purposes
- Highlight any possible deficits in practice, which require review.

Difference between extravasations from other conditions is given in Table 6.15.

Table 6.15: Distinguishing extravasations from other conditions

Characteristics	Flare reaction	Vessel irritation	Venous shock	Extravasations
Presenting symptoms	Itchy blotches or hives; pain and burning uncommon	Aching and tightness	Muscular wall of the blood vessel in spasm	Pain and burning are common at injection site; stinging may occur during infusion
Coloration	Raised red streak, blotches or 'hive-like' erythema along the vessel; diffuse or irregular pattern	Erythema or dark discoloration along vessel		Erythema around area of needle or around the venipuncture site
Timing	Usually appears suddenly and dissipates within 30–90 minutes	Usually appears within minutes after injection; coloration may only appear later in the process	Usually appears right after injection	Symptoms start to appear right after injection, symptoms endure
Swelling	Unlikely	Unlikely	None	Occurs often; does not dissolve for several days
Blood return	Usually, but not always intact	Usually, but not always intact	Often absent	Usually absent or sluggish

Poorly Managed Extravasation

Poorly managed extravasations leads to:
- Pain from the necrotic site
- Physical defect
- Increase in cost of hospitalization
- Delay in the treatment of disease
- Psychological distress.

Preparation and Administration

Equipment

- Clean tray or receiver in which to place drug and equipment
- Use 21 G needle(s) to ease reconstitution and drawing up, 23 G needle if from a glass ampule
- Ordered intravenous fluid
- Syringe(s) of appropriate size for amount of drug to be given
- Swabs saturated with 70% isopropyl alcohol
- Sterile topical swab, if drug is presented in ampule form
- Drug(s) to be administered
- Patient's prescription chart, to check dose, route, etc.
- Recording sheet or book as required by law or hospital policy

- Personal protective equipments (cap, mask, apron, industrial gloves, eye goggles)
- Drug labels.

Procedure

Extravasations procedure is given in Table 6.16.

Table 6.16: Procedure for extravasation

Sl No	Care action	Rationale
1.	Wash hands	To reduce risk of microbial contamination
2.	Put on a pair of disposable sterile gloves	To prevent the skin contact
3.	Wear cap, mask, apron with full sleeves and eye goggles	To prevent contact with skin/clothes in case of accidental spill
4.	Follow the six rights of drug administration	To prevent medication error
5.	Vials containing drugs requiring reconstitution should be vented	To reduce the internal pressure; this reduces the probability of spraying and spillage
6.	Use disposable syringe to draw the solvent from the solvent vial	To reduce risk of microbial contamination
7.	The external surface of the vial should be wiped with an alcohol swab	To reduce risk of microbial contamination
8.	The contents should be transferred aseptically into drug vial	To reduce risk of microbial contamination and to prepare the drug
9.	When opening the glass ampule, wrap and then snap at the break point using an alcohol swab; hold ampule away from your face	To reduce the possibility of injury and risk of contamination
10.	Reconstitution should be carried out within a laminar hood provided	To prevent skin contact
11.	Syringes and intravenous (IV) bottles containing cytotoxic drug should be labeled with patient identity, drug name, dose, date and time of starting; the prepared solutions should be stored separately from other medications	To prevent the administration error
12.	Explain the action, dose and expected adverse effect of the drug to the patient; administer the medicine	Patient has the rights to know the treatment
13.	Record the administration on appropriate charts	To maintain accurate records, provide point of reference in the event of any queries and prevent any duplication of treatment
14.	Contaminated needles, syringes, IV tubings, gloves, mask and cap should be disposed according to biomedical wastage policy; vials should be replaced in black cover and linen contaminated with drugs, patient excreta or body fluids should be handled separately; it must be sealed	To prevent aerosol generation and injury

CARE FOR NEUTROPENIC

Low Count Measures

- Proper handwashing before and after touching the patient and procedure
- Pulse/Temperature monitoring every 4th hourly; may need to be more frequent
- Mouth care: Hexidine/Listerine mouthwash after each feed/thrice a day
- Candid mouth painting twice daily
- Betadine scrub in axilla/groin and peripheral region and sitz bath daily
- Fucidin ointment in both nostrils twice a day (bd)
- Central venous catheter care if any (dressing to be changed in the alternative days)
- Sterile food (freshly cooked hot food and double boiled) from hospital preferably
- No fruits (unpeeled)/flowers
- No intramascular (IM) injections/enema/per rectal (PR) examination
- Weight recording once daily
- Neosporin powder in axilla and groin bd
- Limited visitors
- Complete blood count (CBC), renal parameter as applicable daily and liver function test (LFT) thrice a week
- Wash the hands before examining the patient, blood products to be given through the leukocyte filters only
- Use N95 mask for the patient (to prevent further infection)
- Use alcohol swab before using any port
- Use clave connecter for all lines
- Use sterile gloves, mask, cap and apron for each procedure.

MODIFIED EARLY WARNING SIGNS

Terms and Definition

Scoring systems were developed in response to studies that showed patients, who suffered in-hospital cardiac arrest, often had abnormal physiologic values charted in the preceding hours. Modified early warning signs (MEWS) provided in Table 6.17.

Table 6.17: Modified early warning signs

Score	3	2	1	0	1	2	3	Total
Glasgow coma scale				15	14	9–13	Less than or equal to 8	

Contd...

Contd...

Score	3	2	1	0	1	2	3	Total
Respiratory rate (breath per minute)		Less than 8		9–14	15–20	21–29	Greater than 30	
Heart rate (beats per minute)		Less than 40	40–50	51–100	101–110	111–130	Greater than 130	
Systolic blood pressure (mm Hg)	Less than 70	71–80	81–100	101–180	181–200	201–220	Greater than 220	
Temperature (°F)	Less than 93.2	93.2–95		95.18–99.5	99.68–101.3	101.48–104	Greater than 104	
Oxygen saturation with appropriate oxygen therapy (%)	Less than 90	91–93		94–100				
Urine output (mL/h)	Less than 10	Less than 20						
Total score								

Any single score of 3 in any category or a total score of 4 indicate the need to initiate 'rapid response call (MET)'.

Rapid response call alert is the call given by the unit/ward nurses to the medical emergency team (MET) for early decision and management (Fig. 6.1).

Purpose

To decrease unexpected mortality by early recognition of a patient's condition and intervene before the patient either goes to arrests or requires transfer to intensive care unit (ICU).

Aim

To empower nurses to call rapid response for whatever level of help is required.

Most Common Abnormalities in Ward to ICU

- Tachypnea and an altered level of consciousness
- Also derangement of heart rate, arterial blood pressure, arterial oxygen saturation and urinary output.

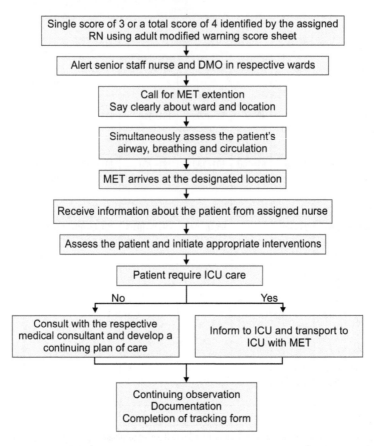

FIGURE 6.1: Modified early warning signs and rapid response (DMO, duty medical officer; ICU, intensive care unit; MET, medical emergency team; RN, registered nurse).

Criteria to Call the MET

- Respiratory rate of more than 25 or less than 10 breaths per minute
- Arterial systolic blood pressure of less than 90 mm Hg
- Heart rate of more than 110 or less than 55 beats per minute
- Not fully alert and oriented
- Oxygen saturation of less than 90%
- Urine output over the last 4 hours of less than 100 mL
- Respiratory rate more than 35 breaths or a heart rate more than 140 beats per minute.

Rapid Response Call Team Members

1. Specialist on call for service: Assesses, collaborates and initiates appropriate interventions.
2. Intensive care unit nurse: Guides and assists the primary nurse in the assessment and nursing management for the patient.

3. Respiratory therapist: Assesses, collaborates and initiates appropriate respiratory interventions.

Interpretation

- The greater the physiologic deviation from the normal parameters, the higher the point scores
- Clinical deterioration is subsequently detected and medical intervention can be implemented at an early stage in the patient's illness.

BASIC LIFE SUPPORT

Definition

Cardiopulmonary resuscitation (CPR) is a basic emergency procedure of manual external cardiac message and artificial respiration.

Basic life support (BLS) acts to slow down the deterioration of the brain and the heart until defibrillation or advanced cardiac life support (ACLS) can be provided.

Chain of Survival

The chain of survival refers to a series of actions that, when put into action, reduce the mortality associated with cardiac arrest. The four interdependent links in the chain of survival are explained in Figure 6.2.

Working of CPR

The air we breathe in travels to our lung, where oxygen is picked up by our blood and then pumped by the heart to tissue and organs. When a person experiences cardiac arrest whether due to heart failure in adults and the elderly or an injury such as near drowning, electrocution or severe trauma in a child, the heart goes from a normal best to an arrhythmic pattern and eventually ceases to beat altogether.

This prevents oxygen from circulating throughout the body, rapidly killing cells and tissue in essence, cardio (heart) pulmonary (lung) resuscitation (revive, revitalize) serves as an artificial heart beat and artificial respiration.

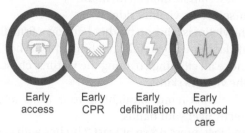

Early access   Early CPR   Early defibrillation   Early advanced care

FIGURE 6.2: Chain of survival for cardiac arrest (CPR, cardiopulmonary resuscitation).

The CPR may not save the victim even when performed properly, but if started within 4 minutes of cardiac arrest and defibrillation is provided within 10 minutes it is possible to save one's life.

The CPR consist of four main components:
1. Circulation.
2. Airway.
3. Breathing.
4. Defibrillation.

Before you start any rescue efforts you must remember to check the responsivenss by taping the victims shoulder and shout 'are you okay'.

For infants: Tap the infant's foot and shout, if the victim has no response activates emergency response system.

Circulation

After checking response, locate the carotid pulse.

Steps to locate the carotid artery pulse
The steps to locate the carotid artery pulse in adults are the following:
- Maintain a head tilt with one hand on the victim's forehead
- Locate the trachea using two or three fingers into the other hand
- Slide these two or three fingers into the groove between the trachea and the muscle at the side of the neck, where you can feel the carotid pulse
- Palpate the artery for at least 5 seconds and not more than 10 seconds.

Steps to locate the brachial artery pulse
The steps to locate the brachial artery pulse in infants as follows:
- Place two or three fingers on the inside of the upper arm, between the infants elbow and shoulder
- Press the index and middle fingers gently on the upper arm for at least 5 second and not more than 10 second when attempting to feel the pulse.

Chest compression technique
If no pulse, start cycle of:
- In 1 and 2: Rescuer adult and child CPR
- Ratio: Comperession of 30:2
- Rate: 100/min
- Depth: At least 2 inches.

Steps to perform chest compression on an adult
1. Position yourself at the victim's side.
2. Make sure the victim is lying on his/her back on a firm, flat surface. If the victim is lying face down, carefully roll him into his/her back.
3. Move or remove all clothing covering the victim's chest. You need to be able to see the victim's skin.
4. Put the heel of first-hand. Straighten your arms and position your shoulder directly over your hands.
5. Push hard and fast, press down at least 2 inches with each compression make sure you push straight down on the victim's breastbone.

6. At the end of each compression, make sure you allow the chest recoil or re-expand completely. Full chest recoil will reduce the blood flow created by chest compression.

7. Deliver compression in a smooth fashion at a rate of 100 compression per minute.

Steps to perform chest compression on an infant

- In 1: Rescuer infant CPR
- Ratio: Comperession 30:2
- Rate:100/min
- Depth: At least 1.5 inches
- Draw an imaginary line between the nipples place two fingers on the breastbone just below this line. This will allow you to compress on the lower half of the breastbone. Do not press on the xiphoid process.

Rescue infants CPR (2 thumb-encircling hands technique)

Steps includes the following:

1. Draw an imaginary line between the nipples. Place both thumbs side by side in the center of the infant's chest on the breastbone, just below this line. This will allow you to compress on the lower half of the breastbone. Do not press on the xiphoid. The thumps may overlap in very small infants.

2. Encircle the infant's chest and support the infants back with the fingers of both hands.

3. With your hands encircling the chest, use both thumbs to depress the breast approximately at least 1.5 inches the depth of the infant's chest. As you push down with your thumbs, squeeze the infant's chest with your fingers.

4. After each compression completely release the pressure on the breastbone and chest and allow the chest to fully recoil.

5. Deliver compression in a smooth fashion at a rate of 100 compression per minute.

6. After every 15 compression, pause briefly for the second rescuer to open the airway with head tilt-chin lift and give two breaths. Coordinate compression and ventilation to avoid simultaneous deliver and to ensure adequate ventilation and chest expansion, especially when the airway is unprotected.

Airway

1. After giving the chest compression you need to make sure that his airway is clear of any obstruction. The breath may be faint and shallow.

2. Look, listen and feel for any signs of breathing. If you determine that the victim is not breathing then something may be blocking the air passage. The tongue is the most common airway obstruction in an unconscious person.

3. Open the victims airway with a head tilt-chin lift maneuver and look for the chest rise and fall, place your ear near the victim's mouth and nose

and listen for air escaping during exhalation, feel for flow of air against your cheek.

4. If the victim is not breath adequately, use a barrier device to give two breath or by mouth–to-mouth resuscitation.

Steps to give mouth-to-mouth breath to adults
- Hold the victim's airway open with a head tilt-chin lift
- Pinch the nose closed with our thumb and index finger
- Take a regular breath and seal your lips around the victim's mouth, creating an airtight seal
- Give one breath (blow for 1 second) watch for the chest to rise as you give the breath
- Give the second breath like the same as above.

Steps to give mouth-to-mask breath to adults
- Position yourself at the victim's side
- Place the mask on the victim's face using the bridge of the nose as a guide for correct position
- Seal the mask against the face
- Using your hand that is closer to the top of the victim's head that closer to the top of the victim's head, place the index finger and thumb along the border of the mask
- Place the thumb of your other hand along the lower margin of the mask
- Place the remaining fingers of your hand closer to the victim's neck along the bony margin of the jaw and lift to open the airway
- While you lift the jaw, press firmly and completely around the outside margin of the mask to seal the mask against the face.

Techniques for giving mouth-to-mouth breath to infants
- Hold the victim's airway open with a head tilt-chin lift
- Place your mouth over the infants mouth and nose create an airtight seal
- Give one breath (blow for 1 second) watch for the chest to rise as you give the breath
- Give the second breath like the same as above.

Steps to give mouth-to-mask breath to infants
- Same maneuver for adult.

Procedure

Procedure of CPR (basic life support) is given in Table 6.18.

Table 6.18: Procedure for cardiopulmonary resuscitation

SI No	Care action	Rationale
1.	Note time of arrest	Lack of cerebral perfusion for approximately 3–4 minutes can lead to irreversible brain damage

Contd...

Sl No	Care action	Rationale
2.	Call for help; if second nurse is available can call for cardiac arrest team	Cardiopulmonary resuscitation (CPR) is more effective if two rescuer is present One is responsible for inflating the lung and the other is giving chest compression
3.	Place cardiac table under the patient	Effective cardiac massage can be performed only on a hard surface
4.	If the patient is in bed, remove head end rail and ensure adequate space between back of bed and wall	To allow easy access of patients head in order to facilitate ventilation
5.	Check for the carotid pulse with two or three fingers	To know circulation is present or not
6.	If the circulation is not present place the heel of one hand in the center of the sternum and place the other on top, ensuring that the hand is on the center of the sternum and only the heel of the dominant hand is touching the sternum	To ensure the cardiac compression and reduce the delay in commencing cardiac compression
7.	The sternum should be depressed sharply 4–5 cm; cardiac compression should be forceful and sustained at a rate of 100 per min	This produced a cardiac output by applying direct downward force of compression
8.	Maintain cardiac compression and ventilation ratio 30:2, this must be continue until the cardiac output returns or handed over the patient to advanced cardiac life support (ACLS) team	To maintain circulation and ventilation Thus reducing the risk of damage to vital organs
9.	Ensure a clear airway this is best achieved by head tilt-chin lift maneuver	To establish and maintain airway, thus facilitate ventilation
10.	If breath is not present give artificial respiration	For adequate oxygenation and ventilation
11.	When the cardiac arrest team arrives, it will assume responsibility for the arrest in coordination with ward staff	To ensure an effective team coordinates the resuscitation
12.	Attach patient to electrocardiogram (ECG) monitor using three electrodes defibrillator patches	To obtain adequate ECG signal Accurate recording of cardiac rhythm will determine the appropriate treatment
Intubation		
13.	Continue to ventilate and oxygenate the patient before intubation	The risk of cardiac arrhythmias due to hypoxia is decreased
14.	Equipment for intubation should be checked before handing to appropriate medical or nursing staff	To provide continuity of care

Contd...

Contd...

Sl No	Care action	Rationale
15.	Recommence ventilation and oxygenation once intubation is completed	Intubation should be interrupt resuscitation only for a maximum of 16 seconds to prevent the occurrence of cerebral anoxia
16.	Once the patient intubated, chest compression at the rate of 100/min, should continue and ventilation should continue at 10–12 breath per minute	Uninterrupted compression result in a substantially higher mean coronary perfusion pressure A pause in chest compression allows the coronary pressure to fall
Intravenous access		
17.	Venous access must be established through the large vein as soon as possible	To administer cardiac drug and fluid replacement
18.	Asepsis should be maintained throughout the procedure	To prevent local and systemic infection
19.	The correct rate of infusion is required	To ensure maximum drug and solution effectiveness
20.	Document in detail the proceedings in the CPR track sheet and in the nurse's record and document the condition of the patient with time, medications used, response and interventions done	To monitor differences and detect trends; any irregularities should be brought to the attention of the appropriate senior nursing and medical teams

ADVANCED CARDIAC LIFE SUPPORT

In ACLS, the specific treatment of a given dysrhythmias or condition depends on the patient's hemodynamic status.

Patient Assessment

In general, patients can be divided into four categories to determine treatment priorities:
1. Asymptomatic.
2. Stable symptomatic.
3. Unstable symptomatic.
4. Pulseless.

Asymptomatic patients do not receive treatment, but should be monitored for changes in condition. Any patient with symptoms (even apparently mild symptoms such as palpitations) should be assessed to determine if they are stable or unstable. Determination of a patient's level of hemodynamic compromise can include several factors.

General Appearance

The first indication of hemodynamic status comes from a patient's general appearance, including skin signs, level of activity and work of breathing. If a patient shows signs of compensation (e.g. pale cool or diaphoretic skin) or acute distress, they are unstable.

Level of Consciousness

Interaction with the patient allows the provider to evaluate the patient's level of consciousness based on the patient's activity, awareness of their surroundings and ability to provide information. If a patient shows any level of mental deficit, family or friends should be consulted to determine if this state differs from the patient's baseline. If the mental deficit is acute, the patient should be considered unstable.

Vital Signs

Vital signs provide a diagnostic evaluation of the patient. Blood pressure is the primary indicator. A systolic blood pressure above 90 mm Hg usually indicates that the patient is stable (although the provider should be alert for changes in blood pressure that might indicate an unstable patient even if blood pressure is normal).

Other vital signs may be useful, but should not be relied upon exclusively. Pulse oximetry can be useful, especially if it rises or falls, but providers should remember that various conditions (such as CO_2 poisoning) can make changes in blood oxygen levels and that high O_2 saturation may be present in unstable patients (such as those in shock). Additionally, heart rate is of no use in determining if a patient is stable or unstable; a patient with a heart rate of 80 can be severely unstable, while a patient with a heart rate of 210 can be stable if they are still perfusing well.

Assessment Findings

If a patient's general appearance, level of consciousness and vital signs are all normal, the patient is stable. If possible, treatment should be rendered starting with the least invasive that is appropriate for that patient's hemodynamic status. In ACLS, the preferential treatment is symptomatic, but a stable patients is generally medications, while the preferential treatment for unstable patients is generally electrical therapy.

Once treatment is rendered, the provider must reassess the patient. If the patient remains symptomatic, the appropriate treatment (medications or electricity) should be given again depending on the patient's heart rhythm and current hemodynamic status (thus, if a patient was stable before, but becomes unstable after administration of a drug, the patient should receive electrical therapy to continue treating the dysrhythmia rather than additional doses of a medication).

If a patient's general appearance indicates that they may be unconscious, then should check for responsiveness. If the patient is unresponsive, get help [send someone to call 911 and bring back an external defibrillator (AED), call a code, etc.]. The BLS algorithm should then be followed—open the airway, check for breathing, and assess circulation. If the patient is apneic, rescue breathing should be started; if the patient is pulseless, rescuers should begin CPR.

Once you determine that a patient is pulseless, an automated AED or ECG monitor should be attached as soon as possible. CPR should be continued with minimal interruptions. After each rhythm check, the patient should be defibrillated if appropriate [for ventricular fibrillation (V-Fib or VF) and pulseless ventricular tachycardia (V-Tach or VT)]. Regardless of the heart rhythm, medications should be given as soon as possible after CPR is resumed (the specific medication determined by the patient's exact status and heart rhythm).

Algorithm Review of ACLS

Always start with the CABD survey. CABD stands for circulation, airway, breathing, defibrillation.

Acute Coronary Syndromes

Algorithm: Consider MONA for patients with suspected acute coronary syndrome (ACS) [angina or acute myocardial infarction (AMI)]:
- Morphine
- Oxygen
- Nitroglycerine
- Aspirin.

Bradycardia

Algorithm: Steps given below:
1. Atropine 0.5 mg intravenous pyelogram (IVP) for sinus bradycardia and 1°, 2° type I arteriovenous (AV) Block.
2. Transcutaneous pacing (preferred for 2° type II and 3° heart block); do not delay pacing in symptomatic patients (even those in sinus bradycardia or low-degree heart blocks).
3. Dopamine 5–10 µg/kg/min (if patient unresponsive to atropine/pacing).
4. Epinephrine drip 2–10 µg/min (if patient unresponsive to atropine/pacing).

Note: Atropine is not indicated for 2° type II and 3° heart blocks, proceed directly to pacing if the patient is symptomatic, although atropine can be considered if pacing is delayed.

Tachycardia

Algorithm: Tachycardia with pulses. If the patient is unstable, go directly to synchronized cardioversion. Otherwise:
1. For regular narrow complex tachycardia [probable supraventricular tachycardia (SVT)]:
   - Obtain 12-lead ECG; consider expert consultation
   - Attempt vagal maneuvers
   - Adenosine 6 mg rapid IV push. If no conversion, give up to two more doses at 12 mg each.

2. For irregular narrow complex tachycardia [probable artrial fibrillation (A-Fib)]:
   - Obtain 12-lead ECG; consider expert consultation
   - Control rate with diltiazem or beta blockers.
3. For regular wide complex tachycardia (probable V-Tach):
   - Obtain 12-lead ECG; consider expert consultation
   - Convert rhythm using amiodarone—150 mg over 10 minutes
   - Elective cardioversion.
4. For irregular wide complex tachycardia:
   - Obtain 12-lead ECG; consider expert consultation
   - Consider antiarrhythmics
   - If torsades de pointes, give magnesium sulfate 1–2 g over 5–60 minutes.

Ventricular Fibrillation/Pulseless Ventricular Tachycardia

Algorithm: Pulseless arrest (shockable).

Stage I
1. CPR: Start immediately. Push hard and push fast.
2. Shock: Analyze rhythm and shock if in VF/pulseless VT.
3. CPR: Resume CPR immediately after shock delivery. Continue for 5 cycles/2 minutes.
4. Vasopressor: Epinephrine 1 mg q 3–5 min (can replace 1st or 2nd dose of epinephrine with 40 units vasopressin). Give as soon as possible after resuming CPR, circulate with chest compressions.

Stage II
1. Shock: Analyze rhythm, and shock if in VF/pulseless VT.
2. CPR: Resume CPR immediately after shock delivery. Continue for 5 cycles/2 minutes.
3. Antiarrhythmic: Amiodarone 300 mg IV/IO or lidocaine 1–1.5 mg/kg up to 3 mg/kg. Give as soon as possible after resuming CPR, circulate with chest compressions.

Stage III
1. Shock: Analyze rhythm and shock if in VF/pulseless VT.
2. CPR: Resume CPR immediately after shock delivery. Continue for 5 cycles/2 minutes.

Note: Minimize interruptions to chest compressions; do not check a pulse or evaluate the heart rhythm after a shock. After each shock, resume CPR immediately and continue for 5 cycles prior to rhythm analysis and possible pulse check. After a second dose of epinephrine, a second antiarrhythmic dose (amiodarone 150 mg or lidocaine 0.5–0.75 mg/kg) may be given after the next rhythm check.

Pulseless Electrical Activity

Algorithm: Pulseless arrest (not shockable) [pulseless electrical activity (PEA)]:
1. Possible causes (consider the 6 H's and 5 T's).
2. Epinephrine 1 mg q 3–5 min (can replace 1st or 2nd dose of epinephrine with 40 units vasopressin). Give as soon as possible after resuming CPR, circulate with chest compressions.

3. Atropine 1 mg intravenous/introsseous (IV/IO) q 3–5 min to maximum 3 mg (only if electrical rate is < 60). Give as soon as possible after resuming CPR, circulate with chest compressions.

Note: In PEA, the electrical system of the heart is functioning, but there is a problem with the pump, pipes or volume—a mechanical part of the system is not working. You can use the 6 H's and 5 T's to remember the most common reversible causes of PEA.

H's
- Hypovolemia
- Hypo- or hyper-kalemia
- Hydrogen ion (acidosis)
- Hypothermia
- Hypoxia
- Hypoglycemia.

T's
- Tension pneumothorax
- Tamponade (cardiac)
- Trauma
- Toxins
- Thrombosis (coronary or pulmonary).

Asystole

Algorithm: Pulseless arrest (not shockable) (Dead?):
1. Determine whether to initiate resuscitation.
2. Epinephrine 1 mg q 3–5 min (can replace 1st or 2nd dose of epinephrine with 40 units vasopressin). Give as soon as possible after resuming CPR, circulate with chest compressions.
3. Atropine, 1 mg IV/IO q 3–5 min to maximum 3 mg. Give as soon as possible after resuming CPR, circulate with chest compressions.
4. Differential diagnosis or discontinue resuscitation: Are they still dead? Consider the 6 H's and 5 T's (refer above); check blood glucose; check core temperature; consider Naloxone, etc.

Electrocardiogram and Electrical Therapy Review

The ECG tracing represents electrical activity through the heart. The P-wave represents depolarization of the atria; the QRS complex represents depolarization of the ventricles and the T-wave represents the later stage of repolarization of the ventricles. The interval from the first deflection of the P-wave to the beginning of the QRS complex is the PR interval (PRI) and should be between 0.12 and 0.20 seconds. A normal QRS complex has duration of 0.12 seconds or less, a longer duration (wide QRS) indicates delayed conduction through the ventricles, often as the result of a ventricular pacemaker focus.

The horizontal axis of the ECG strips measures time. Each large box represents 0.20 seconds; each small box represents 0.04 seconds.

To obtain a 3-lead ECG tracing, place the white [right arm (RA)] electrode on the right chest just below the clavicle, the black electrode [left arm (LA)] on the left chest just below the clavicle and the red electrode [left leg (LL)] laterally on the lower left abdomen. Pacer pads go in the anterior/posterior positions. Defibrillation pads go on the upper right chest and lower left abdomen, although on children and other small patients the pads may need to be placed in the middle of the anterior and posterior chests.

Rhythm disturbances treat the patient, not the dysrhythmia. Always assess your patient for pulses, perfusion and level of consciousness—is the patient stable, unstable or pulseless? Next, assess the rhythm—is it fast or slow? Is it life-threatening? As you treat the patient, try to discover the cause of the dysrhythmia, for many patients, their only chance of survival is if you can identify and treat a reversible cause. There are many possible causes of rhythm disturbances or PEA. Common causes include sympathetic stimulation, stress, hypoxia, ischemia, drugs/toxins and electrolyte disturbances. Although laboratory draws can be useful, a history of the patient and the current event obtained from a family member or caregiver is often more useful.

Defibrillation (Unsynchronized Shock)

Fibrillation is a disorganized rhythm that, if present in the ventricles, is life-threatening. Immediate CPR combined with early defibrillation is critical to survival from sudden cardiac arrest. Defibrillation terminates all electrical activity in the pulseless heart, hopes that it will resume beating in a coordinated fashion. A shock should be delivered about once every 2 minutes if the patient remains in ventricular fibrillation. With a monophasic monitor, the recommendation is to deliver a single shock at 360 joules. If a biphasic monitor is used, the recommended dosage is machine dependent and should appear on the front of the monitor. If optimal shock dosage is not known, the consensus is to defibrillate at 200 J.

Synchronized Cardioversion

Synchronized cardioversion is the preferred treatment for unstable patients with a tachycardia such as atrial fibrillation, V-Tach with a pulse or supraventricular tachycardia (SVT). The shock is timed by the monitor to be delivered in coordination with the QRS complex of the heart. If the patient is conscious, consider sedation prior to cardioversion; however, synchronized cardioversion should not be delayed while waiting for sedation in severely symptomatic patients.

With a monophasic monitor, the initial shock is delivered at 100 J; if the rhythm does not terminate, deliver additional shocks in stepwise fashion (200 J, 300 J and 360 J for subsequent shocks). With a biphasic monitor, dosage and steps are device dependent; if optimal doses are unknown, begin at 100 J and step up from there.

Transcutaneous Pacing

External cardiac pacing is the recommended treatment for symptomatic bradycardia. If the patient is conscious, consider sedation; however, pacing should not be delayed while waiting for sedation. Begin pacing at zero milliampere, slowly increasing until capture is achieved. Then, set the rate at 20 beats per minute (bpm) above the monitored heart rate, with a minimum rate of 50 bpm.

Medications Review of ACLS

This information on medications meets the standard set by the 2005 American Heart Association (AHA) for advanced cardiac life support. It does not supersede local protocols or medical control; consult with your medical director for the most up-to-date guidelines on medication administration where you work.

Intravenous/intraosseous medications should be administered in a peripheral line during CPR, as soon as possible after a rhythm check. It is recommended that you flush with 20 mL of fluid after each drug administration and elevate the extremity. Always use large bore catheters if possible.

A note on endotracheal administration of medications: This route of medication administration is being de-emphasized by the AHA; the IV or 10 routes are preferred. However, the endotracheal (ET) route can still be used if providers are unable to gain access by IV/IO. Use the mnemonic 'NAVEL' to remember, which drugs can be administered via this route:

- Narcan
- Atropine
- Vasopressin
- Epinephrine
- Lidocaine.

If using the ET route, the drug dosage must be increased, typically 2–2.5 times the IV/IO bolus dosage (although there is no consensus on epinephrine or vasopressin dosing via this route), followed by a 10 mL normal saline flush.

Adenosine

Class: Endogenous nucleoside.

Indicated for: Paroxysmal supraventricular tachycardia (PSVT)/Regular narrow complex tachycardia.

Intravenous bolus dosage: Includes the following:
- Rapid IV push 6 mg—1st dose
- Rapid IV push 12 mg—2nd dose
- Rapid IV push 12 mg—3rd dose.

Notes: Doses are followed by a saline flush. Two subsequent doses of 12 mg each may be administered at 1–2 minutes intervals. Use the port closest to cannulation. The AHA recommends that the dose be cut by half if administering through a central line or in the presence of dipyridamole or carbamazepine. Larger doses may be required in the presence of caffeine or theophylline.

Amiodarone

Class: Antiarrhythmic.

Indicated for: V-Fib/pulseless V-Tach.

Intravenous/Intraosseous bolus dosage: Are as follows:
- 300 mg—1st dose
- 150 mg—2nd dose.

Arrhythmias: Dosage are the following:
- 360 mg over 6 hours (slow)
- 150 mg over 10 minutes (rapid) infusion dose
- 540 mg IV/IO over 18 hours (0.5 mg/min).

Notes: Cumulative doses more than 2.2 g/24 hours are associated with significant hypotension. Do not administer with other drugs that prolong QT interval (i.e. procainimide). Terminal elimination is extremely long half-life lasts up to 40 days. During arrest, IV bolus should be delivered slowly, over 1–3 minutes.

Aspirin

Class: Non-steroidal anti-inflammatory drug (NSAID).

Indicated for: Chest pain/acute coronary syndrome (ACS).

Per os (PO) dosage (no IV/IO): 160–325 mg.

Suppository dose: 300 mg.

Notes: In suspected ACS, Aspirin can block platelet aggregation and arterial constriction. Also helps with pain control. May cause or exacerbate gastrointestinal (GI) bleeding.

Atropine

Class: Parasympathetic blocker.

Indicated for: Bradycardia, asystole and slow PEA.

Intravenous/Intraosseous bolus dosage: Includes the following:
- 0.5 mg every 3–5 minutes as needed
- 1 mg every 3–5 minutes (up to 3 mg).

Notes: Used only in symptomatic bradycardia or in PEA with heart rate less than 60 (not indicated in 2° type II or 3° heart block). Doses less than 0.5 mg may result in paradoxical slowing of the heart. ET route discouraged, but can be used if IV/IO access not available.

Dextrose/Glucose

Class: Carbohydrate.

Indicated for: Hypoglycemia.

Intravenous/Intraosseous bolus dosage: 25 g (50 mL) of dextrose 50% in water (D50W).

Notes: Used to reverse documented hypoglycemia in patients with symptomatic bradycardia or during cardiac arrest. Should not be used routinely during cardiac arrest.

Dopamine

Class: Catecholamine.

Indicated for: Symptomatic bradycardia hypotension.

Intravenous infusion: These are the following:
- 2–10 μg/kg/min, cardiac dose
- 10–20 μg/kg/min, vasopressor dose.

Notes: Titrate to patient response. Correct hypovolemia with volume replacement before initiating dopamine. It may cause tachyarrhythmias. Do not mix with sodium bicarbonate.

Epinephrine

Class: Catecholamine.

Indicated for: Pulseless arrest.

Intravenous/Intraosseous bolus dosage: 1 mg (1:10,000) every 3–5 minutes.

Symptomatic bradycardia infusion: 1 mg in 500 mL of D5 W or NaCl at 1 μg/min titrated to effect.

Notes: First line drug in all pulseless rhythms. Increases myocardial oxygen demand and may cause myocardial ischemia or angina. ET route is discouraged, but if used give 2–2.5 mg of a 1:1,000 solution diluted in 10 mL normal saline.

Fluid Administration

Example: Normal saline/NaCl.

Class: Fluid volume.

Indicated for: Hypovolemia.

Intravenous/Intraosseous bolus dosage: 250–500 cc bolus (repeat as needed).

Notes: Use to treat specific reversible causes such as hypovolemia. Routine administration of fluids during a resuscitation is not indicated, as it can reduce coronary perfusion pressure.

Heparin (Unfractionated)

Class: Anticoagulant.

Indicated for: ST-segment elevation acute myocardial infarction (STEMI) (AMI).

Intravenous/Intraosseous bolus dosage: These are as follows:

Initial dose: 60 IU/kg (maximum 4,000 IU).

Infusion: 12 IU/kg/h (maximum 1,000 IU/h).

Notes: Do not use in patients with active bleeding or bleeding disorders, severe hypertension or recent surgery. Monitor activated partial thromboplastin time (aPTT) and platelet count, while administering.

Lidocaine

Class: Antiarrhythmic.

Indicated for: V-Fib/pulseless V-Tach, stable V-Tach.

Intravenous/Intraosseous bolus dosage: 1–1.5 mg/kg (1st dose).

Infusion: 1–4 mg/min (30–50 µg/kg/min).

Notes: May repeat at 0.5–0.75 mg/kg every 5–10 minutes to a maximum dose of 3 mg/kg. Use with caution in presence of impaired liver; discontinue if signs of toxicity develop. Prophylactic use in AMI is contraindicated. ET route discouraged, but can be used if IV/IO access not available.

Magnesium Sulfate

Class: Electrolyte.

Indicated for: Torsades de pointes or hypomagnesemia.

Intravenous/Intraosseous bolus dosage: 1–2 g in 10 mL D5W over 5–20 minutes.

Notes: A fall in blood pressure may be noted with rapid administration. Dose is given over 5–20 minutes during cardiac arrest, 5–60 minutes in living patients. Use with caution in renal failure.

Morphine Sulfate

Class: Opiate/Analgesic.

Indicated for: Chest pain and pulmonary edema.

Intravenous/Intraosseous bolus dosage: 2–4 mg every 5–30 minutes.

Notes: Administer slowly and titrate to effect; may cause hypotension. May cause respiratory depression; be prepared to support ventilations. Naloxone is the reversal agent.

Nitroglycerin

Class: Vasodilator.

Indicated for: Chest pain/ACS.

Intravenous bolus dosage: 12.5–25 μg in D5W or NaCl.

Sublingual dose: 0.3–0.4 mg.

Notes: Most commonly given sublingually as tablet or spray, repeat up to 3 doses at 5 minute intervals. Hypotension may occur. Do not use with Viagra or other phosphodiasterase inhibitors; with severe bradycardia or tachycardia; or in presence of right ventricular (RV) infarction or inferior MI. Do not mix with other drugs.

Sodium Bicarbonate

Class: Buffer.

Indicated for: Acidosis, hyperkalemia.

Intravenous bolus dosage: 1 mEq/kg.

Notes: Not recommended for routine use in cardiac arrest patients. If available, use arterial blood gas analysis to guide bicarbonate therapy.

Vasopressin

Class: Hormone.

Indicated for: Pulseless arrest.

Intravenous/Intraosseous bolus dosage: 40 U IV/IO.

Notes: Only given one time to replace the first or second dose of epinephrine; epinephrine dosing can continue 3–5 minutes after vasopressin is administered. Vasopressin should not replace antiarrhythmics (such as amiodarone). May cause cardiac ischemia and angina. Not recommended for responsive patients with coronary artery disease. ET route discouraged, but can be used if IV/IO access not available.

Verapamil

Class: Calcium channel blocker.

Indicated for: A-Fib/A-flutter, paroxysmal supraventricular tachycardia (PSVT).

Intravenous bolus dosage: 2.5–5 mg over 2–5 minutes.

Notes: Alternative drug after adenosine to terminate PSVT with adequate blood pressure and preserved left ventricular (LV) function can cause peripheral vasodilatation and hypotension. Use with extreme caution in patients receiving oral beta blockers.

GLASGOW COMA SCALE

Definition

Glasgow coma scale (GCS) is a standardized neurological scale that aims to give a reliable, objective way of recording the conscious state of a patient following a traumatic brain injury for initial as well as subsequent assessment.

Purposes

1. Gives an overview of the patient's level of consciousness (LOC).
2. The GCS allows health practitioner to quickly and easily communicate the severity of a patient's head injury in the1st hours or days after the trauma.
3. The GCS is a good prognostic indicator to identify the patient condition.
4. To assess the level of consciousness in any patient, who has altered sensorium.
5. To track the prognosis of patients, who have been admitted with altered sensorium.

Equipments

- Glasgow coma scale scoring sheet (Table 6.19)
- Pen torch.

Table 6.19: Glasgow coma scale sheet

Activity	Response	Score
Eye opening		
None	Even to supraorbital pressure	1
To pain	Pain from sternum/limb/supraorbital pressure	2
To speech	Non-specific response, not necessarily to command	3
Spontaneous	Eyes open, not necessarily aware	4
Motor response		
None	To any pain; limbs remain flaccid	1
Extension	Shoulder adducted and shoulder and forearm internally rotated	2
Flexor response	Withdrawal response or assumption of hemiplegic posture	3
Withdrawal	Arm withdraws to pain, shoulder abducts	4
Localizes pain	Arm attempts to remove supraorbital/chest pressure	5
Obeys commands	Follows simple commands	6
Verbal response		
None	No verbalization of any type	1
Incomprehensible sound	Moans/groans, no speech	2
Inappropriate	Intelligible, no sustained sentences	3
Confused	Converses but confused, disoriented	4
Oriented	Converses and oriented	5

Contd...

Contd...

Activity	Response	Score
Total score		3–15
Mild head injury 13–15 Moderate head injury 9–12 Severe head injury (coma) 8 or less		

Procedure

Glasgow coma scale procedure is given in Table 6.20.

Table 6.20: Procedure for Glasgow coma scale

Sl No	Action	Rationale
1.	Keep the patient in a comfortable position	To evaluate responses accurately
2.	Score response in the Glasgow coma scale sheet	Grades the level of conscious of the patient

Assisting Procedures

ABDOMINAL PARACENTESIS

Definition

Paracentesis is a procedure to take out fluid that has collected in the abdomen (peritoneal fluid). The fluid is taken out using a long, thin needle put through the abdomen. Paracentesis also may be done to take the fluid out to relieve belly pressure or pain in people with cancer or cirrhosis.

Purposes

1. Find the cause of fluid buildup in the abdomen.
2. Diagnose an infection in the peritoneal fluid.
3. Check for certain types of cancer such as liver cancer.
4. Remove a large amount of fluid that is causing pain or difficulty in breathing or that is affecting how the kidneys or the intestines (bowel) are working.
5. Check for damage after an abdominal injury.

Equipments

- Sterile abdominal paracentesis set
- Sterile dressing pack
- Sterile specimen container
- Tincture benzoin
- Xylocaine injection (2%)
- Disposable needle and syringe
- Sterile gloves
- Tape measure
- Weighing machine
- Disposable plastic apron
- Mask
- Mackintosh
- Appropriate antiseptic solution (Betadine)
- Underpad/Disposable clean pad
- Adhesive plaster
- Clean intravenous (IV) bottle.

Procedure

Procedure of abdominal paracentesis is given in Table 7.1.

Table 7.1: Procedure of abdominal paracentesis

Sl No	Care action	Rationale
1.	Explain the procedure to the patient/patient's relative	Ensure that the patient and the relative understand the procedure, and to get the valid consent
2.	Before starting the procedure, check whether the patient is on anticoagulant therapy	To prevent the complication of bleeding after the procedure
3.	Arrange all the needed articles near the bedside	To prevent unnecessary contamination and easy to perform the procedure
4.	Tell the patient to empty his/her bladder before the procedure	To prevent the puncture of the bladder, while doing the trocar insertion
5.	Place the mackintosh under patient's back and hip	To prevent soiling of the linen
6.	Check abdominal girth and weigh patient before and after the procedure and record the readings	This provides an indication of fluid shift and how much fluid has reaccumulated
7.	Place patient in supine position with head elevated 20°–30°; select and mark a position on the abdominal wall for puncture	Helps for the removal of fluid from the abdomen by gravity
8.	Drape the patient appropriately and expose the abdomen puncture site	To make the patient feel privacy and comfortable
9.	Wear sterile gown, gloves and mask	To prevent the contamination
10.	Use skin preparation solution to cleanse skin over the proposed puncture site and drape to define a sterile field	To prepare sterile environment for the procedure
The following procedure will be done by the doctor; the nurse will assist		
11.	Anesthetize the skin over the proposed puncture site with the Xylocaine drawn up in the 5 cc syringe with the attached 25 gauge needle Anesthetize down to the peritoneum Aspirate periodically; if ascitic fluid returns, withdraw the needle slightly to re-enter tissue before further anesthetic is infiltrated	To prevent the local/systemic infection
12.	Insert the 18 gauge needle/trocar perpendicularly through the anesthetized abdominal wall, and advance until hub of needle is 5 mm to1cm from the skin surface	To prevent injury to the abdominal wall
13.	Ascitic fluid is collected (20–200 mL as per the requirement of therapeutic/diagnostic purpose/both)	If necessary to diagnose the cause of ascitis

Contd...

Contd...

SI No	Care action	Rationale
14.	Once the fluid is withdrawn, collect it in the appropriate specimen container. Once a biopsy is taken, transfer the biopsy specimen into a container with 10%–12% formalin	To preserve tissue status
	Collect sample in the labeled container	To ensure correct identity of the specimen
15.	If for therapeutic purpose, a large volume of fluid has to be drained in the drainage bottle	To promote comfort by reducing the fluid pressure
Nurse's responsibilities		
16.	Check the vital status of the patient (BP*, pulse, respiration, temperature, SpO_2†)	To assess any signs of complication
17.	To change vacuum bottles, as they become full, close the clamp on the tubing gently and remove full bottle, and reinsert into empty bottle; reopen clamp to start fluid flow again	To prevent misplacement of the needle in the abdomen
18.	Once the paracentesis is done, simply remove needle from abdominal wall; place a small pressure dressing on puncture site and instruct the patient to remain supine for 2–4 hours	To arrest leak of abdominal fluid
19.	Comfort patient and replace all equipments used	To make them ready for the next usage
20.	Wash the hands	To prevent the risk of cross infection
21.	Document the procedure in the nurse's record in detail	To maintain accurate records, provide a point of reference in the event of any queries

*BP, blood pressure; †SpO_2, peripheral oxygen saturation.

THORACENTESIS

Definition

Thoracentesis is a procedure to take out fluid that has collected in the pleural cavity of the lungs (plural fluid). The fluid is taken out using a long, thin needle put through the thoracic cavity.

Purposes

1. It is used diagnostically to establish the cause of a pleural effusion.
2. To relieve pneumothorax, hemothorax and pyothorax.
3. Diagnose an infection in the pleural fluid.
4. Remove a large amount of fluid that is causing pain or difficulty in breathing.

Equipments

- Sterile thoracentesis set (trocar and cannula)
- Sterile dressing pack
- A 3–way adopter
- Sterile specimen container
- Drainage bottle
- Tincture benzoin
- Xylocaine injection (2%)
- Disposable needle and syringe
- Sterile gloves
- Disposable plastic apron
- Mask
- Mackintosh
- Appropriate antiseptic solution (Betadine)
- Underpad/Disposable clean pad
- Adhesive plaster.

Procedure

The procedure of thoracentesis is detailed in Table 7.2.

Table 7.2: Procedure for thoracentesis

Sl No	Care action	Rationale
1.	Explain the procedure to the patient	Ensure that the patient understand the procedure and to get the valid consent
2.	Tell the patient to empty his/her bladder before the procedure	To avoid interruption during the procedure
3.	Arrange all the needed articles near the bedside	To prevent unnecessary contamination; and to easily perform the procedure
4.	Place the mackintosh under the patient's back and hip	To prevent the soiling of the linen
5.	Assess the respiratory rate and depth; symmetry of chest on inspiration and expiration; cough and sputum	To obtain the baseline data
6.	Place patient in sitting position with head leaning forward on the cardiac table (Fig. 7.1), lateral decubitus or supine with head elevated 45°; select and mark a position on the chest wall for puncture	Helps for the removal of fluid from the lungs by gravity and increase the intercostal space
7.	Drape the patient appropriately and expose the chest puncture site	To make the patient feel privacy and comfortable
8.	Wear sterile gown, gloves and mask	To prevent the contamination

Contd...

Contd...

Sl No	Care action	Rationale
9.	Use skin preparation solution to cleanse skin over the proposed puncture site and drape to define a sterile field	To prepare sterile environment for the procedure
The following procedure will be done by the doctor; the nurse will assist		
10.	Anesthetize the skin over the proposed puncture site with the Xylocaine drawn up in the 5 cc syringe with the attached 25 gauge needle	To prevent local/systemic infection
11.	Insert the 18 gauge needle/trocar through the anesthetized chest wall	To remove the excess fluid in the thoracic cavity
12.	Connect the 3-way adapter with the trocar and collect the required quantity of pleural fluid in the specimen container	To send it to the laboratory
13.	If for therapeutic purpose, a large volume of fluid has to be drained in the drainage bottle	To promote comfort by normal lung function
Nurse's responsibilities		
14.	Check the vital status of the patient (BP*, pulse, respiration, temperature)	To assess any signs of complication
15.	Observe for sudden shortness of breath, tracheal deviation and decreased oxygen saturation	It indicates the complication
16.	Once the thoracentesis is done, simply remove needle from chest wall; place a small pressure dressing on puncture site; instruct the patient to remain supine for 2–4 hours	To arrest leak of abdominal fluid
17.	Remove the mackintosh from the patient side	To make the patient comfortable
18.	Wash and replace the equipments; send the specimen to the laboratory with all patient details	To make them ready for the next usage
19.	Document the procedure and patient parameters (during and after the procedure) in the nurse's record	To maintain accurate records, provide a point of reference in the event of any queries

*BP, blood pressure.

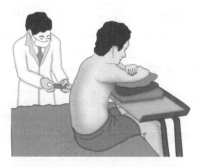

FIGURE 7.1: Position for thoracentesis

ASSISTING WITH LUMBAR PUNCTURE

Definition

A lumbar puncture is a diagnostic and at times therapeutic procedure that is performed in order to collect a sample of cerebrospinal fluid (CSF) for biochemical, microbiological and cytological analysis or very rarely as a treatment (therapeutic lumbar puncture) to relieve increased intracranial pressure (ICP).

Purposes

- To detect possible infection in the CSF
- To measure the pressure in the CSF
- To measure the level of chemicals in the CSF
- To collect CSF for diagnostic purposes
- To detect the spinal subarachnoid block.

Equipments

- A sterile tray [lumbar puncture (LP) set]
- Antiseptic skin cleaning agents (e.g. Betadine or chlorhexidine)
- Local anesthetic (Xylocaine injection)
- Sterile gloves
- Appropriate size of lumbar puncture needles
- Sterile specimen bottles (these bottles should be labeled as bottle 1, 2, 3 with patient's profile)
- Tincture benzoin
- Mackintosh
- Adhesive plaster.

Procedure

The procedure of lumbar puncture assisting is described in Table 7.3.

Table 7.3: Procedure of lumbar puncture

Sl No	Care action	Rationale
1.	Explain the procedure to the patient	To get valid consent from the patient/patient's relatives
2.	Ensure that the patient passed urine before starting the procedure	To ensure comfort of the patient
3.	Arrange needed articles near the bedside	Easy to perform the procedure and to prevent unnecessary contamination
4.	Place the mackintosh and draw sheet under the lumbar region	To prevent the soiling of the linen

Contd...

Contd...

Sl No	Care action	Rationale
5.	Position the patient in lateral knee-chest position at the edge of the cot (universal flexion)	To ensure maximum expand of the intervertebral spaces and thus easier access to the subarachnoid space; easy to perform the procedure
6.	Place the pillow under the head and between the knees	To maintain the position and comfort of the patient and avoid sudden movement by the patient
7.	Drape the patient properly	To provide privacy to the patient
8.	Wash the hands	To minimize the infection
9.	Provide sterile gloves to the consultant	To prevent infection, as it is an invasive procedure
10.	Assist the doctor during the procedure	
11.	Communicate the patient in between the procedure and observe the hemodynamic level during the procedure	To give psychological support to the patient and identify the early signs of abnormalities
12.	The following step will be done by the doctors: • Prepare and drape the area after identifying landmarks; use anesthetic agent to anesthetize the skin and the deeper tissues under the insertion site • Insert Quincke needle bevel up through the skin and advance through the deeper tissues between the second and third lumbar vertebrae, and into the subarachnoid space • When CSF* flows, attach the 3-way stopcock and manometer; measure ICP† • Collect the suitable specimens of CSF for analysis and filling collection tubes 1–3 with 1–2 mL of CSF each • If intrathecal medication is to be instilled, drug and dose must be checked and administered safely	Anesthetic agent prevents pain sensation
13.	As soon as the needle is removed, assist the doctor in applying tincture benzoin seal or Healex spray and put the dressing on the punctured area	To prevent the leakage of the CSF fluid
14.	Make the patient in supine position without pillow at least for 4–6 hours	To avoid complication such as headache and reduction in CSF pressure
15.	Monitor the vital signs of the patient	To identify the abnormalities immediately
16.	Remove the mackintosh form the patient side	To make the patient comfortable
17.	Wash and replace the equipments	To make them arranged for next usage
18.	Send the specimen to the laboratory with all patient details	To do the analysis
19.	Document the procedure and patient parameters (during and after the procedure) in the nurse's record	For follow-up care of the patient

*CSF, cerebrospinal fluid; †ICP, intracranial pressure.

Points to Note

* Monitor the vital signs of the patient every 15 minutes for the first 1 hour, followed by every ½ hour for 6 hours.
* Encourage fluid intake as per physician order.
* Observe for the complications such as headache, nausea, vomiting and loss of sensation or movement in lower limbs.
* Check puncture site frequently for CSF leakage.

LIVER BIOPSY

Definition

Liver biopsy is the removal of small sample of tissue from the liver.

Methods

* Percutaneous needle biopsy
* Laparoscopic or open surgical biopsy.

Purposes

* Investigation of suspected diffuse liver disease
* Investigation of focal liver disease, e.g. hepatoblastoma, sarcoma
* Management of liver transplant.

Contraindications

* A patient who is too unstable or critically ill to undergo this procedure
* Significant coagulopathy
* Significant thrombocytopenia
* Ascites.

Equipments

* A sterile tray (liver biopsy set)
* Antiseptic skin cleaning agents (e.g. Betadine or chlorhexidine)
* Local anesthetic (Xylocaine injection)
* A 5 mL syringe and needle
* Sterile gloves
* Appropriate size of liver biopsy needles
* Sterile specimen bottles (these bottles should be labeled as bottle 1, 2, 3 with patient's profile)
* Tincture benzoin
* Adhesive plaster
* Mackintosh.

Procedure

The procedure of liver biopsy is given in Table 7.4.

Table 7.4: Procedure of liver biopsy

Sl No	Care action	Rationale
1.	Explain the procedure to the patient; obtain informed consent from the patient	To get valid consent from the patient/patient relatives
2.	Make sure whether the patient has completed 6 hours fasting	To prevent gastrointestinal complications during procedure
3.	Obtain and check the coagulation studies and blood glucose levels	To prevent the complication of bleeding and hypoglycemia after the procedure
4.	Arrange all the needed articles near the bedside	Easy to perform the procedure and to prevent unnecessary contamination
5.	Tell the patient to empty his/her bladder before the procedure	To ensure comfort of the patient
6.	Obtain a premedication order and give sedation	To avoid interruption during the procedure
7.	Place the patient in a supine position	To ensure comfort during the procedure
8.	Use skin preparation solution to cleanse skin over the liver biopsy site and drape to define a sterile field	To prevent infection and to make the patient feel privacy and comfortable
9.	Wear sterile gown, gloves and mask	To prevent infection, as it is an invasive procedure
The procedure will be done by the doctor; the nurse will assist		
10.	Anesthetize the skin over the proposed biopsy site with the Xylocaine drawn up in the 5 cc syringe with the attached 25 gauge needle	To prevent the local/systemic infection
11.	Ask the patient to hold the breath and insert the liver biopsy needle through the anesthetized abdominal wall	To prevent injury to the liver tissue
12.	Biopsy is taken as per the requirement	To send it to the lab for histopathological examination
13.	Once the biopsy is taken, place it in the appropriate medium; normally it is a very small amount of sterile normal saline in a sterile specimen container	To prevent the growth of microorganisms
Nurse's responsibilities		
14.	Check the vital status of the patient (blood pressure, pulse, respiration, temperature)	To identify the abnormalities immediately
15.	Once the biopsy is done, simply remove needle from abdominal wall; place several layers of pressure dressing on puncture site Instruct the patient to roll on to the right side and advise him to remain in the same position for 1–2 hours	To prevent bleeding and bile leakage complications

Contd...

Contd...

Sl No	Care action	Rationale
16.	Remove the mackintosh from the patient side	To make the patient comfortable
17.	Wash and replace the equipments	To make them arranged for next usage
18.	Send the specimen to the laboratory with all patient details	To do the analysis
19.	Document the procedure and patient parameters (during and after the procedure) in the nurse's record	To maintain accurate records; provide a point of reference in the event of any queries

BONE MARROW ASPIRATION AND BIOPSY

Definition

A bone marrow aspiration involves the removal of a small amount of marrow, the liquid material from the bone. Bone marrow biopsy takes a small sample of bone and bone marrow using a needle.

Purposes

To diagnose the conditions and diseases that can affect our bone marrow, which include:
1. Anemia or a low red blood cell count.
2. Bone marrow diseases such as myelofibrosis or myelodysplastic syndrome.
3. Blood cell conditions such as leukopenia or polycythemia.
4. Cancers of the bone marrow or blood such as leukemias or lymphomas.
5. Hemochromatosis, a genetic disorder in which iron builds in the blood.

Equipments

- A sterile tray (bone marrow aspiration set)
- Antiseptic skin cleaning agents (e.g. Betadine or chlorhexidine)
- Local anesthetic (Xylocaine injection)
- Sterile gloves
- Appropriate size of bone marrow biopsy needle
- Sterile specimen bottles and slides (these bottles should be labeled as bottle 1, 2, 3 with patient's profile)
- Tincture benzoin
- Adhesive plaster
- Mackintosh.

Procedure

Procedure of the bone marrow aspiration and biopsy is detailed in Table 7.5.

Table 7.5: Procedure of the bone marrow aspiration and biopsy

Sl No	Care action	Rationale
1.	Explain the procedure to the patient; explain to client that pain may occur when the bone marrow is aspirated	To get valid consent from the patient/patient's relatives
2.	Arrange all the needed articles near the bedside	Easy to perform the procedure and to prevent unnecessary contamination
3.	Tell the patient to empty his/her bladder before the procedure	To ensure comfort of the patient
4.	Obtain a premedication order and give sedation	To avoid interruption during the procedure
5.	Assist client in maintaining correct position (Fig. 7.2)	To ensure comfort during the procedure
6.	Drape the patient appropriately and expose the bone marrow aspiration site	To make the patient feel privacy and comfortable
7.	Wear sterile gown, gloves and mask	To prevent infection, as it is an invasive procedure
8.	Use skin preparation solution to cleanse skin over the proposed bone marrow aspiration site and drape to define a sterile field	To prevent infection and to make the patient feel privacy and comfortable
The procedure will be done by the doctor; the nurse will assist		
9.	Anesthetize the skin over the proposed puncture site with the Xylocaine drawn up in the 5 cc syringe with the attached 25 gauge needle	To prevent the local/systemic infection
10.	Insert the bone marrow aspiration needle through the anesthetized pelvic wall	To prevent sensation of pain
11.	Bone marrow fluid is aspirated as per the requirement	To send it to the laboratory for investigation
12.	Once the fluid is withdrawn, collect in an appropriate labeled specimen container	To send it to the laboratory
Nurse's responsibilities		
13.	Check the vital status of the patient (BP*, pulse, respiration, temperature, SpO$_2$†)	To identify the abnormalities immediately
14.	Once the bone marrow aspiration is done, simply remove needle from pelvic wall and place a small pressure dressing on puncture site; instruct the patient to remain supine for 2–4 hours	To prevent bleeding
15.	Remove the mackintosh from the patient side	To make the patient comfortable
16.	Wash and replace the equipments	To make them arranged for next usage
17.	Send the specimen to the laboratory with all patient details	To do the analysis
18.	Document the procedure and patient parameters (during and after the procedure) in the nurse's record	To maintain accurate records, provide a point of reference in the event of any queries

*BP, blood pressure; †SpO$_2$, peripheral oxygen saturation.

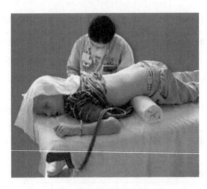

FIGURE 7.2: Position of the patient for bone marrow aspiration and biopsy

KIDNEY BIOPSY

Definition

A biopsy is a procedure performed to remove tissue or cells from the body for examination under a microscope. During a kidney biopsy, tissue samples are removed with a special needle to determine if cancer or other abnormal cells are present, or to determine how well the kidney is working.

Types of Kidney Biopsy

There are two types of kidney biopsies:
1. Needle biopsy: After a local anesthetic is given, the doctor inserts the special biopsy needle into the kidney to obtain a sample. Ultrasound (high-frequency sound waves) or computerized tomography (CT) scan may be used to guide the biopsy needle insertion. Most kidney biopsies are performed using this technique.
2. Open biopsy: After a general anesthetic is given, the doctor makes an incision in the skin and surgically removes a piece of the kidney.

Purposes

- Determine the reason for poor kidney function
- Determine if a tumor in the kidney is malignant (cancerous) or benign
- Evaluate how well the transplanted kidney is working.

Equipments

- A sterile tray (kidney biopsy set)
- Antiseptic skin cleaning agents (e.g. Betadine or chlorhexidine)
- Local anesthetic (Xylocaine injection)
- Sterile gloves
- Appropriate size of renal biopsy needle
- Sterile specimen bottles (these bottles should be labeled as bottle 1, 2, 3 with patient's profile)

- Tincture benzoin
- Adhesive plaster
- Mackintosh.

Procedure

Procedure of kidney biopsy is described in Table 7.6.

Table 7.6: Procedure of kidney biopsy

Sl No	Care action	Rationale
1.	Explain the procedure to the patient; obtain informed consent from the patient	To get valid consent from the patient/patient relatives
2.	Make sure whether the patient has completed 6 hours fasting	To prevent gastrointestinal complications during procedure
3.	Obtain and check the coagulation studies	To prevent the complication of bleeding after the procedure
4.	Arrange all the needed articles near the bedside	Easy to perform the procedure and to prevent unnecessary contamination
5.	Tell the patient to empty his/her bladder before the procedure	To ensure comfort of the patient
6.	Obtain a premedication order and give sedation	To avoid interruption during the procedure
7.	Place the patient in a prone position	To reach the kidney easily
8.	Use skin preparation solution to cleanse skin over the liver biopsy site and drape to define a sterile field	To prevent infection and to make the patient feel privacy and comfortable
9.	Wear sterile gown, gloves and mask	To prevent infection, as it is an invasive procedure
The procedure will be done by the doctor; the nurse will assist		
10.	Anesthetize the skin over the proposed biopsy site with the Xylocaine drawn up in the 5 cc syringe with the attached 25 gauge needle	To prevent the local/systemic infection
11.	Ask the patient to hold the breath and insert the kidney biopsy needle through the anesthetized abdominal wall	To prevent the movement of the diaphragm during the procedure
12.	Biopsy is taken as per the requirement	To send it to the laboratory for histopathological examination
13.	Once the biopsy is taken, place it in the appropriate medium; normally it is a very small amount of sterile normal saline in a sterile specimen container	To prevent the growth of microorganism
Nurse's responsibilities		
14.	Check the vital status of the patient (blood pressure, pulse, respiration, temperature)	To identify the abnormalities immediately

Contd...

Contd...

SI No	Care action	Rationale
15.	Once the biopsy is done, simply remove needle from abdominal wall; place a several layers of pressure dressing on puncture site and instruct the patient to lie down in a supine position and advise to remain in the same position for 1–2 hours	To prevent bleeding
16.	Remove the mackintosh from the patient side	To make the patient comfortable
17.	Wash and replace the equipments	To make them arranged for next usage
18.	Send the specimen to the laboratory with all patient details	To do the analysis
19.	Observe the urine	To check for bleeding
20.	Document the procedure and patient parameters (during and after the procedure) in the nurse's record	To maintain accurate records, provide a point of reference in the event of any queries

ASSISTING FOR CENTRAL VENOUS CATHETERIZATION

Definition

A central venous catheter (central line, CVC, central venous line or central venous access catheter) is a catheter placed into a large vein in the neck (internal jugular vein), chest (subclavian vein or axillary vein) or groin (femoral vein). It is used to administer medication or fluids, obtain blood sample for the tests (specifically the mixed venous oxygen saturation), and directly obtain cardiovascular measurements such as the central venous pressure (CVP).

Purposes

- Venous access is needed for IV fluids or antibiotics
- For CVP measurement
- For the administration of certain chemotherapeutic drugs or total parenteral nutrition (TPN)
- For hemodialysis or plasmapheresis.

Equipments

- A sterile tray (CVP set)
- Antiseptic skin cleaning agents (e.g. Betadine or chlorhexidine)
- Local anesthetic (Xylocaine injection)
- Sterile gloves
- Appropriate size of central line catheters
- Labeled specimen container
- Tincture benzoin
- Adhesive plaster
- Mackintosh.

Procedure

The procedure of central venous catheterization is given in Table 7.7.

Table 7.7: Procedure of central venous catheterization

Sl No	Care action	Rationale
1.	Explain the procedure to the patient	To get valid consent from the patient/patient's relatives
2.	Ensure that the patient passed urine before starting the procedure	To ensure comfort of the patient
3.	Arrange needed articles near the bedside	Easy to perform the procedure and to prevent unnecessary contamination
4.	Place the mackintosh and draw sheet under the head and neck	To prevent the soiling of the linen
5	Remove the pillow; place the patient in prolonged Trendelenburg position (15°–30° head down) and turn the head in the opposite direction of the insertion site	To ensure easy to identify the visible veins and easy to perform the procedure To reduce the chance of an air embolism
6.	Place a rolled towel or sheet between the shoulder blades and place the arms to the sides of the patient	To make the clavicles more prominent
7.	Wash the hands	To minimize the infection
8.	Provide sterile gloves to the consultant	To prevent infection, as it is an invasive procedure
9.	Assist the doctor during the procedure	
10.	Observe the hemodynamic level during the procedure	To identify the early signs of abnormalities
11.	The following step will be done by the doctors: • Prep and drape the area after identifying landmarks; use anesthetic agent to anesthetize the skin and the deeper tissues under the insertion site • Use 22 gauge needle (seeker needle) on a 3 cc syringe to locate the vein, aspirating as the needle is advanced until a flush of blood returns • Use 18 gauge needle on a 5 cc syringe to follow the path of the seeker needle, aspirating as the needle is advanced; entry into the vein is marked by a flush of blood • Stabilizing the needle with the thumb and forefinger, remove the syringe and immediately occlude the hub of the needle • Thread the J wire into the 18 gauge needle leaving about half of the wire extruding from the needle • Secure the J wire with a fingertip and remove the 18 gauge needle over the exposed, remaining portion of the J wire • Make a small cut in the skin adjacent to the entry site of the J wire using a scalpel, thread the silastic dilator over the wire • Advance the dilator fully into the chest and remove the dilator, while still leaving the J wire in place • Remove the hub from the long central catheter; thread the long central catheter over the wire into the vein	To prevent local and systemic infection and pain

Contd...

Contd...

SI No	Care action	Rationale
	• Leave 5–10 cm of the catheter outside the skin and carefully remove the J wire • Attach intravenous (IV) tubing to the catheter; lower the IV bag below the level of the patient to observe for blood return	
12.	As soon as possible, position the catheter; assist the doctor for suturing the line	To prevent the misplacement of the catheter
13.	Discontinue the Trendelenburg position and make the patient to lying down	To ensure the comfort of the patient
14.	Collect the needed blood sample in the labeled container	For analysis
15.	Monitor the vital signs of the patient	To identify the abnormalities immediately
16.	Remove the mackintosh form the patient side	To make the patient comfortable
17.	Wash and replace the equipments	To make them arranged for next use
18.	Send the specimen to the laboratory with all patient details	To do the analysis
19.	Document the procedure and patient parameters (during and after the procedure) in the nurse's record	To follow-up care for the patient

> **Points to Note**
>
> ✦ The rolled towel, which is used for the clavicles position, should not over accentuate this position, since it might move the clavicle closer to the first rib, making cannulation of the subclavian vein more difficult.

ASSISTING WITH ENDOTRACHEAL INTUBATION

Definition

Endotracheal intubation is a medical procedure in which a tube is placed into the windpipe (trachea) through the mouth or the nose. In most emergency situations, it is placed through the mouth.

Purposes

- Protection from gastric aspiration and secretions
- Access and maintenance in difficult airway and difficult surgical positions/procedures
- Provide positive pressure ventilation can be done for shorter periods with a mask or Oxylog
- Oxygenation to provide a controlled concentration of oxygen up to 100%, also provides for complete scavenging
- Secretions facilitates removal of secretions via suctioning.

Equipments

- Cardiac monitor
- Pulse oximeter
- Laryngoscope (check light)
- Adult blades No. 3 and No. 4
- Magill forceps
- Lubricant
- Connector: Body/Elbow (may be required)
- Flexible introducer
- Syringe 10 mL
- Clamp
- Appropriate size of airway
- Tape for ties
- Licorice stick
- Appropriate endotracheal tubes:
  - Size of tube is dependent on size of patient
  - The 'universally accepted' size is 7.5 mm for an unknown victim
  - Men are comparatively taller, therefore 8.0 mm tube may be appropriate
  - Females are usually smaller, therefore 7.0 mm tube may be appropriate.
- Means of inflating lungs: Air Viva, anesthetic machine
- Suction apparatus with Yankauer nozzle and endotracheal suction catheter
- Container for used laryngoscope, face mask
- Sterile gloves
- Mask
- Mackintosh and drawsheet.

Procedure

The procedure of endotracheal intubation is given in Table 7.8.

Table 7.8: Procedure of endotracheal intubation

Sl No	Care action	Rationale
1.	Explain the procedure to the patient's relatives	To get valid consent from the patient's relatives
2.	Determine whether the patient requires endotracheal (ET) intubation	For baseline assessment
3.	Assemble required equipment near the bedside	To prevent unnecessary contamination
4.	Place the mackintosh and draw sheet under the head and neck	To prevent the soiling of the linen
5.	If patient is in bed, remove head end rail; make sure there is adequate space between the back of bed and wall	To allow easy access to patient's head in order to facilitate intubation

Contd...

Contd...

Sl No	Care action	Rationale
6.	Position of the patient: • Supine • Pillow under head • Flexion of the neck	To complete direct visualization of the vocal cords
7.	Open the mouth by separating the lips and pulling on the upper jaw with the index finger	To get direct visualization of the vocal cords
8.	Check for any loose teeth or dentures; if found, remove with Magill forceps	To prevent the obstruction during the procedure
9.	Suction the patient (no longer than 12 second)	To maintain a patent airway
10.	Oxygenate patient for 1 minute with 100% oxygen using the Ambu bag	To prevent hypoxia
11.	Provide the laryngoscope to the doctor (switched on)	To visualize the larynx and the epiglottis
12.	Hold the laryngoscope in the left hand and insert the laryngoscope into the mouth with blade directed to the right tonsils; once the right tonsil is reached, sweep the blade to the midline, keeping the tongue on the left	To insert the ET tube easily and visualize the larynx and the epiglottis clearly
13.	Advance the laryngoscope blade till it reaches the angle between the base of the tongue and the epiglottis Insert the ET tube through the cords only till the cuff is just below the cords First inflate the ET tube cuff and check for any air leak; if no leak is present, deflate the ET tube cuff Inflate the cuff of the ET tube with 10 mL of air	To prevent leakage of the tube and misplacement of the tube
14.	Auscultate, listen/feel for airflow through the tube and observe for bilateral chest movements	To identify any displacement of the tube
15.	Connect the Ambu bag with oxygen to the ET tube and continue bagging	To prevent hypoxia
16.	Fix the ET tube in position by adhesive strips, securing the ET tube over the bridge of the nose/cheek	To prevent dislodgement of the tube
17.	Connect to ventilator	To prevent hypoxia
18.	Document the procedure in the nurse's record in detail	To maintain accurate records, provide a point of reference in the event of any queries

APPLICATION OF SKIN TRACTION

Definition

Skin traction is the traction on a body part maintained by an apparatus affixed by dressings to the body surface. Skin traction requires pressure on the skin to maintain the pulling force across the bone.

Purposes

- Helps to reduce the fracture
- Helps to reduce the muscle spasm
- To keep the suitable alignment of an injured part
- Helps to prevent the deformities
- Helps to stretch the muscles and obtain more working space within the joint prior to the total hip replacement surgery.

Equipments

- Cotton roll
- Roller bandages
- Spreader
- Rope
- Pulley
- Required weight
- Bed blocks
- Appropriate size of adhesive plaster
- Tincture benzoin
- Disposable gloves
- Kidney tray
- Mackintosh and draw sheet.

Procedure

The skin traction procedure is detailed in Table 7.9.

Table 7.9: Procedure of skin traction

SI No	Care action	Rationale
1.	Explain the procedure to the patient	To ensure that the patient should understand the procedure and give valid consent
2.	Arrange all the needed articles near the patient bedside	Easy to perform the procedure and minimize unnecessary contamination
3.	Wash the hands	To reduce the cross infection
4.	Place the mackintosh and draw sheet under the limb area	To prevent the soiling of the linen
5.	Wear gloves and clean the area with soap and water, and dry it	To reduce the infection and contamination
6.	Collect the history from the patient whether he/she have any adhesive tape allergy before applying; measure the appropriate length of adhesive strapping and place it on a level surface with the adhesive side up	Helps to support the part entirely

Contd...

Contd...

SI No	Care action	Rationale
7.	Place a square wooden spreader of about 7.5 cm (with a central hole) in the middle of the adhesive strapping	Helps to maintain the traction position correctly
8.	Gently elevate the limb off the bed, while applying longitudinal traction; apply the strapping to the medial and lateral sides of the limb, allowing the spreader to project 15 cm below the sole of the foot	Helps to place the traction downward
9.	Pad bony areas with felt or cotton wool; wrap the crepe or ordinary gauze bandage firmly over the strapping	Helps to support the strapping
10.	Elevate the end of the bed and attach a traction cord through the spreader with the required weight; the weight should not exceed 5 kg	To prevent the compartment syndrome
11.	Make the patient comfortable	To ensure the comfort of the patient
12.	Clean and replace the equipments properly	To make them ready for next use
13.	Remove the gloves, discard as per institutional policy and wash the hands	To minimize the contamination
14.	Document the procedure in the nurse's record	To do the follow-up care for the patient

Points to Note

Check the whole system of traction for its work order:
- The rope and pulley are in straight alignment.
- The weight is freely hanging without touching the bed or floor.
- The force of pull is felt by the patient.
- The toes are freely movable.

APPLICATION OF PELVIC TRACTION

Definition

Pelvic traction is applied to the lower spine with a belt around the waist.

Purposes

- The conservative management for prolapsed lumbar intervertebral disk
- To stretch muscle and ligaments
- To separate vertebral bodies in the spine.

Equipments

- Pelvic unit and belt
- Spreader
- Rope
- Required weight
- Bed locks.

Procedure

The application procedure of pelvic traction is detailed in Table 7.10.

Table 7.10: Procedure of pelvic traction

SI No	Care action	Rationale
1.	Explain the procedure to the patient	To ensure that the patient should understand the importance of the procedure and give valid consent
2.	Arrange all the needed articles near the patient bedside	Easy to perform the procedure and minimize unnecessary contamination
3.	Wash the hands	To reduce the cross infection
4.	Wear gloves	To reduce the cross infection
5.	Place the patient in supine position and remove the pillow from the head end	To make the patient comfortable and easy to perform the procedure
6.	Spread the pelvic belt underneath the lumbar region; take the belt to the front on the abdomen and secure it tightly	To maintain the position and to apply the traction easily
7.	Elevate the foot end of the bed, as needed	Helps to hang the weight appropriately
8.	Connect the belt to spreader and pass the rope through the pulley	Helps to maintain the position by placing the weight
9.	Apply the weight as per doctor's order and provide a small pillow under the knee	Helps to support the knee joint
10.	Make the patient comfortable	To ensure the comfort of the patient
11.	Wash and replace the articles	To make them ready for next usage
12.	Remove the gloves, discard as per institutional policy and wash the hands	To minimize the contamination
13.	Document the procedure in the nurse's record	To do the follow-up care for the patient

Points to Note

+ Clear instruction should be given to the patient that, not to fold the lower limbs or turn while on traction for too long period.

ASSISTING FOR SKULL TRACTION

Definition

Use skull traction for traumatic and infectious conditions in the cervical spine. Apply it to the skin using head halter traction, or to the skull bones using Gardner-Wells tongs or a halo device.

Purposes

• To regain normal length and alignment of involved bone
• To reduce the fracture and immobilize a fractured bone.

Equipments

- Spreader
- Rope
- Pulley
- Required weight
- Dressing pack
- Appropriate size of adhesive plaster
- Tincture benzoin
- Disposable gloves
- Kidney tray
- Mackintosh
- Appropriate skull traction set
- Razor
- Antiseptic solution
- Disposable apron.

Procedure

The assisting procedure of skull traction application is given in Table 7.11.

Table 7.11: Procedure of skull traction

SI No	Care action	Rationale
1.	Explain the procedure to the patient/patient's relatives	To ensure that the patient should understand the procedure and give valid consent
2.	Arrange all the needed articles near the patient bedside	Easy to perform the procedure and minimize unnecessary contamination
3.	Wash the hands	To reduce the cross infection
4.	Place the mackintosh and draw sheet under the head	To prevent the soiling of the linen
5.	**Gardner-Wells tongs technique** Place the pins below the brim of the skull in line with the external auditory meatus, 2–3 cm above the top of the pinna	Helps to place the traction in accurate place
6.	Prepare the patient's scalp by shaving the hair and washing the skin with an antiseptic solution	To minimize the infection
7.	Position the tongs correctly and mark the pin entrance points	To perform hole accurately
8.	Infiltrate the pin sites with 1% lidocaine and make stab wounds through the skin and down to the bone; insert the pins by alternately tightening one side and then the other, until 3.6 kg of torque is applied and determine the tightness with a special torque screwdriver or by tightening the pins using two fingers only—to grip the screwdriver	To prevent mobility and misplacement traction

Contd...

Contd...

Sl No	Care action	Rationale
9.	Dress the wounds with sterile gauze and apply the appropriate traction weight; tighten the pins once again on the following day, then leave those alone unless they are loose	To minimize the unnecessary contamination
10.	**Halo traction technique** Determine the ring size by measuring the head circumference or by trial; the clearance should be 1–2 cm at all points	Helps to fit the traction accurately
11.	Cautiously place the patient's head off the end of the bed and hold it with a special head holder or with an assistant; the halo should be just above the eyebrows and ears	Easy to place the traction correctly
12.	Use two pins posterolaterally and two in the lateral third of the forehead; these may be placed as far back as the hairline for cosmetic reasons, but should be anterior to the temporal muscle	Helps to prevent the mobility
13.	Advance the pins to finger tightness while keeping the halo placement symmetrical; ask the patient to keep his/her eyes closed during the procedure	To avoid pulling the skin upward and preventing eye closure, once the pins are tight
14.	Next, tighten the pins sequentially across the diagonals; if a torque screwdriver is available, tighten the screws to 34–45 cm/kg; if not, twist the screws tight by holding the screwdriver with two fingers	To place the traction accurately
15.	Tighten the screws once after 1–2 days and thereafter, only if loose; traction can now be applied or the patient can be placed in a halo jacket	To prevent the mobility
16.	Make the patient comfortable	To ensure the comfort of the patient
17.	Clean and replace the equipments properly	To make them ready for next use
18.	Remove the gloves, discard as per institutional policy and wash the hands	To minimize the contamination
19.	Document the procedure in the nurse's record	To do the follow-up care for the patient

ASSISTING FOR SKELETAL TRACTION

Definition

Apply skeletal traction by placing a metal pin through the metaphyseal portion of the bone and apply weight to the pin.

Purposes

- Helps to reduce overlying space of fractured bones
- Helps to maintain the reduction of the fracture
- Helps to reduce muscle spasms, friction between bony surfaces and pain
- Helps to separate bone surface.

Equipments

- Dressing pack
- Rope
- Pulley
- Required weight
- Bed blocks
- Appropriate size of sterile skeletal traction set
- Disposable gloves
- Kidney tray
- Mackintosh
- Xylocaine injection (2%)
- Disposable syringe.

Procedure

The assisting procedure for skeletal traction given in Table 7.12.

Table 7.12: Assisting procedure for skeletal traction

Sl No	Care action	Rationale
1.	Explain the procedure to the patient	To ensure that the patient should understand the procedure and give valid consent
2.	Arrange all the needed articles near the patient bedside	Easy to perform the procedure and minimize unnecessary contamination
3.	Place the mackintosh and draw sheet under the limb area	To prevent the soiling of the linen
4.	Wash the hands	To reduce the cross infection
5.	Cover the surrounding area with sterile drapes; infiltrate the skin and soft tissues down to the bone with 2% Xylocaine both the entrance and exit sides	To prepare the sterile environment and to minimize the contamination
6.	Make a small stab incision in the skin and introduce the pin through the incision horizontally and at right angles to the long axis of the limb; proceed until the point of the pin strikes the underlying bone	Helps to make the pathway for the hand drill
7.	Insert the pins with a T-handle or hand drill; advance the pin until it stretches the skin of the opposite side and make a small release incision over its point	Helps to apply the traction equally in the area

Contd...

Contd...

SI No	Care action	Rationale
8.	Dressing the skin wounds separately with sterile gauze attach a stirrup to the pin, cover the pin ends with guards and apply traction	To minimize the contamination
9.	Apply countertraction by elevating the appropriate end of the bed or by placing a splint against the root of the limb	To prevent the mobility
10.	Make the patient comfortable	To ensure the comfort of the patient
11.	Clean and replace the equipments properly	To make them ready for next use
12.	Remove the gloves, discard as per institutional policy and wash the hands	To minimize the contamination
13.	Document the procedure in the nurse's record	To do the follow-up care for the patient

ASSISTING FOR PAPANICOLAOU TEST

Definition

Papanicolaou test or the Pap smear is a gynecological examination procedure, where the cells or tissues collected from the cervix are examined under a microscope.

Purposes

- To detect the presence of certain abnormality such as cancer of the cervix
- Helps to confirm or rule out the abnormal changes in the cells and tissues that occur in case of cancer.

Equipments

- Dressing tray
- Vaginal speculum
- Wooden spatula or cotton swab
- Slide: One slide with office clips
- Preservatives (alcohol 50 mL)
- Permanent marker
- Spotlight
- Mackintosh and draw sheet
- Antiseptic solution
- Kidney tray.

Procedure

Pap smear test procedure is given in Table 7.13.

Table 7.13: Procedure of Pap smear

SI No	Care action	Rationale
1.	Explain the procedure to the patient	To get valid consent from the patient/patient's relatives
2.	Ensure that the patient passed urine before starting the procedure	To ensure comfort of the patient
3.	Arrange needed articles near the bedside	Easy to perform the procedure and to prevent unnecessary contamination
4.	Place the mackintosh and draw sheet under the buttocks	To prevent the soiling of the linen
5.	Wash the hands	To reduce the cross-contamination
6.	Place the patient in lithotomy position	Easy to visualize the part and perform the procedure
7.	Drape the patient appropriately	To ensure the privacy for the patient
8.	Assist the doctor during the procedure	
9.	Communicate with patient in between the procedure	To give psychological support to the patient
10.	Collect the specimen in labeled container	For analysis
11.	Make the patient comfortable	To ensure the comfort of the patient
12.	Check the vitals of the patient	Helps to identify any subnormal parameter early
13.	Send the specimen to the laboratory	To do the analysis
14.	Wash and replace the equipments	To make them arrange for the next use
15.	Document the procedure and patient parameters (during and after the procedure) in the nurse's record	To follow-up care for the patient

ASSISTING FOR DILATATION AND CURETTAGE

Definition

Dilatation and curettage is a surgical procedure usually performed under local anesthesia in which the cervix is dilated and the endometrial lining of the uterus is scraped with a curette; it is performed to obtain tissue samples, to stop prolonged bleeding, to remove small tumors, to remove fragments of placenta after childbirth or as a method of abortion.

Purposes

1. To identify the causes of dysfunctional uterine bleeding.
2. To obtain the specimen for biopsy with incomplete abortion, hydatidiform mole, inevitable abortion, dysfunctional uterine bleeding, polyps, misplaced intrauterine contraceptive devices, medical termination of pregnancy.

Equipments

- Big dressing tray or dressing bin
- Small towel
- Posterior vaginal wall Sims' speculum
- Vulsellum
- Uterine sound
- Graduated cervical canal dilators (Hegar's dilator)
- Ovum forceps
- Anterior vaginal wall retractor
- Uterine curette
- Thumb forceps
- Sedative as per doctor's order
- Disposable syringe
- A sterile gown
- Sterile hand towels
- Sterile leggings
- Sterile big towel
- Antiseptic solution, spirit swab.

Procedure

Procedure of dilatation and curettage is described in Table 7.14.

Table 7.14: Procedure of dilatation and curettage

SI No	Care action	Rationale
1.	Explain the procedure to the patient and patient's relatives	To get valid consent from the patient/ patient's relatives
2.	Wash the hands	To reduce the infection
The following steps will be performed by the doctor		
3.	After adequate anesthesia has been administered, the patient's legs are parted and flexed, and comfortably put up on a stirrup in a position that is called 'lithotomy' position	This ensures a good view of the genital area for the surgeon or gynecologist to operate
4.	The vagina and cervix are scrubbed with an antibacterial solution; that maybe iodine or chlorhexidine	To reduce the infection
5.	The cervix is visualized using speculum Lights are adjusted to visualize the cervix, so that its upper lip can be grasped with 'vulsellum'	Helps to stabilize and bringing the cervix down toward the vaginal opening to ease with rest of the procedure
6.	Dilatation is next done using sequential metal, round, tapered dilators and the opening to the uterus is gradually widened to about the size of a large pencil	Easy to visualize and perform the procedure
7.	The spoon-like curette is inserted into the uterine cavity and is used to gently scrape the lining of the uterus	Helps to remove the tissue or part from the uterus

Contd...

Contd...

SI No	Care action	Rationale
8.	When the surgeon feels the gritty layer of cells just above the muscle of the uterus, then he/she knows that the scraping has gone deep enough to sample the tissue adequately	If any part remained inside, it may cause the infection
9.	This scraping is done throughout the uterus and the tissue that is removed, sent to a pathologist for microscopic examination	To do the analysis and identify any abnormalities
10.	Depending on the indication for the procedure, the surgeon terminates the procedure once he/she feels that enough tissue has been obtained or that the entire cavity has been sampled or scrapped	For therapeutic purposes
11.	Collect the specimen in an appropriate labeled sample container if needed	To do the analysis
12.	Monitor the patient's hemodynamic level or any signs of bleeding	To identify the complications or abnormalities in an early stage
13.	Transfer the patient to the bed and make comfortable	To ensure the comfort of the patient
14.	Send the specimen to the laboratory	To do the analysis
15.	Wash and replace the articles	To make them ready for next usage
16.	Document the procedure and patient's parameters (during and after the procedure) in the nurse's record	To follow-up care for the patient

ASSISTING FOR SUPRAPUBIC CATHETERIZATION

Definition

A urinary bladder catheter inserted through the skin about 1 inch above the symphysis pubis. It is inserted under a general or local anesthetic. It is used for closed drainage and may be left in place for a time, sutured to the abdominal skin.

Purposes

1. To lower the incidence of urinary tract infection.
2. To turn away the flow of urine from the urethra in case of traumatic and pathological condition of the bladder and urethra is observed.
3. After gynecological surgery, wherein bladder dysfunction is likely to occur.

Equipments

A tray containing:
- Antiseptic solution
- Sterile catheterization set
- Gloves
- Disposable syringe and needle

- Water for injection or sterile water
- Sterile suturing set
- Xylocaine injection (2%)
- Appropriate size of Foley catheter and urosac set
- Sterile specimen container (if needed)
- Mackintosh and draw sheet
- Kidney tray
- Measuring jar
- Adhesive tape and scissors.

Procedure

Procedure of suprapubic catheterization is detailed in Table 7.15.

Table 7.15: Procedure of suprapubic catheterization

SI No	Care action	Rationale
1.	Explain the procedure to the patient	To get valid consent from the patient/patient's relatives
2.	Arrange needed articles near the bedside	Easy to perform the procedure and to prevent unnecessary contamination
3.	Shave the suprapubic area if the patient is hairy	To avoid the entry of the hair, while doing the insertion
4.	Place the mackintosh and draw sheet under the back and buttocks	To prevent the soiling of the linen
5.	Place the patient in lying down position	Easy to perform the procedure
6.	Drape the patient appropriately	To provide privacy to the patient
7.	Wash the hands	To minimize the infection
8.	Provide sterile gloves to the consultant	To prevent infection, as it is an invasive procedure
9.	Assist the doctor during the procedure	
10.	Communicate the patient in between the procedure and observe the hemodynamic level during the procedure	To give psychological support to the patient and identify the early signs of abnormalities
11.	The following step will be done by the doctors: • Provide adequate parenteral analgesia with or without sedation • Clean the lower abdominal wall by applying an antiseptic solution from the pubis to the umbilicus; repeat the application of the antiseptic solution more than two times and allow the area to dry • Apply sterile drapes and verify the insertion site by palpating the anatomic landmark • Fill the 10 mL syringe with a local anesthetic agent and use the 25 gauge needle to raise a skin at the insertion site	To prevent local and systemic infection and pain

Contd...

Contd...

SI No	Care action	Rationale
	• Advance the needle through the skin, subcutaneous tissue, rectus sheath and retropubic space, while alternating injection and aspiration, until urine enters the syringe; note the direction and depth required to enter the bladder • By using No. 11 blade, make a 4-mm stab incision at the insertion site with the blade facing inferiorly • Insert the needle obturator into the Malecot catheter and lock it into the port by twisting it, so that the needle tip projects 2.5 mm from the distal end of the catheter • Connect the 60 mL syringe to the port of the needle obturator • Place the tip of the catheter-obturator unit into the skin incision and direct it caudally and at a 20°–30° angle from true vertical toward the patient's legs • The practitioner's non-dominant hand should be placed on the lower abdominal wall, and the unit should be stabilized between the thumb and index fingers • The dominant hand should be used to advance the unit, while aspirating, until urine enters the syringe • Once urine enters the syringe, advance the unit 3–4 additional centimeters into the bladder • While securing the unit with the non-dominant hand, unscrew the obturator from the catheter • Advance the catheter approximately 5 additional centimeters over the obturator and then completely withdraw the obturator needle • Connect the extension tubing to the catheter and connect the tubing to a urinometer or a leg bag • Gently withdraw the catheter to lodge the wings against the bladder wall • Apply drain dressings around the catheter at the insertion site • Tape the catheter to the skin (leaving a mesentery between the skin and catheter) or stitch the catheter to the skin	
12.	Collect the specimen in a labeled container if needed	For analysis
13.	Make the patient in comfortable position	To ensure the patient's comfort
14.	Monitor the vital signs of the patient	To identify the abnormalities immediately
15.	Remove the mackintosh form the patient side	To make the patient comfortable
16.	Wash and replace the equipments	To make them ready for the next use
17.	Send the specimen to the laboratory with all patient details	To do the analysis
18.	Document the procedure and patient parameters (during and after the procedure) in the nurse's record	To follow-up care for the patient

Points to Note

- To observe for hematuria, bladder or abdominal distension.
- Check for kinks and patency of the tubings.
- Instruct the patient to avoid tension on the catheter site.

Infection Control Procedures

HAND HYGIENE

Definition

The art of cleansing the hands with water or other liquid, with or without the inclusion of soap or other detergent, for the purpose of removing soil, dirt or microorganism.

Standard Handwashing Procedure

According to Occupational Safety Health Administration (OSHA) standards regarding bloodborne pathogens, handwashing should be performed, at a minimum:

- Before and after every patient contact
- After removing gloves and other protective wear
- After handling blood or other body fluids
- When visibly contaminated with blood or tissues
- Before leaving the patient area
- Before and after eating, applying makeup, using the bathroom
- Handling contact lenses, handling equipment.

Purposes

- To remove visible soiling from hands
- To prevent transfer of bacteria from the home to the hospital
- To prevent transfer of bacteria from the hospital to the home
- Preventing the risk of cross infection
- Protecting the patients, visitors, healthcare workers from healthcare-associated infection (HAI)
- Importance of handwashing to reduce nosocomial infections
- Reduces spread of disease from patient-to-patient
- Reduces spread of disease from patient to healthcare professional
- Reduces spread of disease from healthcare professional to patient
- Reduces spread of disease from healthcare professional to other healthcare professionals
- Reduce spread of disease to visitors in the healthcare facility.

Procedure

Step 1: Palm-to-palm (Fig. 8.1A).

Step 2: Right palm over left dorsum and left palm over right dorsum (Fig. 8.1B).

Step 3: Palm-to-palm fingers interlocked (Fig. 8.1C).

Step 4: Back of fingers to opposing palms with fingers interlocked (Fig. 8.1D).

Step 5: Rotational rubbing of right thumb clasped in left palm and vice versa (Fig. 8.1E).

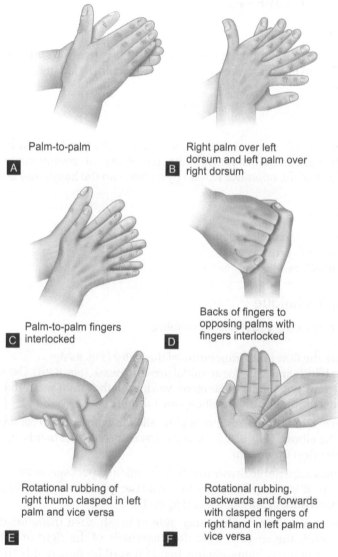

A — Palm-to-palm

B — Right palm over left dorsum and left palm over right dorsum

C — Palm-to-palm fingers interlocked

D — Backs of fingers to opposing palms with fingers interlocked

E — Rotational rubbing of right thumb clasped in left palm and vice versa

F — Rotational rubbing, backwards and forwards with clasped fingers of right hand in left palm and vice versa

FIGURES 8.1A to F: Procedure of handwashing

Step 6: Rotational rubbing back and forwards with clasped fingers of right hand in left palm and vice versa (Fig. 8.1F).

Points to Note

* Keep short nails and pay attention to them when washing hands.
* Avoid wearing rings.
* Do not wear artificial nails, nail polish.
* Remove wrist watches, bracelets, bangles, roll up long sleeves.

SURGICAL SCRUBBING

Definition

The act of washing the fingernails, hands and forearms with a bactericidal soap or solution in a prescribed manner for a specific period before a surgical procedure.

Purposes

1. Surgical scrub is the removal of bacteria from the hands and arms.
2. Surgical scrub helps prevent the possibility of contamination and infection of the operative wound by bacteria on the hands and arms.

Equipments

* Germicidal soap or detergent
* Surgical scrub brush
* Sterile hand towel.

Scrub Up Technique

Step 1: Note the time you started scrubbing.
Step 2:
* Regulate the flow and temperature of the water (Fig. 8.2A)
* Wet the hands and arms for an initial prescrub wash (Fig. 8.2B). Use several drops (5 mL) of surgical detergent, work up lather then wash the hands and arms thoroughly to the elbows for 1 minute.

Step 3: Rinse hands and arms thoroughly, allowing the water to run from the hands to the elbows (Fig. 8.2C). Do not retrace or shake the hands and arms, let the water drip from them.

Step 4: Remove the sterile brush and file from opened package, moisten brush and work up lather. Soap fingertips and clean the spaces under the fingernails of both hands under running water (Fig. 8.2D).

Step 5: Lather fingertips with sponge side of brush, then using bristle side of brush, scrub the spaces under the fingernails of the right or left hand (Fig. 8.2E). When scrubbing, slightly bend forward holding hands and arms above the elbow, and keep arms away from the body.

Step 6: Lather fingers (Fig. 8.2F); wash on all four sides of each finger. Only nails should be brushed as brushing of other areas has been shown to be damaging to the skin surface causing abrasions.

Step 7: Begin with the thumb or little finger on the right or left hand. Wash one hand and arm completely before moving on to the other hand and arm:

1. Lather palm, back of hand, heel of hand and space between thumb, and index finger washing each surface. Move up the forearm, lather then wash to the elbow (subsequent washes should encompass two thirds of the forearm only).
2. Repeat for the other arm. Discard brush and rinse hands and arms without retracing. Allow the water to drip from elbows before approaching gown pack.

Step 8: Slightly bend forward, pick up a hand towel from the top of the gown pack and step back from the table:

1. Grasp the towel and open it; do not allow the towel to touch any unsterile object or unsterile parts of the body.
2. Hold hands and arms higher than the elbows, and keep arms away from the body (Fig. 8.2G).

Step 9: Holding one end of the towel with one hand, dry the other hand and arm with a blotting, rotating motion (Fig. 8.2H).

Step 10: Work from fingertips to the elbow (Fig. 8.2I); do not retrace any area. Dry all sides of the fingers, the forearm and the arms thoroughly (Fig. 8.2J).

Step 11: Grasp the other end of the towel, dry the other hand and arm in the same manner as above.

Step 12: Discard the towel into an appropriate receptacle.

Points to Note

- Rinse as often as possible using one direction only. Start from the hand going to the arm, taking care not to touch the faucet and the sink.
- A person with cut or burn should not scrub because of the high bacterial count.
- The hands and arms can never be rendered sterile no matter how long or how strong the antiseptics.
- Surgical scrub is most effective when firm motion is applied. Short horizontal or circular stroke could be used.
- Use an sufficient supply of antiseptics.
- Since the hands are to be cleaner than any other area, after the initial hand wash, they are held higher than the elbows, during the rest of the procedure to prevent water from running back the scrubbed hands.

Preparation before doing surgical scrub

- Attend to your personal needs.
- Adjusts your cap and mask properly. The hair should be confined inside the cap. The mask should cover the nose, mouth, cheek and chin.
- Roll up sleeves of the uniform 3 inches above the elbow if sleeves are long.
- Check on the liquid soap and brush dispenser.
- Remove your jewelry.
- Check on your fingernails. They must be kept clean and short to reduce the bacteria count and to prevent the puncturing or tearing of gloves.

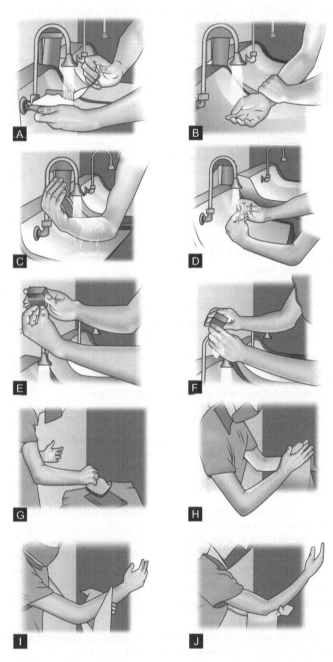

FIGURES 8.2A to J: Scrub up technique. **A.** Regulate the flow and temperature of water; **B.** Prescrub wash; **C.** Allow the water to run from hands to elbow; **D.** Cleaning the finger nails; **E.** Later fingertips with brush; **F.** Cleaning the nails with brush; **G.** Grasping the towel from the gown pack; **H.** Drying the hand with the towel; **I.** Dry the hands from finger tips to elbow; **J.** Dry all sides of the hands and arm.

GOWNING

Definition

Wearing of sterile gown over theater clothing, before assisting surgical patient.

Purpose

The sterile gown is worn in order to permit the wearer to come within the sterile field and carry out sterile technique during an operative procedure.

Equipments

- Gown
- Surgical towel.

Technique

Step 1: With one hand, pick up the entire folded gown from the wrapper by grasping the gown through all layers, being careful to touch only the inside top layer, which is exposed. Step back from the trolley/shelf (Fig. 8.3A).

Step 2: Hold the gown in the manner shown in Figure 8.3B near the gown's neck and allow it to unfold being careful that it does not touch either the body or other unsterile objects. Grasp the inside shoulder seams and open the gown with the armholes facing.

Step 3: Slide arms part way into the sleeves of the gown keeping hands at shoulder level away from the body (Fig. 8.3C).

Step 4: Slide arms further into the gown sleeves and when the fingertips are level with the proximal edge of the cuff, grasp the inside seam at the juncture of gown sleeve and cuff using thumb and index finger (Fig. 8.3D). Be careful that no part of the hand protrudes from the sleeve cuff.

Step 5: The circulating person should assist at this point to position, the gown over the shoulders by grasping the inside surface of the gown at the shoulder joint. They can then adjust the gown over the scrub person's shoulders. The circulating person's hands are only in contact with the inside surface of the gown (Fig. 8.3E).

Step 6: The circulating person then prepares to secure the gown, the neck and back may be secured with a Velcro tab or ties. The circulating person then ties the gown at waist level at the back. This technique prevents the contaminated surfaces at the back of the gown from coming into contact with the front of the gown (Fig. 8.3F).

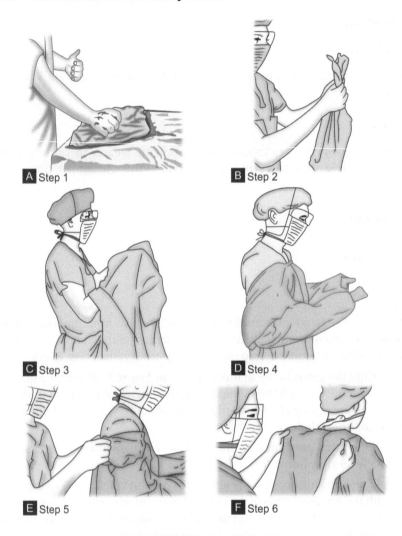

FIGURES 8.3A to F: Gowning technique

Points to Note

- This is done after the surgical scrub.
- Use an oscillating motion pat dry in drying the hands and arms. Start from the hand going to the arms.
- Do not dry hand then arms and return to the same hand.
- In drying the hand and arms, a towel could be used. If a towel is used, dry one hand and arm on one end of the towel and use the opposite end to dry the other hand and arm.
- In serving the gown, do not turn your back on the sterile field to prevent contamination.
- In picking the gown from a sterile linen pack, be careful not to touch any other articles in the pack with.

MASKING

Definition

Wearing a disposable mask over nose and mouth.

Purpose

- To prevent dispersal of droplet from wearer to environment and patient.

Equipment

Disposable or clean mask.

Procedure

To Wear the Mask

- Wash hands
- Hold mask by top two strings or loop, keeping top edge above bridge of nose (Fig. 8.4A)
- Tie both string at the top of back of head firmly above ears (Fig. 8.4B)
- Tie two lower strings snugly at the back of neck (Fig. 8.4C)
- Gently press nose clip of the disposable mask for a snug fit (Fig. 8.4D)
- Change surgical mask when contaminated (Fig. 8.4E)
- Dispose the mask after use (Fig. 8.4F).

To Remove the Mask

- Wash hand
- Untie lower strings first, then top once and pull mask away from face
- Hold mask by string and discard into appropriate receptacle.

GLOVING TECHNIQUE

Gloving is done after the gowning technique.

Purpose

Gloves are worn to complete the sterile dress in order that the one, who wears them may handle sterile equipment.

Technique

Step 1: Open the inner package containing the gloves and pick up one glove by the folded cuff edge with the sleeve-covered hand (Fig. 8.5A).

Step 2: Place the glove on the opposite gown sleeve palm down, with the glove fingers pointing toward the shoulder. The palm of the hand inside the gown sleeve must be facing upward toward the palm of the glove (Figs 8.5B and C).

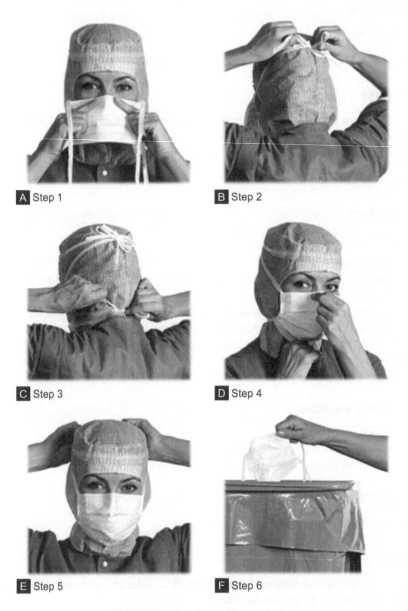

A Step 1   B Step 2

C Step 3   D Step 4

E Step 5   F Step 6

FIGURES 8.4A to F: Masking technique

Step 3: Place the glove's rolled cuff edge at the seam that connects the sleeve to the gown cuff. Grasp the bottom rolled cuff edge of the glove with the thumb and index finger (Fig. 8.5D).

Step 4: While holding the glove's cuff edge with one hand, grasp the uppermost edge of the glove's cuff with the opposite hand (Fig. 8.5E). Take care not to expose the bare fingers, while doing this.

Step 5:

- Continuing to grasp the glove, stretch the cuff of the glove over the hand (Fig. 8.5F)
- Using the opposite sleeve covered hand, grasp both the glove cuff and sleeve cuff seam and pull the glove onto the hand. Pull any excessive amount of gown sleeve from underneath the cuff of the glove.

Step 6: Using the hand that is now gloved put on the second glove in the same manner. When gloving is completed no part of the skin has touched the outside surface of the gloves. Check to make sure that each gown cuff is secured and covered completely by the cuff of the glove. Adjust the fingers of the glove as necessary, so that they fit snugly.

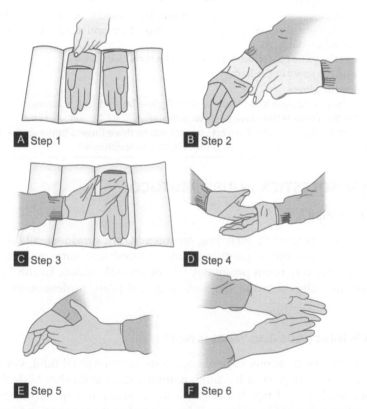

FIGURES 8.5A to F: Gloving technique. **A.** Pick up one glove with thumb and forefinger; **B.** Pull glove on hand; **C.** Slip partially gloved hand under cuff of second glove; **D.** Pull second glove over other hand and pull glove up to gowned wrist; **E.** Slip fingers of completely gloved hand under cuff of first hand, pull glove to gowned wrist; **F.** Gloving procedure completed.

Points to Note

- Not to contaminate the outside surface of the glove.
- In serving the gloves, the nurse must have a wide base of support by putting her foot apart.
- Always serve the right hand glove first.
- In serving, get the right glove with the left and the left hand glove with the right hand.
- Always keep gloved hands at waist level or above.
- Keep gloved hands away from your mask.

Removing the gown and the gloves

- Regardless of whether the scrub nurse assists in a case or contaminated case remove gown first and then the gloves. Wash the gloved hands, if they are grossly contaminated before removing the gown.

Removing the gown

- With the gloves still in, ask the circulating nurse to loosen the ties and the belt.
- Grasp the right shoulder of the gown and slip off the arm allowing use sleeves to turn inside out.
- Repeat the same procedure for the opposite shoulder.
- Discard the gown in the hamper.

Removing the gloves

- With the gloved right hand, remove the left glove by holding it at its outer surface and pull off (this is the glove to glove technique).
- To remove the right glove, insert your thumb or three fingers between the skin and the glove and pull off (this is the skin to skin technique).

POST NEEDLESTICK INJURY PROTOCOL

Who is at Risk?

All healthcare personnel, including emergency care providers, all hospital employees, interns, nursing staff and students, physicians, surgeons, dentists, labour and delivery room personnel, laboratory technicians, health facility sanitary staff, clinical waste handlers and healthcare professionals at all levels.

What is Infectious and What is Not?

Exposure to blood, semen, vaginal secretions, cerebrospinal fluid, synovial, pleural, peritoneal, pericardial fluid, amniotic fluid and other body fluids contaminated with visible blood can lead to infection. Exposure to tears, sweat, saliva, urine and feces is non-infectious unless these secretions contain visible blood.

The risk of acquiring human immunodeficiency virus (HIV) infection following percutaneous needle stick injury and after mucous membrane exposure has been estimated to be 0.3%–0.09%.This is because of the low concentration of virus in the blood of HIV patients.

The risk of acquiring hepatitis B virus (HBV) infection is related to the hepatitis B e-antigen (HBeAg) status of the source person. The risk associated with a single parental exposure to blood from a source patient ranges from 6% in HBeAg negative patients to as high as 40% in HBeAg positive patients.

The average risk of seroconversion following needle stick injury from an hepatitis C virus (HCV) infected patient is about 2%.

Immediate Care

First Aid in Management of Exposure

For skin

If the skin is broken after a needle stick or sharp instrument:
- Immediately wash the wound and surrounding skin with water, soap and rinse
- Do not scrub
- Do not use antiseptics or skin washes (bleach, chlorine, alcohol, Betadine).
  After a splash of blood or body fluids on unbroken skin:
- Wash the area immediately
- Do not use antiseptics.

For the eye
- Irrigate exposed eye immediately with water or normal saline. Sit in a chair, tilt head back and ask a colleague to gently pour water or normal saline over the eye.

For mouth
- Spit fluid out immediately
- Rinse the mouth thoroughly, using water or saline and spit again. Repeat this process several times.

Reporting

All sharps injury (break of skin with any sharp instrument such as hypodermic needle previously used on a patient) and mucosal exposure (blood or body fluids coming into contact with eye, mouth, etc.) should be reported to the hospital infection control nurse, nursing supervisors, floor managers and to the medical superintendent.

Protocol

After needle stick injury or blood/body fluid exposure, follow the below protocols.

Incident

Needle sticks injury or blood/body fluid exposure (exposure means contact with mucous membranes, intact or breached skin).

Procedure

Procedures to be followed after needle stick injury:

- Do not panic
- Do not put pricked finger in mouth
- Do not squeeze wound to bleed
- Wash the hands with soap and water
- Do not use bleach, chlorine, alcohol, Betadine, iodine, any antiseptic or detergent.

Process Flow

- Inform the floor manager/supervisor of the respective department
- File a report within half an hour form needle stick injury (NSI) available at intensive care unit (ICU), accident and emergency department and operation theater (OT)
- Go to the emergency department
- Get assessed by duty medical officer (DMO)/physician within 2–6 hours
- Proceed with the treatment suggested
- Review for the follow-up care as advised.

Instructions for the Staff

Standard Precautions

1. Wash hands after patient contact and after removing gloves.
2. Wash hands immediately, if hands are contaminated with body fluids.
3. Wear gloves when contamination of hands with body substances is anticipated.
4. Protective eyewear and masks should be worn when splashing with body substances is anticipated.
5. All healthcare workers should take precautions to prevent injuries during procedures and when cleaning or during disposal of needles or other sharp instruments.
6. Needles should not be recapped.
7. Needles should not be purposely bent or broken by hand and not removed from disposable syringes nor manipulated by hand.
8. After using disposable syringes and needles, scalpel blades and other sharp instruments should be placed in a puncher resistant container.
9. Healthcare worker who have lesions or dermatitis should refrain form direct patient care and from handling equipment.
10. All needle stick injuries should be reported to the emergency room (ER), who in turn will inform infection control nurse.
11. Handle and dispose of sharps safely.
12. Clean and disinfect blood/body substances spills with appropriate agents.
13. Adhere to disinfection and sterilization standards.
14. Vaccinate all clinical and laboratory workers against hepatitis B.
15. Other measures are double gloving, changing surgical techniques to avoid 'exposure prone' procedures, use of needleless systems and other safe devices.

BIOMEDICAL WASTE MANAGEMENT

Definition

The waste generated during the diagnosis, treatment or immunization of human beings or animals or in research activities pertaining to or in the production of testing biologicals.

Purposes

- Ensure occupational health safety
- Avoid illegal reuse
- Favors recycling
- Reduce the cost of treatment and disposal.

Color Code of Biomedical Waste Management

Details about color code and usage is given in Table 8.1:
- Yellow
- Red
- Black
- Green
- Blue
- Puncture proof container.

Table 8.1: Color code of biomedical waste management

Color	Waste category	Location	Treatment
Yellow	Human anatomical and body parts	Operation theater (OT) and labor room	Incineration/Burial
Red	Infectious gauze, cotton, plastic tubing, syringes, other infected plastics, etc.	All wards/nursing stations	Autoclave
Blue	Vials and bottles	All wards/nursing stations	Autoclave
Puncture proof container	Sharp	All wards/nursing stations	Sharp pit
Green	General wastes	Separately kept from biomedical waste bins	Composing/Handed over to municipal corporation
Black	Cytotoxic drugs, expiry medicines	All wards/nursing stations	Return to original supplier, incineration at high temperatures

Yellow Bag (Infectious)

- Postoperative human body parts
- Placenta
- Pathological waste.

Red Bag (Infectious Plastics)

- All types of intravenous (IV) sets and tubes/bags
- Gloves, blood bags, urine bags
- Disposable syringes (without needle)
- Catheters
- All kinds of drains and aprons (like cotton, swabs and bandages)
- Dialysis kits.

Green Bag (General Waste)

- Paper and plastic packing
- Disposable cups and plates, etc.
- Cans and tins
- Food items.

Black Bag

- Chemotherapy waste
- Acids and alkalis
- Phenol
- Expiry medicines.

Puncture Proof Container (Infectious)

- All kinds of broken glasses, tools and ampules
- All kinds of sharps like scalpels, needles, blades, IV catheters, etc.
- Clinical and pathological slides
- Guide wires
- Venflon needles, etc.

Tips for Safe-sharp Disposal

- Avoid recap
- Empty the sharp container once the fill is three fourth
- The container should be filled with 1% hypochloride solution always
- Avoid the use of burner or needle cutter
- Avoid the store rage of needle in the kidney tray after use. It should be discarded immediately after use.

Treatment Options of Biomedical Waste

Treatment options of biomedical waste is given in Table 8.2.

Table 8.2: Treatment method of biomedical waste

SI No	Waste type	Treatment method
1.	Body parts	Incineration/Deep burial
2.	Bandages/Cotton/Linen	Incineration/Autoclaving/Microwaving
3.	Gloves/Surgical gowns/ Needles/Sharps	Chemicals/Disinfection/Autoclaving/Microwaving
4.	Intravenous (IV) bottles/Plastic tubing/Blood bags/Urine bags/Items used in hemodialysis units	Autoclaving/Microwaving
5.	IV sets/Catheters	Chemicals/Disinfection/Autoclaving
6.	Syringes/Vacutainer tubes	Autoclaving/Chemicals/Disinfection
7.	Unused drugs	Return to manufacturer
8.	Waste chemicals	Incineration
9.	Culture fluids/Lavage fluids/Blood/Urine samples/Other body fluids	Chemicals/Disinfection/Autoclaving
10.	Culture plates/vials	Autoclaving/Microwaving

Index

Page numbers followed by *t* refer to table and *f* refer to figure